AF147513

Percutaneous Coronary Interventions
for Chronic Total Occlusion

Yangsoo Jang
Editor

Percutaneous Coronary Interventions for Chronic Total Occlusion

A Guide to Success

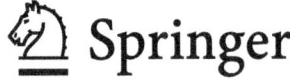 Springer

Editor
Yangsoo Jang
Cardiovascular Hospital
Yonsei University Health System
Seoul
South Korea

ISBN 978-981-10-6025-0   ISBN 978-981-10-6026-7   (eBook)
https://doi.org/10.1007/978-981-10-6026-7

Library of Congress Control Number: 2018961438

© Springer Nature Singapore Pte Ltd. 2019
This work is subject to copyright. All rights are reserved by the Publisher, whether the whole or
part of the material is concerned, specifically the rights of translation, reprinting, reuse of
illustrations, recitation, broadcasting, reproduction on microfilms or in any other physical way,
and transmission or information storage and retrieval, electronic adaptation, computer software,
or by similar or dissimilar methodology now known or hereafter developed.
The use of general descriptive names, registered names, trademarks, service marks, etc. in this
publication does not imply, even in the absence of a specific statement, that such names are
exempt from the relevant protective laws and regulations and therefore free for general use.
The publisher, the authors, and the editors are safe to assume that the advice and information in
this book are believed to be true and accurate at the date of publication. Neither the publisher nor
the authors or the editors give a warranty, express or implied, with respect to the material
contained herein or for any errors or omissions that may have been made. The publisher remains
neutral with regard to jurisdictional claims in published maps and institutional affiliations.

This Springer imprint is published by the registered company Springer Nature Singapore Pte Ltd.
The registered company address is: 152 Beach Road, #21-01/04 Gateway East, Singapore
189721, Singapore

Contents

Contributors

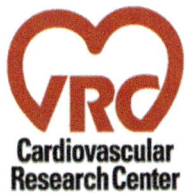 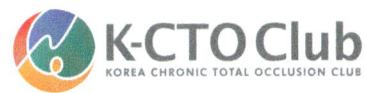

Jung Rae Cho Division of Cardiology, Kangnam Sacred Heart Hospital, Hallym University College of Medicine, Seoul, South Korea

Jin-Ho Choi Samsung Medical Center, Sungkyunkwan University School of Medicine, Seoul, South Korea

Cai De Jin Department of Cardiology, The Affiliated Wuxi No. 2 People's Hospital of Nanjing Medical University, Wuxi, Jiangsu, China

Maoto Habara Department of Cardiology, Toyohashi Heart Center, Toyohashi, Aichi, Japan

Bum-Kee Hong Division of Cardiology, Gangnam Severance Hospital, Yonsei University College of Medicine, Seoul, South Korea

Duck Hyun Jang Korea University Anam Hospital, Seoul, South Korea

Yangsoo Jang Division of Cardiology, Severance Cardiovascular Hospital, Yonsei University College of Medicine, Seoul, South Korea

Byeong-Keuk Kim Severance Cardiovascular Hospital, Yonsei University College of Medicine, Seoul, South Korea

Dong-Bin Kim Department of Cardiology, St. Paul's Hospital, The Catholic University of Korea, Seoul, South Korea

Dong-Kie Kim Inje University Haeundae Paik Hospital, Busan, South Korea

Doo-Il Kim Inje University Haeundae Paik Hospital, Busan, South Korea

Hee-Yeol Kim Department of Cardiology, Bucheon St. Mary's Hospital, The Catholic University of Korea, Bucheon-si, Gyeonggi-do, South Korea

Moo Hyun Kim Department of Cardiology, Dong-A University Hospital, Busan, South Korea

Bong-Ki Lee Division of Cardiology, Department of Internal Medicine, Kangwon National University Hospital, Kangwon National University School of Medicine, Chuncheon, South Korea

Jae-Hwan Lee Chungnam National University Hospital, Daejeon, South Korea

Jang Hoon Lee Department of Internal Medicine, Kyungpook National University Hospital, School of Medicine, Kyungpook National University, Daegu, South Korea

Jong-Young Lee Division of Cardiology, Kangbuk Samsung Hospital, Sungkyunkwan University School of Medicine, Seoul, South Korea

Jun-Won Lee Division of Cardiology, Department of Internal Medicine, Yonsei University Wonju College of Medicine, Wonju Severance Christian Hospital, Wonju, South Korea

Nae Hee Lee Soon Chun Hyang University, Bucheon Hospital, Bucheon, South Korea

Seung-Hwan Lee Division of Cardiology, Department of Internal Medicine, Yonsei University Wonju College of Medicine, Wonju Severance Christian Hospital, Wonju, South Korea

Seung-Whan Lee Department of Cardiology, Asan Medical Center, University of Ulsan College of Medicine, Seoul, South Korea

Kenya Nasu Department of Cardiovascular Medicine, Toyohashi Heart Center, Toyohashi, Aichi, Japan

Hun Sik Park Department of Internal Medicine, Kyungpook National University Hospital, School of Medicine, Kyungpook National University, Daegu, South Korea

Sang Min Park Division of Cardiology, Chuncheon Sacred Heart Hospital, Hallym University College of Medicine, Chuncheon, South Korea

Seung-Woon Rha Korea University Guro Hospital, Seoul, South Korea

Sanghoon Shin National Health Insurance Service Ilsan Hospital, Goyang-si, Gyeonggi-do, South Korea

Jon Suh Soon Chun Hyang University, Bucheon Hospital, Bucheon, South Korea

Satoru Sumitsuji Division of Cardiology for International Education and Research, Graduate School of Medicine, Osaka University, Suita, Japan

Etsuo Tsuchikane Department of Cardiology, Toyohashi Heart Center, Toyohashi, Aichi, Japan

Hoyoun Won Cardiovascular-Arrhythmia Center, Chung-Ang University Hospital, Chung-Ang University College of Medicine, Seoul, South Korea

Chang-Hwan Yoon Division of Cardiology, Department of Internal Medicine, Seoul National University Bundang Hospital, Seongnam, South Korea

Cheol Woong Yu Korea University Anam Hospital, Seoul, South Korea

Yangsoo Jang and Hoyoun Won

1.1 History of CTO Intervention

Currently, chronic total occlusion (CTO) is defined as the complete occlusion of coronary arteries with the duration of more than 3 months. Prevalence of CTO in patients who underwent coronary angiography ranged between approximately 20 and 50% [1, 2]. Total occlusion of coronary artery was firstly described in the 1940s. The role of coronary collateral circulation in chronic total occlusion was found in the late 1960s [3]. In the early period of percutaneous coronary intervention (PCI), PCI had been considered as contraindication in totally occluded vessel. In addition, the concept of CTO had not been established. A term of total coronary artery occlusion was widely used following categorization according to the estimated duration, including more than 12 weeks. The first successful PCI for total coronary occlusion lesion was published in 1984 [4] (Fig. 1.1). Holmes et al. published PCI result in total coronary artery occlusion in the same year [5]. However, all PCI were failed

in patients who had coronary occlusion estimated to be of more than 12 weeks' duration in this study. In the early period (from late 1980s to early 1990s) of PCI for CTO lesion, the success rates were about 50–75% [6–8]. The first Korean report for the result of CTO intervention was published by Shim et al. in 1992 [9]. In this study, 7 of 24 patients had total occluded duration with longer than 4 weeks, and successful PCI rate was 42.9% in these lesions.

After coronary stents emerged, the stenting for CTO lesion had been started with Palmaz-Schatz stent in the early 1990s [10]. Since then, CTO interventions have been more rapidly developed. Wire designs have been improved including changes in core design, tapered tips, hydrophilic coatings, and variable tip stiffness. Historically, non-coated and non-tapered wires with increasing tip stiffness have been used to drill through the CTO. An improvement of the histopathological understanding of CTO lesions has enabled the industries to develop new techniques and equipment for CTO PCI. As gleaned from histopathologic studies, intimal wiring could be done via microchannels or loose tissue tracking, and tapered tip wires, whose tip approaches the size of such channels, have been developed for this purpose.

The first retrograde wiring was performed via a bypass graft in 1990 [11]. However, this attempt was performed not via collateral channel as current retrograde concept. The contemporary retrograde CTO PCI via collateral tracking was

Y. Jang (✉)
Division of Cardiology, Severance Cardiovascular Hospital, Yonsei University College of Medicine, Seoul, South Korea
e-mail: jangys1212@yuhs.ac

H. Won
Cardiovascular-Arrhythmia Center, Chung-Ang University Hospital, Chung-Ang University College of Medicine, Seoul, South Korea

© Springer Nature Singapore Pte Ltd. 2019
Y. Jang (ed.), *Percutaneous Coronary Interventions for Chronic Total Occlusion*,
https://doi.org/10.1007/978-981-10-6026-7_1

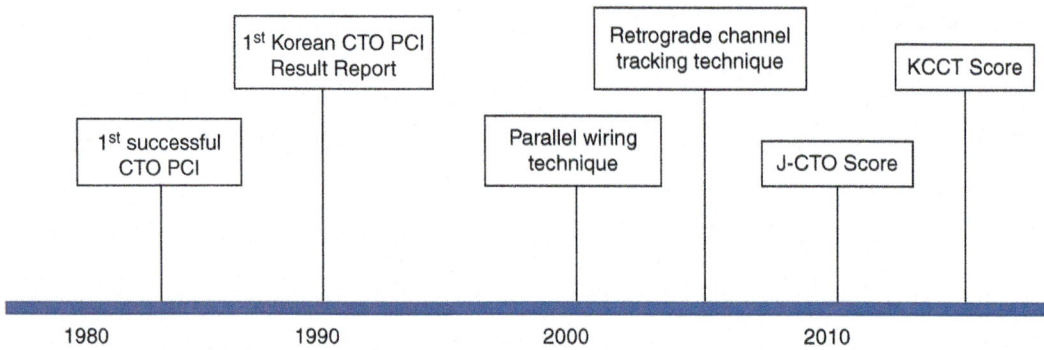

Fig. 1.1 Advance of CTO PCI

performed in the middle of 2000. Katoh et al. introduced the new techniques, so-called retrograde approach-targeted collateral wiring crossing, in 2005 [12]. Since retrograde approach was introduced, the success rate of CTO PCI has dramatically increased and reached over 80% [13].

As the success of CTO PCI was uncertain due to its difficulty and complexity, the predicting success of CTO intervention using scoring system was developed. The first scoring system to grade the difficulty of guidewire crossing was the J-CTO (Multicenter CTO Registry in Japan) score created in 2011 [14]. CTO PCI required integration of contemporary technique including imaging modalities. Computed tomography has been used not only for prediction model, CT-RECTOR score, but for guiding wiring [15–17].

In the past, CTO PCI was the exclusive treatment strategy for only few physicians. However, as patient selection and specialized equipment have become standardized, CTO intervention is an everyday practice in most interventionists worldwide.

1.2 The Benefit of CTO Intervention

Successful revascularization of CTO is related to improved clinical outcomes. Previous studies have shown improvements in angina, myocardial viability, and long-term survival and a reduced requirement for coronary bypass surgery.

1.2.1 Symptom Relief and Improvement in Quality of Life

Successful revascularization of CTO PCI increases myocardial blood flow to ischemic lesion so that CTO PCI showed superiority of symptom improvement in comparison with medical treatment only. In Total Occlusion Angioplasty Study-Societa Italiana di Cardiologia Invasiva (TOAST-GISE) study, 289 patients with successful CTO PCI have significantly improved symptom relief compared to 87 patients with failed CTO PCI (88.7% vs. 75%, $p = 0.008$) [18]. Similarly, in Flow Cardia's Approach to Chronic Total Occlusion Recanalization (FACTOR) study using Seattle Angina Questionnaire (SAQ), successful CTO intervention resulted in significant reduction of chest pain ($p = 0.019$) and improvement in quality of life ($p < 0.001$) [19]. In a multicenter prospective registry, revascularization of CTO had significant improvements in the angina frequency ($p < 0.001$) and quality of life [20].

Even though CTO studies using SAQ have been widely validated, questionnaire studies in CTO PCI have some limitations because it focused on physical limitation. CTO patients tend to adapt to their chest pain and complain of dyspnea on exertion. New methods should be developed to assess other symptoms as well as chest pain in CTO patients with chronic stable angina.

1.2.2 Improvement of Left Ventricular Function

PCI for coronary CTO may provide benefits in terms of myocardial function. Several small studies have investigated the effects of CTO PCI on left ventricular function. In a cardiac magnetic resonance imaging (CMR) study with a small number of CTO patients, hyperemic myocardial blood flow and contractility in treated segment were significantly higher at 24 h and 6 months after PCI in CTO group than the medical treatment group [21]. Thirty-three patients with successful CTO PCI were compared with ten unsuccessful CTO interventions using CMR. Reduction of ischemia after procedure was significant in successful CTO PCI group (79–30%, $p < 0.001$), but no change in unsuccessful PCI (80–70%, $p = 0.3$) [22]. In addition, regional contractility in successful CTO PCI group was significantly improved in the segments with delayed enhancement of <50% ($p = 0.01$). Sixty-nine consecutive patients with successful CTO PCI were examined for ischemia and viability with positron emission tomography (PET) and late gadolinium enhancement CMR [23]. Stress myocardial blood flow in both CTO lesions and remote areas significantly increased after 3 weeks from CTO PCI. Left ventricular ejection fraction also significantly increased, but with only minimal effect ($46.4 \pm 11.0\%$ vs. $47.5 \pm 11.4\%$, $p = 0.01$). The less marked effect of left ventricular function in the overall CTO patients may be associated with normal left ventricular function at baseline.

1.2.3 Decreased Demand of Coronary Bypass Surgery

In early CTO PCI era, Ivanhoe et al. reported that successful CTO PCI group significantly decreased demand of coronary artery bypass surgery (CABG) during the 4-year follow-up, compared to the failed group (13% vs. 36%, $p < 0.001$) [24]. Similarly, CABG is reduced in patients with successful CTO PCI than in those with failed CTO PCI in TOAST-GISE study (2.5% vs. 15.7%, $p < 0.001$) [18]. In Korean

Chronic Total Occlusion (K-CTO) registry, a need for CABG was significantly lower in successful CTO PCI than in failed group (0.2% vs. 2.5%, $p < 0.001$) [25]. Overall, the successful CTO PCI with drug-eluting stents reduced the incidence of subsequent bypass surgery by 90% than in failed CTO PCI (odds ratio 0.10, 95% CI = 0.05–0.21, $p < 0.001$) [26].

1.2.4 Improvement of Long-Term Outcome

2568 patients with CTO lesions from the multi-center K-CTO registry were analyzed to evaluate clinical outcomes. During the median 2-year follow-up, the successful CTO PCI group had a significant lower incidence of cardiac death or myocardial infarction than the failed CTO group (1.7% vs. 3.3%, $p = 0.02$) [25]. From the UK Central Cardiac Audit Database, the success rate of CTO PCI was 70.6% [27]. Overall successful CTO PCI was associated with survival improvement (hazard ratio 0.72, 95% confidence interval (CI): 0.62–0.83, $p < 0.001$) than unsuccessful CTO PCI during follow-up of 2.65 years (Table 1.1).

In a recent meta-analysis with a total of 9 studies involving 7469 CTO patients, successful CTO PCI using drug-eluting stents improved long-term all-cause mortality (odds ratio 0.55, 95% CI: 0.44–0.67, $p < 0.001$) and the occurrence of myocardial infarction (odds ratio 0.45, 95% CI: 0.23–0.74, $p = 0.002$) than failed CTO PCI [26].

1.2.5 Mortality Benefit in Myocardial Infarction with CTO

In patients with acute myocardial infarction (AMI), concurrent presence of CTO is significantly associated with poor prognosis [35, 36]. In COREA-AMI registry, successful CTO PCI for non-infarcted arteries improved clinical outcomes in terms of all-cause mortality (16.7% vs. 32.3%, hazard ratio 0.459, 95% CI 0.251–0.841, $p = 0.012$) and major adverse cardiac events

Table 1.1 Comparison of survival rate according to procedural success

Author	Patients number	Procedural success rate (%)	Follow-up duration (year)	Survival rate of successful CTO PCI (%)	Survival rate of failed CTO PCI (%)	p-value
Valenti et al. [28]	486	71	2	91.6	87.4	0.025
Lee et al. [29]	333	75.4	3.6	96.7	94.7	0.28
Yang et al. [30]	136	64	2	92	79.6	0.036
Borgia et al. [31]	202	78	4	92	86.2	0.23
Niccoli et al. [32]	317	53.9	3	97	92	0.11
Kim et al. [25]	2568	79.6	2	98.8	97.3	0.02
Lee et al. [33]	1173	85.6	4.6	92	92.9	0.92
Toma et al. [34]	2002	83	2.6	84.7	74.1	<0.001

(21.9% vs. 55.2%, hazard ratio 0.311, 95% CI 0.187–0.516, $p < 0.001$) compared with occluded CTO group [37]. Valenti et al. compared 58 patients who underwent successful staged CTO PCI to 111 patients with failed or non-attempted CTO PCI in AMI [38]. At 1 year, cardiac death occurred in only 1.7% of successful CTO PCI group but significantly high in 12% of occluded CTO patients ($p = 0.025$). At 3 years, successful CTO PCI reduced cardiac mortality by 80% (hazard ratio 0.20, 95% CI 0.05–0.92, $p = 0.038$).

1.2.6 The EXPLORE Trial and DECISION-CTO Study

The most CTO PCI data were derived from non-randomized studies with limited study population so far.

The EXPLORE (Evaluating Xience and Left Ventricular Function in Percutaneous Coronary Intervention on Occlusions After ST-Elevation Myocardial Infarction) trial, which is a randomized controlled trial, investigated whether second-stage CTO PCI in non-infarct-related artery within 7 days after primary PCI showed additional benefit compared to non-CTO PCI [39]. A total of 304 patients with STEMI were randomly assigned to CTO PCI group and medical treatment group. LVEF assessed by CMR was not significantly different between two groups (44.1 ± 12.2% vs. 44.8 ± 11.9%, $p = 0.06$) at 4 months (Table 1.2). LV end-diastolic volume

(LVEDV) was also similar in CTO PCI group and non-CTO PCI group (215.6 ± 62.5 mL vs. 212.8 ± 60.3 mL, $p = 0.07$). However, when non-infarct CTO lesion was located at left anterior descending artery (LAD), CTO PCI group showed significant superiority to non-CTO PCI group in terms of LVEF and LVEDV. The EXPLORE study seemed to show no definite overall benefit for CTO PCI in patients with STEMI and concurrent CTO.

But, several confounding factors must be considered to interpret the result. Firstly, improvement in LV function in STEMI patients mostly depends on the extent of culprit lesion and the success of primary PCI, but revascularization of CTO lesion might contribute in part. Secondly, myocardial viability subtended by CTO lesion at baseline was not assessed in all patients. Thirdly, optimal timing of CTO PCI for non-infarct-related artery has not been clearly known.

The DECISION-CTO (Drug-Eluting Stent Implantation Versus Optimal Medical Treatment in Patients with Chronic Total Occlusion) study was the first randomized controlled trial of 834 Asian patients without STEMI to compare the clinical outcomes, which is a composite of all-cause death, MI, stroke, and any repeat revascularization of CTO PCI with medical treatment only at 3 years. The success rate of CTO PCI with stenting was 91.1%. A composite endpoint at 3 years in intention-to-treat population was similar between CTO PCI and medical group (19.6% vs. 20.6%, $p = 0.008$ for

Table 1.2 The results of EXPLORE trial

	CTO PCI ($N = 136$)	Non-CTO PCI ($N = 144$)	Difference (95% CI)	P-value
LVEF, %	44.1 (12.2)	44.8 (11.9)	−0.8 (−3.6 to 2.1)	0.60
LVEDV, mL	215.6 (62.5)	212.8 (60.3)	2.8 (−11.6 to 17.2)	0.70
Major adverse cardiac events	($N = 148$)	($N = 154$)		
Cardiac death	4 (2.7)	0 (0.0)		0.056
Myocardial infarction	5 (3.4)	3 (1.9)		0.49
Periprocedural	4 (2.7)	1 (0.6)		
Spontaneous or recurrent	2 (1.4)	2 (1.3)		
CABG operation	–	1 (0.6)		–
MACE	8 (5.4)	4 (2.6)		0.25

Table 1.3 The results of DECISION-CTO study

	Optimal medical treatment ($N = 398$)	CTO PCI ($N = 417$)	Hazard ratio (95% CI)	p-value
Primary endpoint				
A composite of death, MI, stroke, any repeat revascularization	19.6	20.6	0.95 (0.74–1.22)	0.67
All-cause death	4.4	3.0	1.5 (0.75–3.03)	0.25
MI	8.4	10.7	0.77 (0.49–1.19)	0.24
Stroke	1.3	1.0	2.56 (0.80–8.17)	0.11
Repeat revascularization	8.6	10.4	0.81 (0.52–1.28)	0.38

non-inferiority) (Table 1.3). There were no differences in quality of life measured by the Seattle Angina Questionnaire at 1 year and among pre-specified subgroups. Conversely, 18% of patients allocated to medical group were crossed over into CTO PCI group. In the per-protocol and as-treated population analysis, the non-inferiority margin was not met for CTO PCI. Event rates were numerically higher in medical treatment group than in CTO PCI group (22.3% vs. 19.0%, $p = 0.15$ for non-inferiority). Authors carefully suggested medical treatment only as the initial treatment strategy for CTO lesion compared to CTO PCI. However, there was some criticism after coming up with the results.

To properly interpret this result, we need to understand it more deeply. First, although estimated study population was 1284, only 834 patients were included due to difficulties in enrolling patients. Furthermore, most of the patients were actively enrolled in a single center. Second, periprocedural MI, defined as five-time increase of cardiac biomarker, included as a part of the primary endpoint, gave a burden to the CTO PCI arm. Third, although intention-to-treat anal-

ysis was performed, overall death was lower in CTO PCI group than in medical group (3.0% vs. 4.4% at 3 years, 4.5% vs. 7.9% at 5 years, crude hazard ratio 1.5, 95% CI 0.75–3.03, $p = 0.25$). Particularly, cardiac death was much lower in CTO PCI group than in medically treated group (1.9% vs. 3.6%, $p = 0.22$). Although these differences were not significant, the final results could be changed if more patients were completely followed up.

1.3 Conclusion

CTO PCI has rapidly evolved. CTO PCI was previously performed only by few experts, but has expanded to more interventionists with new strategies and devices. The success rate is increasing while complication risk is decreasing. The benefit of CTO PCI includes symptom relief, improvement of left ventricular function, decreased demands of bypass surgery, and improved long-term outcome. There is no doubt that more research is required to better understand the benefit of CTO PCI.

References

1. Fefer P, Knudtson ML, Cheema AN, Galbraith PD, Osherov AB, Yalonetsky S, Gannot S, Samuel M, Weisbrod M, Bierstone D, Sparkes JD, Wright GA, Strauss BH. Current perspectives on coronary chronic total occlusions: the Canadian Multicenter Chronic Total Occlusions Registry. J Am Coll Cardiol. 2012;59:991–7.

2. Kahn JK. Angiographic suitability for catheter revascularization of total coronary occlusions in patients from a community hospital setting. Am Heart J. 1993;126:561–4.

3. Rees JR. The myocardial collateral circulation. Br Heart J. 1969;31:1–4.

4. Stein JH, Weiss MB, Ro JH, Herman MV. Percutaneous transluminal coronary angioplasty of a coronary artery with a total occlusion. Arch Intern Med. 1984;144:1875–7.

5. Holmes DR Jr, Vlietstra RE, Reeder GS, Bresnahan JF, Smith HC, Bove AA, Schaff HV. Angioplasty in total coronary artery occlusion. J Am Coll Cardiol. 1984;3:845–9.

6. Safian RD, McCabe CH, Sipperly ME, McKay RG, Baim DS. Initial success and long-term follow-up of percutaneous transluminal coronary angioplasty in chronic total occlusions versus conventional stenoses. Am J Cardiol. 1988;61:23G–8G.

7. Stone GW, Rutherford BD, McConahay DR, Johnson WL Jr, Giorgi LV, Ligon RW, Hartzler GO. Procedural outcome of angioplasty for total coronary artery occlusion: an analysis of 971 lesions in 905 patients. J Am Coll Cardiol. 1990;15:849–56.

8. Hoye A, van Domburg RT, Sonnenschein K, Serruys PW. Percutaneous coronary intervention for chronic total occlusions: the Thoraxcenter experience 1992–2002. Eur Heart J. 2005;26:2630–6.

9. Shim WH, Kim HS, Jang YS, Cho SY, Lee WK. Percutaneous transluminal coronary angioplasty in total coronary artery occlusion. Korean Circ J. 1992;22:532–49.

10. Maiello L, Colombo A, Almagor Y, Bouzon R, Thomas J, Zerboni S, Finci L. Coronary stenting with a balloon-expandable stent after the recanalization of chronic total occlusions. Catheter Cardiovasc Diagn. 1992;25:293–6.

11. Kahn JK, Hartzler GO. Retrograde coronary angioplasty of isolated arterial segments through saphenous vein bypass grafts. Catheter Cardiovasc Diagn. 1990;20:88–93.

12. Surmely JF, Tsuchikane E, Katoh O, Nishida Y, Nakayama M, Nakamura S, Oida A, Hattori E, Suzuki T. New concept for CTO recanalization using controlled antegrade and retrograde subintimal tracking: the CART technique. J Invasive Cardiol. 2006;18:334–8.

13. Rathore S, Katoh O, Matsuo H, Terashima M, Tanaka N, Kinoshita Y, Kimura M, Tsuchikane E, Nasu K, Ehara M, Asakura K, Asakura Y, Suzuki T. Retrograde percutaneous recanalization of chronic total occlusion of the coronary arteries: procedural outcomes and predictors of success in contemporary practice. Circ Cardiovasc Interv. 2009;2:124–32.

14. Morino Y, Abe M, Morimoto T, Kimura T, Hayashi Y, Muramatsu T, Ochiai M, Noguchi Y, Kato K, Shibata Y, Hiasa Y, Doi O, Yamashita T, Hinohara T, Tanaka H, Mitsudo K, J-CTO Registry Investigators. Predicting successful guidewire crossing through chronic total occlusion of native coronary lesions within 30 minutes: the J-CTO (Multicenter CTO Registry in Japan) score as a difficulty grading and time assessment tool. JACC Cardiovasc Interv. 2011;4:213–21.

15. Opolski MP, Achenbach S, Schuhback A, Rolf A, Mollmann H, Nef H, Rixe J, Renker M, Witkowski A, Kepka C, Walther C, Schlundt C, Debski A, Jakubczyk M, Hamm CW. Coronary computed tomographic prediction rule for time-efficient guidewire crossing through chronic total occlusion: insights from the CT-RECTOR Multicenter Registry (Computed Tomography Registry of Chronic Total Occlusion Revascularization). JACC Cardiovasc Interv. 2015;8:257–67.

16. Kim BK, Cho I, Hong MK, Chang HJ, Shin DH, Kim JS, Shin S, Ko YG, Choi D, Jang Y. Usefulness of intraprocedural coronary computed tomographic angiography during intervention for chronic total coronary occlusion. Am J Cardiol. 2016;117:1868–76.

17. Yu CW, Lee HJ, Suh J, Lee NH, Park SM, Park TK, Yang JH, Song YB, Hahn JY, Choi SH, Gwon HC, Lee SH, Choe YH, Kim SM, Choi JH. Coronary computed tomography angiography predicts guidewire crossing and success of percutaneous intervention for chronic total occlusion: Korean Multicenter CTO CT Registry Score as a tool for assessing difficulty in chronic total occlusion percutaneous coronary intervention. Circ Cardiovasc Imaging. 2017;10:e005800.

18. Olivari Z, Rubartelli P, Piscione F, Ettori F, Fontanelli A, Salemme L, Giachero C, Di Mario C, Gabrielli G, Spedicato L, Bedogni F, TOAST-GISE Investigators. Immediate results and one-year clinical outcome after percutaneous coronary interventions in chronic total occlusions: data from a multicenter, prospective, observational study (TOAST-GISE). J Am Coll Cardiol. 2003;41:1672–8.

19. Grantham JA, Jones PG, Cannon L, Spertus JA. Quantifying the early health status benefits of successful chronic total occlusion recanalization: results from the FlowCardia's approach to chronic total occlusion recanalization (FACTOR) trial. Circ Cardiovasc Qual Outcomes. 2010;3:284–90.

20. Wijeysundera HC, Norris C, Fefer P, Galbraith PD, Knudtson ML, Wolff R, Wright GA, Strauss BH, Ko DT. Relationship between initial treatment strategy and quality of life in patients with coronary chronic total occlusions. EuroIntervention. 2014;9:1165–72.

21. Cheng AS, Selvanayagam JB, Jerosch-Herold M, van Gaal WJ, Karamitsos TD, Neubauer S, Banning AP. Percutaneous treatment of chronic total coronary occlusions improves regional hyperemic myocardial blood flow and contractility: insights from quantitative cardiovascular magnetic resonance imaging. JACC Cardiovasc Interv. 2008;1:44–53.

22. Pujadas S, Martin V, Rossello X, Carreras F, Barros A, Leta R, Alomar X, Cinca J, Sabate M, Pons-Llado G. Improvement of myocardial function and perfusion after successful percutaneous revascularization in patients with chronic total coronary occlusion. Int J Cardiol. 2013;169:147–52.

23. Stuijfzand WJ, Biesbroek PS, Raijmakers PG, Driessen RS, Schumacher SP, van Diemen P, van den Berg J, Nijveldt R, Lammertsma AA, Walsh SJ, Hanratty CG, Spratt JC, van Rossum AC, Nap A, van Royen N, Knaapen P. Effects of successful percutaneous coronary intervention of chronic total occlusions on myocardial perfusion and left ventricular function. EuroIntervention. 2017;13:345–54.

24. Ivanhoe RJ, Weintraub WS, Douglas JS Jr, Lembo NJ, Furman M, Gershony G, Cohen CL, King SB 3rd. Percutaneous transluminal coronary angioplasty of chronic total occlusions. Primary success, restenosis, and long-term clinical follow-up. Circulation. 1992;85:106–15.

25. Kim BK, Shin S, Shin DH, Hong MK, Gwon HC, Kim HS, Yu CW, Park HS, Chae IH, Rha SW, Lee SH, Kim MH, Hur SH, Jang Y. Clinical outcome of successful percutaneous coronary intervention for chronic total occlusion: results from the multicenter Korean chronic total occlusion (K-CTO) registry. J Invasive Cardiol. 2014;26:255–9.

26. Gao L, Wang Y, Liu Y, Cao F, Chen Y. Long-term clinical outcomes of successful revascularization with drug-eluting stents for chronic total occlusions: a systematic review and meta-analysis. Catheter Cardiovasc Interv. 2017;89:574–81.

27. George S, Cockburn J, Clayton TC, Ludman P, Cotton J, Spratt J, Redwood S, de Belder M, de Belder A, Hill J, Hoye A, Palmer N, Rathore S, Gershlick A, Di Mario C, Hildick-Smith D, British Cardiovascular Intervention Society, National Institute for Cardiovascular Outcomes Research. Long-term follow-up of elective chronic total coronary occlusion angioplasty: analysis from the U.K. Central Cardiac Audit Database. J Am Coll Cardiol. 2014;64:235–43.

28. Valenti R, Migliorini A, Signorini U, Vergara R, Parodi G, Carrabba N, Cerisano G, Antoniucci D. Impact of complete revascularization with percutaneous coronary intervention on survival in patients with at least one chronic total occlusion. Eur Heart J. 2008;29:2336–42.

29. Lee SW, Lee JY, Park DW, Kim YH, Yun SC, Kim WJ, Suh J, Cho YH, Lee NH, Kang SJ, Lee CW, Park SW, Park SJ. Long-term clinical outcomes of successful versus unsuccessful revascularization with drug-eluting stents for true chronic total occlusion. Catheter Cardiovasc Interv. 2011;78:346–53.

30. Yang ZK, Zhang RY, Hu J, Zhang Q, Ding FH, Shen WF. Impact of successful staged revascularization of a chronic total occlusion in the non-infarct-related artery on long-term outcome in patients with acute ST-segment elevation myocardial infarction. Int J Cardiol. 2013;165:76–9.

31. Borgia F, Viceconte N, Ali O, Stuart-Buttle C, Saraswathyamma A, Parisi R, Mirabella F, Dimopoulos K, Di Mario C. Improved cardiac survival, freedom from MACE and angina-related quality of life after successful percutaneous recanalization of coronary artery chronic total occlusions. Int J Cardiol. 2012;161:31–8.

32. Niccoli G, De Felice F, Belloni F, Fiorilli R, Cosentino N, Fracassi F, Cataneo L, Burzotta F, Trani C, Porto I, Leone AM, Musto C, Violini R, Crea F. Late (3 years) follow-up of successful versus unsuccessful revascularization in chronic total coronary occlusions treated by drug eluting stent. Am J Cardiol. 2012;110:948–53.

33. Lee PH, Lee SW, Park HS, Kang SH, Bae BJ, Chang M, Roh JH, Yoon SH, Ahn JM, Park DW, Kang SJ, Kim YH, Lee CW, Park SW, Park SJ. Successful recanalization of native coronary chronic total occlusion is not associated with improved long-term survival. JACC Cardiovasc Interv. 2016;9:530–8.

34. Toma A, Gick M, Minners J, Ferenc M, Valina C, Loffelhardt N, Gebhard C, Riede F, Neumann FJ, Buettner HJ. Survival after percutaneous coronary intervention for chronic total occlusion. Clin Res Cardiol. 2016;105:921–9.

35. Claessen BE, van der Schaaf RJ, Verouden NJ, Stegenga NK, Engstrom AE, Sjauw KD, Kikkert WJ, Vis MM, Baan J Jr, Koch KT, de Winter RJ, Tijssen JG, Piek JJ, Henriques JP. Evaluation of the effect of a concurrent chronic total occlusion on long-term mortality and left ventricular function in patients after primary percutaneous coronary intervention. JACC Cardiovasc Interv. 2009;2:1128–34.

36. Claessen BE, Dangas GD, Weisz G, Witzenbichler B, Guagliumi G, Mockel M, Brener SJ, Xu K, Henriques JP, Mehran R, Stone GW. Prognostic impact of a chronic total occlusion in a non-infarct-related artery in patients with ST-segment elevation myocardial infarction: 3-year results from the HORIZONS-AMI trial. Eur Heart J. 2012;33:768–75.

37. Choi IJ, Koh YS, Lim S, Choo EH, Kim JJ, Hwang BH, Kim TH, Seo SM, Kim CJ, Park MW, Shin DI, Choi YS, Park HJ, Her SH, Kim DB, Park CS, Lee JM, Moon KW, Chang K, Kim HY, Yoo KD, Jeon DS, Chung WS, Ahn Y, Jeong MH, Seung KB, Kim PJ. Impact of percutaneous coronary intervention for chronic total occlusion in non-infarct-related arteries in patients with acute myocardial infarction (from the COREA-AMI registry). Am J Cardiol. 2016;117:1039–46.

38. Valenti R, Marrani M, Cantini G, Migliorini A, Carrabba N, Vergara R, Cerisano G, Parodi G, Antoniucci D. Impact of chronic total occlusion revascularization in patients with acute myocardial infarction treated by primary percutaneous coronary intervention. Am J Cardiol. 2014;114:1794–800.

39. Henriques JP, Hoebers LP, Ramunddal T, Laanmets P, Eriksen E, Bax M, Ioanes D, Suttorp MJ, Strauss BH, Barbato E, Nijveldt R, van Rossum AC, Marques KM, Elias J, van Dongen IM, Claessen BE, Tijssen JG, van der Schaaf RJ, EXPLORE Trial Investigators. Percutaneous intervention for concurrent chronic total occlusions in patients with STEMI: the EXPLORE trial. J Am Coll Cardiol. 2016;68:1622–32.

Review of Histopathology of CTO for CTO Success

Satoru Sumitsuji and Jung Rae Cho

2.1 Introduction

Despite technical advancement in the percutaneous coronary intervention for coronary artery disease, there is still room for improvement of success rate. To achieve this goal, deeper understanding of the histopathology of CTO segment is essential. In this chapter, we summarized the current concept of CTO histopathology and its clinical impact for the CTO success in the contemporary interventional practice.

2.2 Definition of CTO

In the earlier literature, CTO has been defined as (1) obstruction of coronary artery with no luminal continuity, (2) Thrombolysis in Myocardial Infarction (TIMI) flow grade 0 or 1, and (3) duration of occlusion >30 days estimated from clinical events (myocardial infarction or worsening of ischemic symptom) or proven by previous angiography [1]. Indication of PCI for CTO includes

S. Sumitsuji (✉)
Division of Cardiology for International Education and Research, Graduate School of Medicine, Osaka University, Suita, Japan
e-mail: satoru@sumi2g.sakura.ne.jp

J. R. Cho
Division of Cardiology, Kangnam Sacred Heart Hospital, Hallym University College of Medicine, Seoul, South Korea

(1) medically refractory angina, (2) large area of ischemia by noninvasive study, and (3) favorable angiographic morphologies. Favorable angiographic morphologies included tapered proximal stump, functional occlusion, no side branch at occlusion site, and absence of bridging collaterals, whereas non-favorable ones included blunted proximal stump, total occlusion, side branch at occlusion site, and presence of bridging collaterals [1]. Because of its feasibility, this classification has been widely used as a guide for the CTO operators to predict technical success rate. From the recent expert consensus, the duration of occlusion generally more than 3 months and only TIMI flow grade 0 are regarded as true CTO [2].

2.3 Components Inside CTO Segments

All the arteries have three layers including intima, media, and adventitia. In usual atherosclerotic plaque, circulating LDL particle is captured and deposited underneath intimal layer leading to a bigger, established plaque which is not distinguishable between plaque and media by IVUS (so-called plaque-media complex). On the other hand, because the CTO segment has no luminal space, CTO plaque is regarded as located in the intimal position ("intimal plaque"), which is the unique concept of CTO histopathology. The space between media and adventitia is regarded

© Springer Nature Singapore Pte Ltd. 2019
Y. Jang (ed.), *Percutaneous Coronary Interventions for Chronic Total Occlusion*,
https://doi.org/10.1007/978-981-10-6026-7_2

Fig. 2.1 Schema of "inside of CTO segment" and "outside of CTO segment"

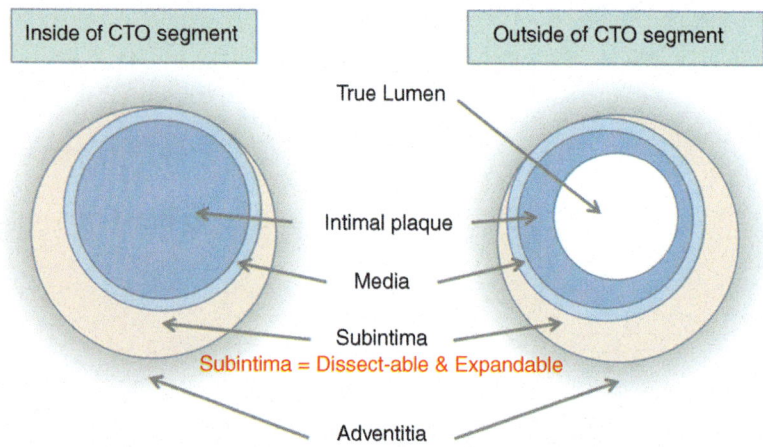

as subintimal space; with its most important feature as expandability, which is clearly seen by IVUS when intramural hematoma develops during CTO-PCI (Fig. 2.1). Because histopathologic evaluation of CTO segment during CTO-PCI is almost impossible to perform, real-time IVUS examination has been used as an alternative in vivo assessment for the similar purpose and has broadened our understanding of CTO. IVUS can distinguish true lumen, plaque-media complex, subintimal space, and extra-coronary hematoma when coronary artery was perforated or ruptured. All of which are essential components of CTO, and it provides important information during CTO-PCI (Fig. 2.2). Pre-procedural cardiac computed tomography (CT) also has become the standard gadget for many CTO operators. Unlike IVUS which is more focusing on cross-sectional image, cardiac CT well visualizes the entire segment of CTO including its course, location, amount of calcium, etc. (Fig. 2.3). The role of pre-procedural CT in the CTO-PCI is that it can help operators make a big picture of how the procedure has to be done. In this regard, imaging of CTO segment could be a feasible alternative to histopathologic examination.

There are scanty number of histopathologic reports of CTO segment in the literature. In the earlier postmortem study among patients having CTO, loose fibrous tissue with small vascular channel was seen inside CTO segment [3]. Besides, intraluminal plaque as well as calcifications could be seen in the CTO segment. Based on

these findings, current understanding of the progression of CTO is postulated like this: (1) obstruction of coronary artery with fresh thrombus, (2) thrombus formation develops proximally and distally, (3) thrombus formation develops up to the side branch ostium and the originally occluded area turns into fibrotic plaque with calcified lesions and finally develops, and (4) aged CTO with fibrotic plaque and calcified lesions including proximal and distal fibrous cap (Fig. 2.4) [4].

2.4 Procedural Impact

2.4.1 Issues Related to Antegrade Approach

In the mature CTO segment, proximal fibrous cap tends to be harder than distal fibrous cap which is not easily penetrated by conventional workhorse guidewires. In case of aged CTO, heavyweight guidewires (Miracle, Conquest, Gaia, all from *Asahi Intecc, Japan*) with proper microcatheter backup (Corsair, Caravel, *Asahi Intecc, Japan*; Finecross, *Terumo, Japan*) are essential to penetrate the proximal cap of CTO. If the operator wants to track down the loose tissue, intermediate-weight hydrophilic guidewire (PILOT 50, *Abbott, USA*; SION black, Fielder-XT, *Asahi Intecc, Japan*) with microcatheter backup can be considered during wire manipulation.

Although the guidewire successfully crossed the proximal cap of CTO segment, another issue

Fig. 2.2 Correlation with histopathology and IVUS findings of CTO (inside and outside of CTO segment)

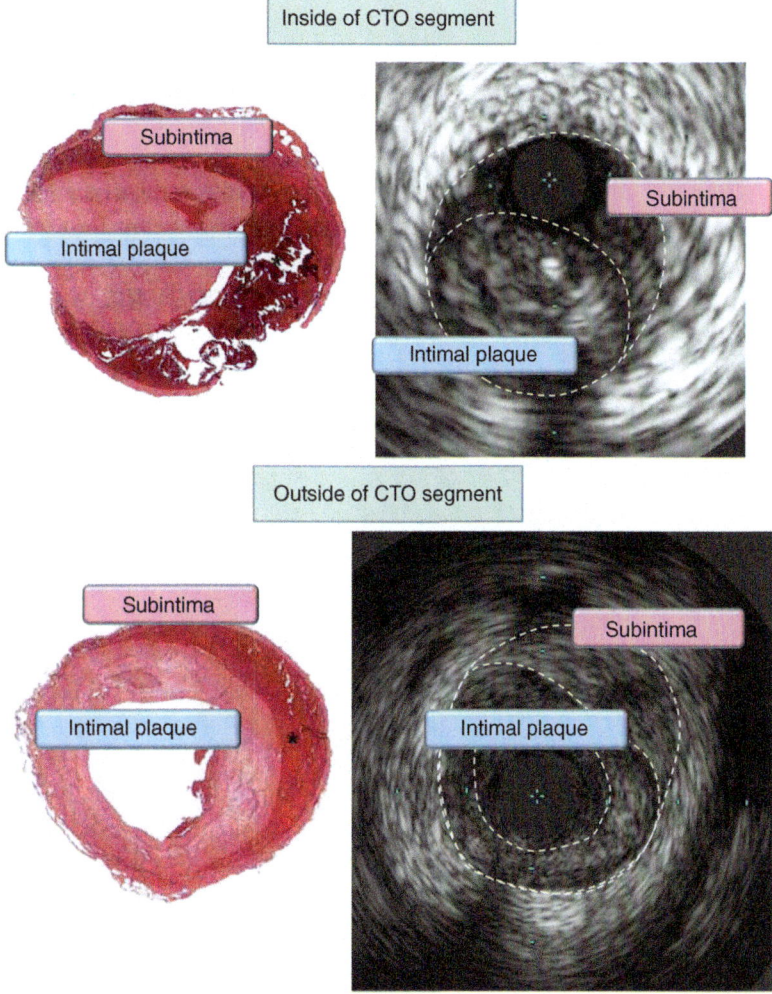

is the calcium. Recently, calcium in the CTO segment can be easily assessed by cardiac CT usually performed before starting CTO-PCI as a pre-procedural evaluation. It is of importance to check the location, morphology, and amount of calcium chunk inside CTO in cross section; all of these information cannot be obtained from simple coronary angiogram or fluoroscopy (Fig. 2.5). Whenever the antegrade guidewire is stuck inside the CTO segment or only subintimal tracking of wire is highly suspected (such as "S-shaped wire configuration by fluoroscopy") (Fig. 2.6), the operator needs to judge whether to keep going with the same guidewire or change to a different strategy according to the lesion characteristics and the location of the guidewire. In an autopsy case of patient who underwent unsuccessful CTO-PCI and who eventually died from retroperitoneal hemorrhage [4], extensive subintimal hematoma with subsequent collapse of distal true lumen was clearly demonstrated, indicating that the main reason for the failed CTO-PCI is the subintimal guidewire passage which did not go back to the distal true lumen. From the histopathologic perspectives, trying every effort to keep the guidewire in the intraplaque position during wire crossing from proximal all the way down to the distal true lumen (i.e., "intimal plaque tracking") is of utmost importance for antegrade wiring (Fig. 2.7). During an antegrade approach where the first guidewire ended up in the seemingly subintimal space, several options can be

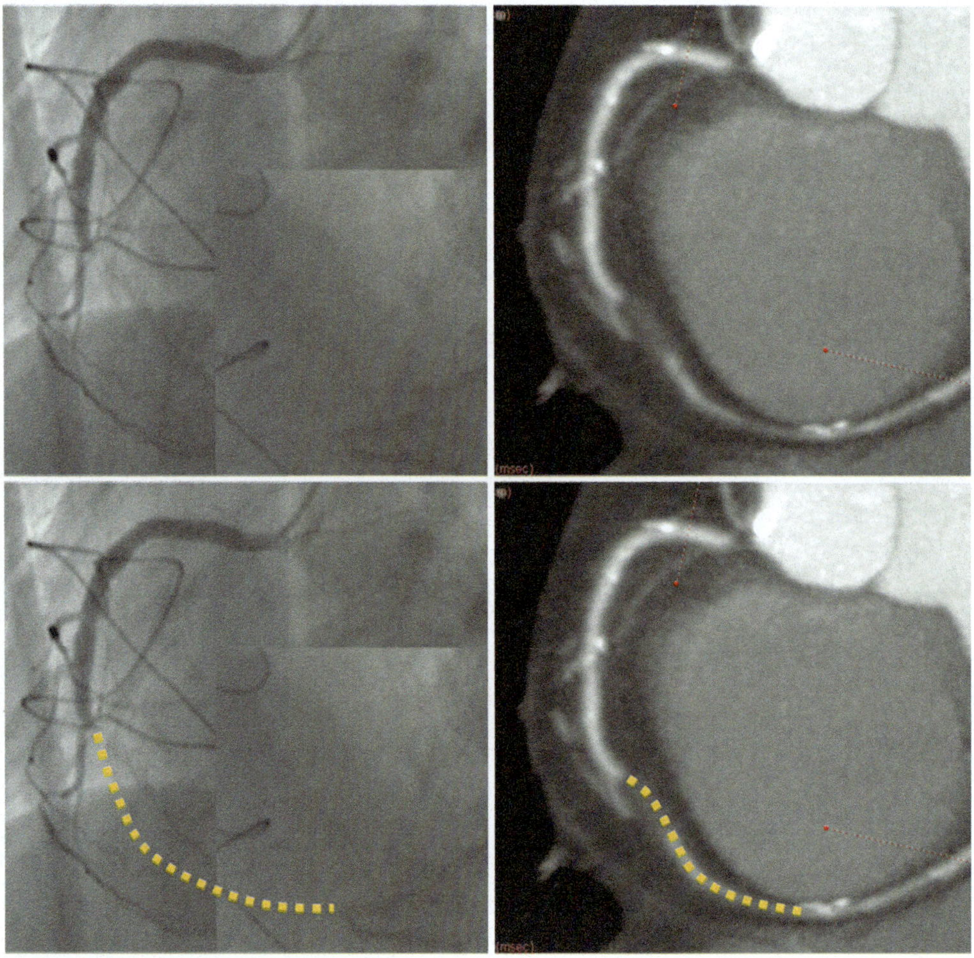

Fig. 2.3 Intimal plaque route in angiogram and CT

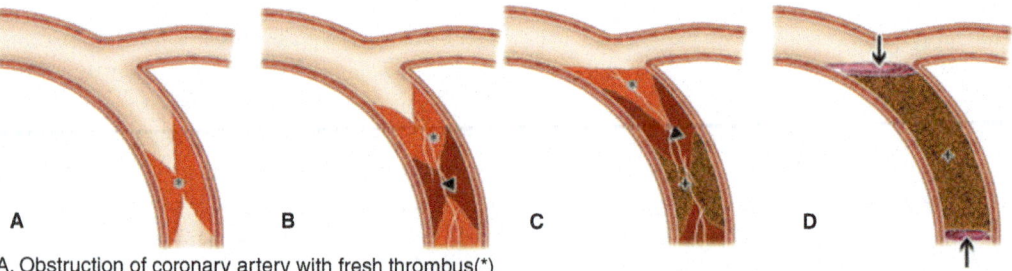

A. Obstruction of coronary artery with fresh thrombus(*)

B. Thrombus formation develops proximally(*) and distally

C. Thrombus formation develops up to the side branch ostium. The originally occluded area turns into fibrotic plaque
   with calcified lesions(+)

D. Aged CTO with fibrotic plaque and calcified lesions(+). Each arrows indicates proximal & distal fibrous cap

Fig. 2.4 Progression of chronic total occlusion. (**a**) Obstruction of coronary artery with fresh thrombus (*). (**b**) Thrombus formation develops proximally (*) and distally. (**c**) Thrombus formation develops up to the side branch ostium. The originally occluded area turns into fibrotic plaque with calcified lesions (+). (**d**) Aged CTO with fibrotic plaque and calcified lesions (+). Each arrow indicates proximal and distal fibrous cap

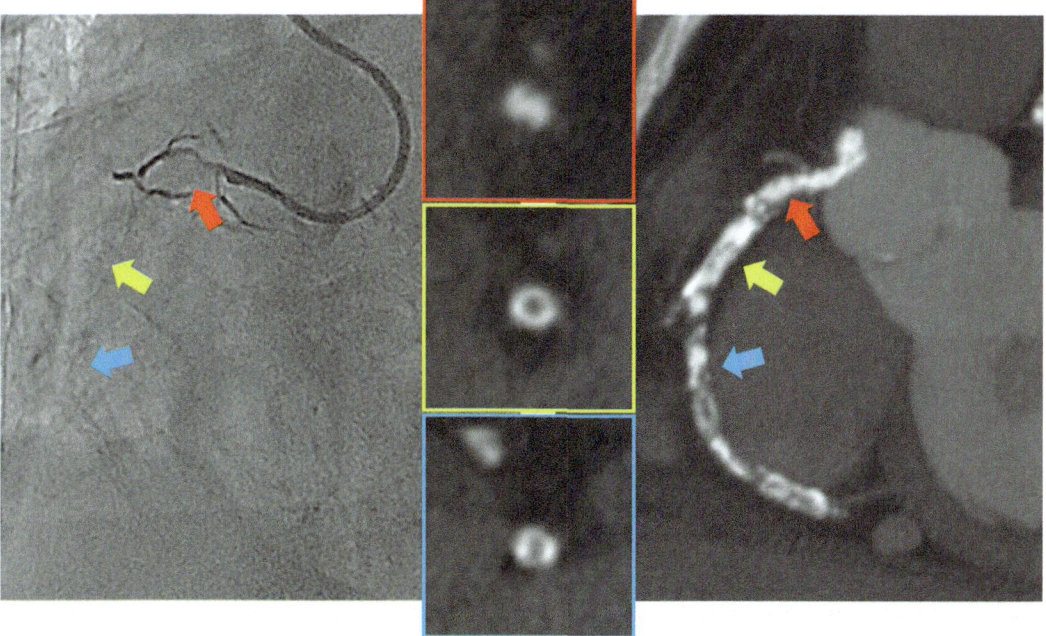

Fig. 2.5 Cross-sectional assessment for calcium by CT

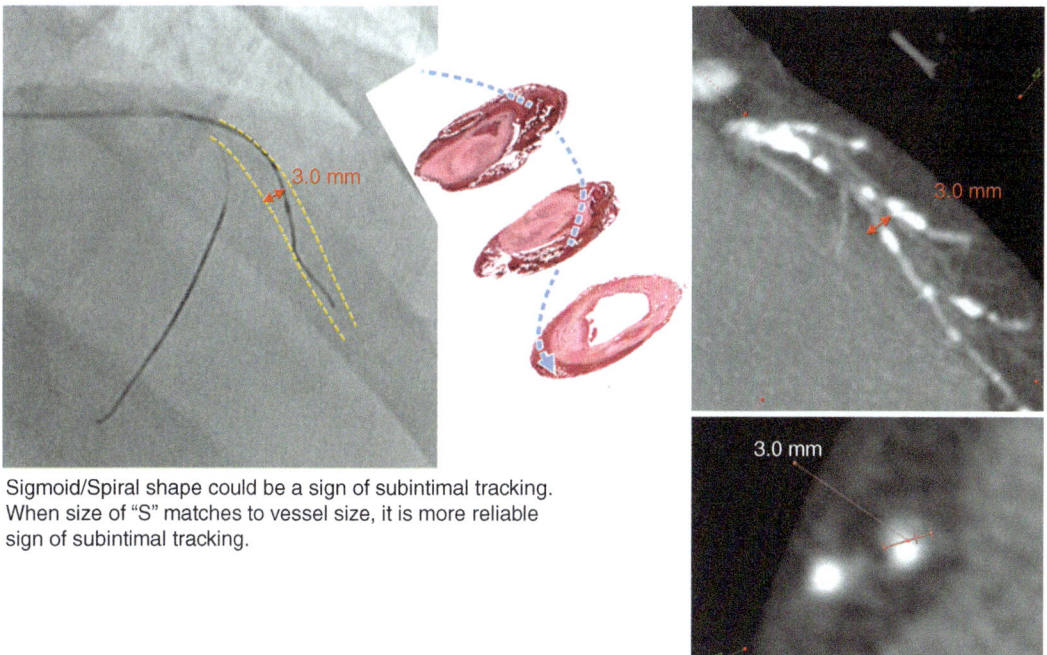

Sigmoid/Spiral shape could be a sign of subintimal tracking. When size of "S" matches to vessel size, it is more reliable sign of subintimal tracking.

Fig. 2.6 S-shaped configuration of guidewire suggestive of its subintimal passage. Sigmoid/spiral shape could be a sign of subintimal tracking. When size of "S" matches to vessel size, it is a more reliable sign of subintimal tracking

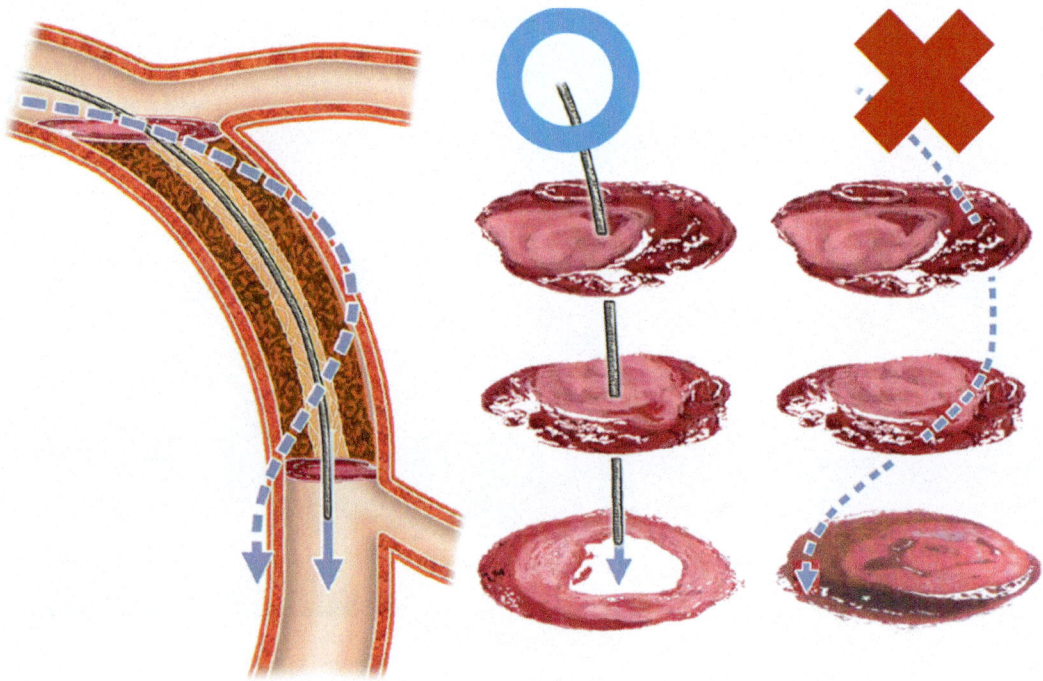

Fig. 2.7 Tracking guidewire inside intimal plaque is the key to success in antegrade wiring

considered. If IVUS catheter could be advanced around the tip of the guidewire, IVUS-guided reentry—deflecting and advancing the wire tip into intimal plaque and distal true lumen—might be a good option. However, if the tip of the guidewire already reached to the subintimal space at the distal true lumen, antegrade dissection reentry (ADR) using CrossBoss/Stingray system (*Boston Scientific*, *USA*) can be considered. Otherwise, we can either keep the first guidewire and advance second guidewire to the intraplaque location as much as possible (a.k.a. "parallel wire technique") or keep the first guidewire and try retrograde approach.

2.4.2 Issues Related to Retrograde Approach

As already mentioned, distal fibrous cap is less rigid than proximal one which is better penetrable and traceable inside intimal plaque by current CTO-dedicated guidewires. There are several variations of combined antegrade/retrograde techniques (CART, reverse CART, kissing wire cross, etc.) designed by Japanese CTO experts. The main purpose of these techniques is to assure wire cross, to shorten procedure time, and to minimize the length of subintimal guidewire passage. Whenever the guidewire position is unclear during retrograde wiring procedure, IVUS examination is highly recommended to make sure of the wire position and provide solutions. The current concept of retrograde approach includes advancing both antegrade and retrograde wire to meet each other in the same space at a certain point. Therefore, four different types of wire configuration by IVUS are possible: (1) antegrade, intimal plaque; retrograde, intimal plaque; (2) antegrade, subintimal; retrograde, intimal plaque; (3) antegrade, intimal plaque; retrograde, subintimal; and (4) antegrade, subintimal; retrograde, subintimal (Fig. 2.8). In case both guidewires inside intimal plaque position (1), antegrade balloon dilation accompanied by retrograde wire penetration into the balloon-dilated space is mostly recommended. When both wires are located in the subintimal space (4), balloon dilation is requested to make a connection between

Fig. 2.8 Four different types of antegrade/retrograde wire configuration

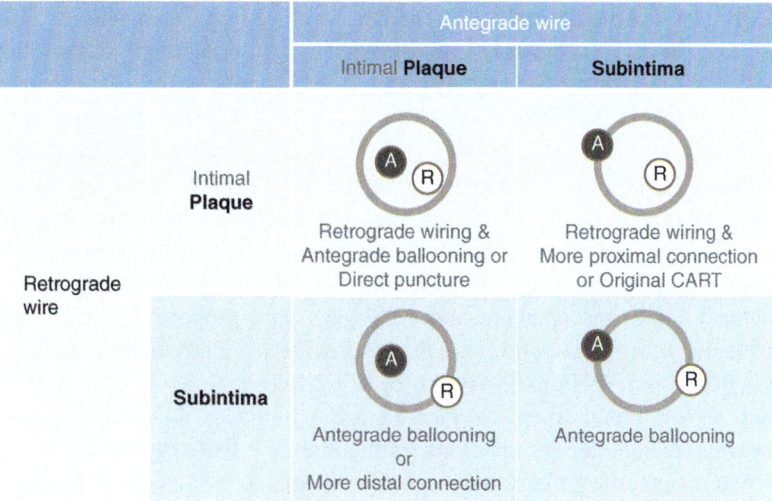

antegrade and retrograde wires, but in this situation required balloon size and dilatation pressure should not be so big and high because subintimal space is quite easy to be dissected and expanded. In case of antegrade, intimal plaque; retrograde, subintimal (3), there are two options. First option is advancing antegrade wire to distal and change configuration of wire position to (1) or (4). After changing configuration, wire cross could be achieved as above. If antegrade wire cannot be advanced, we can choose the second option: reverse CART with bigger size balloon, and deliver higher pressure to make intentional medial dissection, which is necessary for wire cross. Because of making intentional medial dissection in this case, the length of subintimal tracking becomes longer than the first option. In case of the antegrade, subintimal; retrograde, intimal plaque (2) configuration, simple reverse CART never works out because antegrade ballooning dilates subintimal space only and never makes connection to retrograde wire position in intimal plaque. So, in the situation, what we should do is (1) advancing retrograde wire to proximal and change configuration to (1), (3), or (4). If we cannot advance retrograde wire, final option is original CART: advancing balloon with retrograde wire and try to make intentional medial dissection to connect antegrade wire lumen and retrograde wire lumen.

2.5 In-Stent CTO

In-stent CTO is mostly less challenging because stent strut helps to keep guidewire position in intimal plaque. The best situation is both proximal and distal end of CTO located inside the stented segment. Because in-stent material is not expandable like subintimal space, guidewire is always under control and tends to be easily taken into true lumen. However, even the original CTO segment confined in the in-stent CTO segment may extend beyond either or both ends of CTO located outside of the stented segment. In this situation, CTO segment extended to non-stented CTO segment leads to increase the risk of subintimal tracking during wire manipulation. Another difficult issue of in-stent CTO is that the procedural outcome is often depending upon histologic feature and stented location of previous stent. From the autopsy report of patients with in-stent CTO [5], medial tear accompanying in-stent thrombotic occlusion has been suggested as a major etiology of in-stent CTO. However, maturated thrombus with subsequent collagen deposition sometimes mimics hard, very stiff wire, and strong backup force is needed for the secure puncture. In case of subintimal stenting in previous PCI, retrograde extra-stent wiring or ADR is needed to achieve wire cross.

2.6 CTO Segment in Patients Who Previously Underwent Coronary Artery Bypass Graft (CABG)

Although CABG has been regarded as the standard treatment for CTO in the past decade, CABG has a negative impact on the histopathologic composition of CTO segment. In the autopsy study by Sakakura and colleagues on patients with CTO who underwent previous CABG or not, CTO patients with prior CABG has shown more atherosclerotic change with heavier calcium deposit than those without prior CABG, suggesting that CABG accelerates atherosclerosis [6]. For the CTO patients who are eligible for CTO-PCI without much difficulty, it can be better done before performing CABG due to its less calcium accumulation.

2.7 Implications from Peripheral CTO

The observation from the peripheral CTO segment could give a clue to the coronary CTO. In the in vivo angioscopic evaluation of peripheral CTO segment from proximal and distal occlusion sites, thrombus was visible at distal fibrous cap suggesting that CTO segment may evolve and extend distally with thrombosis, suggesting the benefit of early interventional treatment and antithrombotic therapy [7]. The presence of thrombus at the distal cap might be another clue of feasibility of retrograde guidewire advancement.

2.8 Summary

Earlier reports from postmortem study and surgical specimens gave us the better histopathologic understanding of the CTO segment. From the procedural standpoint, IVUS has become the alternative method to assess in vivo histopathology, especially visualizing cross-sectional images of each component of vascular wall including CTO plaque. Cardiac CT has advantage in pre-procedural assessment of intimal plaque route and calcification inside CTO segment. This information has a considerable impact on strategy making steps and procedural outcome in a patient who undergoes CTO-PCI. With the help of these image guidance, we could choose proper strategies and adequate devices for improving the success rate of CTO-PCI.

References

1. Yokoyama N, Yamamoto Y, Suzuki S, Suzuki M, Konno K, Kozuma K, Kaminaga T, Isshiki T. Impact of 16-slice computed tomography in percutaneous coronary intervention of chronic total occlusions. Cathet Cardiovasc Interv. 2006;68(1):1–7.
2. Ybarra LF, Piazza N, Brilakis E, Grantham JA, Stone GW, Rinfret S. Clinical endpoints and key data elements in percutaneous coronary intervention of coronary chronic Total occlusion studies: a call to the academic research consortium for standardized definitions. JACC Cardiovasc Interv. 2017;10(21):2185–7.
3. Katsuragawa M, Fujiwara H, Miyamae M, Sasayama S. Histologic studies in percutaneous transluminal coronary angioplasty for chronic total occlusion: comparison of tapering and abrupt types of occlusion and short and long occluded segments. J Am Coll Cardiol. 1993;21(3):604–11.
4. Sumitsuji S, Inoue K, Ochiai M, Tsuchikane E, Ikeno F. Fundamental wire technique and current standard strategy of percutaneous intervention for chronic total occlusion with histopathological insights. JACC Cardiovasc Interv. 2011;4(9):941–51.
5. Mori H, Lutter C, Yahagi K, Harari E, Kutys R, Fowler DR, Ladich E, Joner M, Virmani R, Finn AV. Pathology of chronic total occlusion in bare-metal versus drug-eluting stents: implications for revascularization. JACC Cardiovasc Interv. 2017;10(4):367–78.
6. Sakakura K, Nakano M, Otsuka F, Yahagi K, Kutys R, Ladich E, Finn AV, Kolodgie FD, Virmani R. Comparison of pathology of chronic total occlusion with and without coronary artery bypass graft. Eur Heart J. 2014;35(25):1683–93.
7. Yamaji K, Ueno M, Yamamoto H, Ikeda T, Suga T, Ikuta S, Kobuke K, Iwanaga Y, Miyazaki S. Backyards of chronic total occlusion: scenery revealed through angioscope. Circulation. 2014;129(25):2715–6.

Interpretation of Coronary Angiography Before CTO Intervention

Jong-Young Lee and Bum-Kee Hong

3.1 Introduction

Diagnostic coronary angiography of chronic total occlusion (CTO) lesions plays an important role in establishing the initial treatment strategy by assessing the indications of interventional treatment and the potential problems which might arise during the procedure. However, coronary angiography for the evaluation of CTO lesions should be in some respects different from usual lesions. Although recent advances in computed tomography (CT) have proven to be helpful in many cases before and after the procedure, we have to deal with guide wire during the procedure by the information obtained from coronary angiography. In addition, even with the same coronary angiography image, there is much difference in the information that an operator can obtain according to the operator's expertise.

Therefore, prior to the CTO lesion intervention, treatment plan should be determined through the thorough understanding of CTO lesion, such as lesion characteristics and stereotypic vessel course by previously taken angiographic images. To achieve this goal, it is necessary to acquire well-examined angiography images, with spending sufficient time to thoroughly assess the lesion, which can play a very important role in determining the success of the CTO procedure. Experienced or high-volume operators with expertise are willing to invest enough time to identify overall information of CTO lesions.

3.1.1 Duration of Occlusion

It is well known that the success rate of CTO largely depends on the duration of occlusion and lesion morphology (Table 3.1). It is difficult to accurately estimate the duration of the lesion occlusion in diagnostic coronary angiography, and the time of occlusion can be roughly predicted considering the history of chest pain or myocardial infarction. Sometimes previous electrocardiograms performed at remote hospital visit may provide clues. In any case, detailed history taking is crucial in determining treatment strategies. If the patient have had a coronary angiogram, the operator needs to check the previous images to help estimate the duration of occlusion. However, if there is a lot of bridge collateral, it usually means long-term occlusion. In this case, the operators must be careful in the selection of guideline because of high risk of perforation or dissection.

J.-Y. Lee
Division of Cardiology, Kangbuk Samsung Hospital, Sungkyunkwan University School of Medicine, Seoul, South Korea

B.-K. Hong (✉)
Division of Cardiology, Gangnam Severance Hospital, Yonsei University College of Medicine, Seoul, South Korea
e-mail: bkhong@yuhs.ac

© Springer Nature Singapore Pte Ltd. 2019
Y. Jang (ed.), *Percutaneous Coronary Interventions for Chronic Total Occlusion*,
https://doi.org/10.1007/978-981-10-6026-7_3

3.1.2 Anatomical Description of CTO Morphology

It is important to determine the shape of the branch at the entrance of the coronary artery to select the proper guiding catheter. Unlike conventional coronary intervention, in CTO lesion intervention, the guiding catheter must have a reliable "backup" role to handle the guide wire in a stable fashion.

Because the probability of success may vary depending on the lesion shape in the angiography, several categories are mentioned, but the most commonly mentioned is the figure below (Fig. 3.1).

3.1.2.1 Left Main Coronary Artery

The left main coronary artery is more often deviated toward the posterior side from the usual location. In this case, the left main trunk (LMT) runs at an acute angle, so an Amplatz catheter for sufficient "backup" is recommended. There is no problem if the ascending aorta is vertical, but if it is close to horizontal, it is difficult to obtain sufficient backup with Judkins left, so physician must choose Amplatz and EBU (extra backup) for sufficient backup. In addition, taking the diameter of ascending aorta into consideration also plays an important role in the selection of the guiding catheter.

3.1.2.2 Right Coronary Artery

Coronary artery anomalies are common in the right coronary artery. Among them, anterior takeoff of the right coronary artery is relatively common. In this case, the right coronary artery

Table 3.1 Guideline for chronic total occlusion

	Class 1	Class 2	Class 3		Class 4
Occlusion duration	1–3 months	More than 3 months	More than 3 months	More than 3 months	More than 3 months
Lesion length	All	<2 cm	<2 cm	≥2 cm	≥2 cm
Lesion morphology	All	Tapered	Abrupt	All	Abrupt
Lesion tortuosity	None	None	None	None	None
Success rate (%)	70–90	50–80	40–70	40–70	25–50

Fig. 3.1 Anatomical classification of CTO lesion

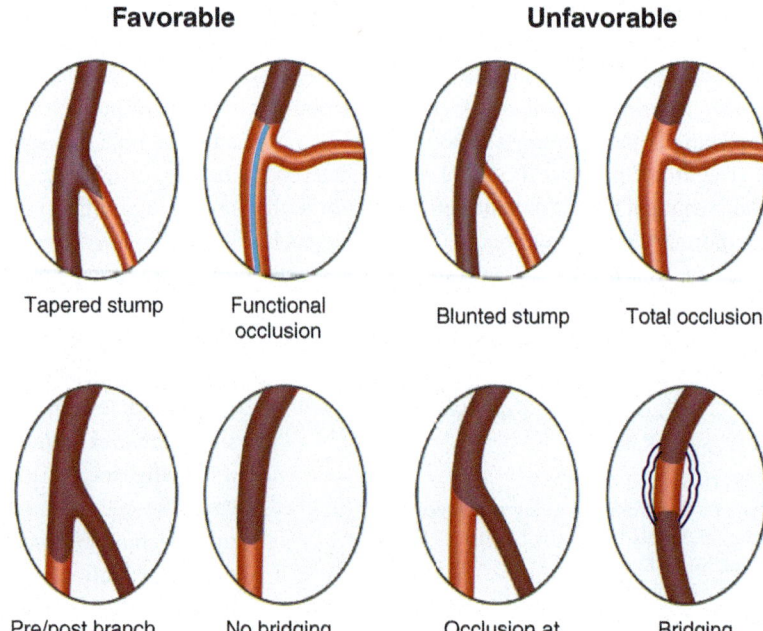

Favorable   Unfavorable

Tapered stump   Functional occlusion   Blunted stump   Total occlusion

Pre/post branch occlusion   No bridging collaterals   Occlusion at side branch   Bridging collaterals

bends rightward after exiting the aorta and travels along the aortic wall. Because it is difficult to insert deeply into the guiding catheter, it is best to choose Amplatz with a strong "backup"; otherwise it is difficult to obtain sufficient "backup" in the usual Judkins right. In addition, if the ascending aorta is vertical, there is no problem, but if it is close to horizontal, Amplatz and Ikari R should be selected because the angle formed by the ascending aorta and the right coronary artery becomes acute and cannot be sufficiently inserted into Judkins right. Also, in case of "Shepherd's crook" right coronary artery and the long horizontal portion of the entrance, Judkins right often fails to obtain sufficient "backup" for CTO lesions. The ascending aortic diameter should also be considered the same as the left coronary artery during guiding catheter selection.

3.1.3 CTO Proximal Lesion, Vascular Bending, and Tortuosity

As mentioned earlier, the coronary arterial branching pattern (entrance position, branching direction, and running) is important for the choice of guiding catheter. If the proximal lesion includes the entrance site, guiding catheter causes ischemia and coronary artery dissection. Therefore, it should be understood sufficiently before procedure. In the right coronary artery, the guiding catheter may need to be inserted deeply. Sometimes, the stent is inserted first by expanding the entrance and proximal lesions; according to the circumstances, not only the complication such as coronary artery dissection can be prevented, but also manipulation of guide wire could be easier. In addition, when the proximal blood vessel of the CTO is severely tortuous or curved, it is difficult to manipulate the guide wire in the CTO lesion. Therefore, physician can use a micro-catheter (TRANSIT, FINECROSS, Corsair, etc.) or OTW [over the wire] balloon to achieve adequate backup support for the advancement of guide wires.

3.1.4 Interpretation of Angiogram About CTO Lesion

3.1.4.1 Proximal Cap of CTO Lesion

Proximal occlusion pattern of CTO lesion is significantly related to CTO success rate. Depending on the type of proximal end occlusion, the tip may be divided into two types: tapered type and abrupt type. In the tapered type (Fig. 3.2), it is easy to find the entry point of the CTO, but in the abrupt type (Fig. 3.3), it is often difficult to find the entry point. However, if you carefully observe the contrast image in many directions, you may find an entry point dimple as an entry point. Therefore, we should observe the contrast image in one frame by one frame in many directions.

In some cases, a "recanalization channel" (microchannel) may be found within the CTO lesion after careful observation of the lesion (Fig. 3.4). At this time, the lesion can be passed from the beginning with a relatively smooth and well-guided wire without the use of a hard guide wire. In the case of bridge collateral development, vasa vasorum connected with bridge collateral may be difficult to differentiate between expanded vessel lumen and recanalization channel. If the wire advances deeply into the bridge collateral by mistake, the possibility of perforation and subsequent hemorrhage might be increased. In this regard, wiring close to bridging collaterals needs extra caution.

Normally, abrupt-type inlet is hard. In order to penetrate this, the operator should use heavyweight guide wire with sufficiently high tip stiffness and adequate "backup" force. The abrupt-type CTO lesion with side branch is the most difficult to perform, because it is difficult to identify the CTO entry point, as well as the manipulation of the guide wire is way more difficult because of its higher chances of penetrating into the branch.

In this situation, the IVUS-guided procedure is widely adopted by many experienced operators. IVUS can be used to improve the procedure success rate by grasping the puncture site as well as anatomical structure in CTO entry.

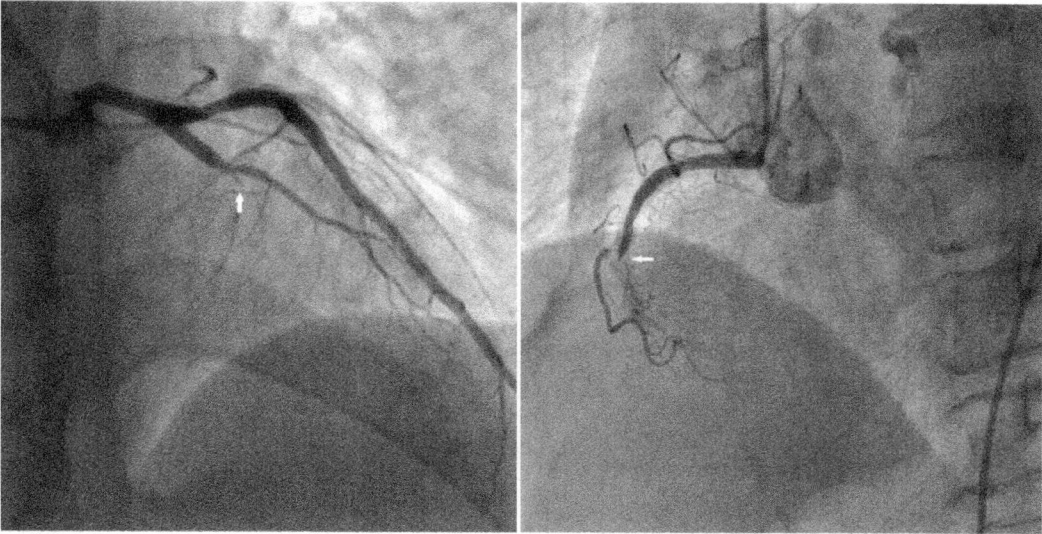

Fig. 3.2 Examples of tapered-type proximal end (white arrow, LAD, and RCA)

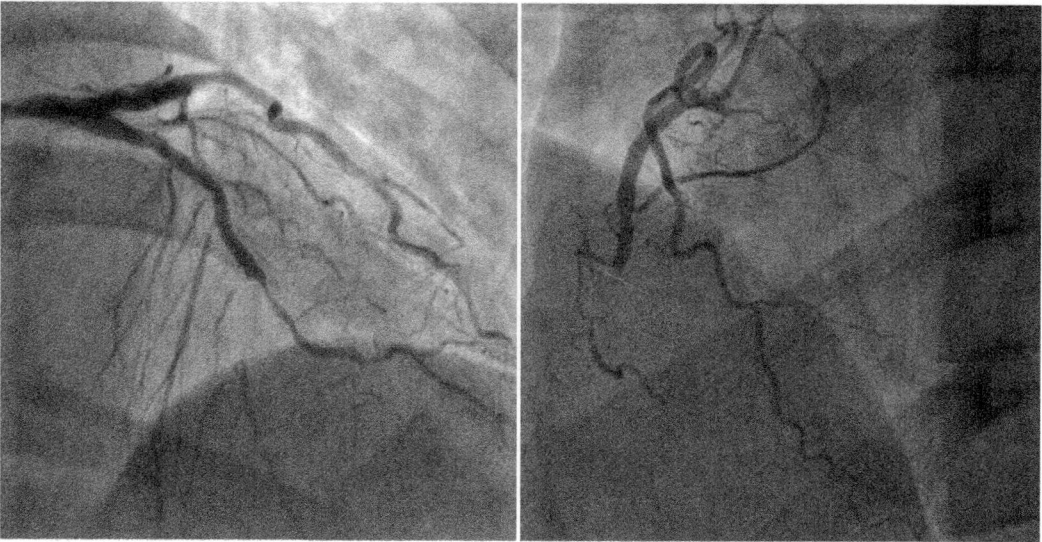

Fig. 3.3 Examples of abrupt type proximal end (white solid line, LAD, and RCA)

3.1.4.2 Vascular Bending in CTO Lesion

Consideration should also be given to vascular bending in CTO lesions. In a long CTO of the right coronary artery or left circumflex coronary artery, it may be very difficult to predict a flexed run. We should always look at the contrast image with the bending of the right coronary artery segment 1, the S-curve of the segment 3, the flexion of the left segment 11–13, and the peripheral segment of the left segment 7. In addition, if the ves-

sel alignment between the proximal and distal ends of the CTO lesion continuously disrupts in accordance with the heartbeat, the course of the CTO lesion will run in a meandering way, so careful image interpretation should be needed for successful guide wire passage.

3.1.4.3 CTO Lesion Calcification

Calcification may be helpful in estimating vascular course. Calcification is usually seen in the

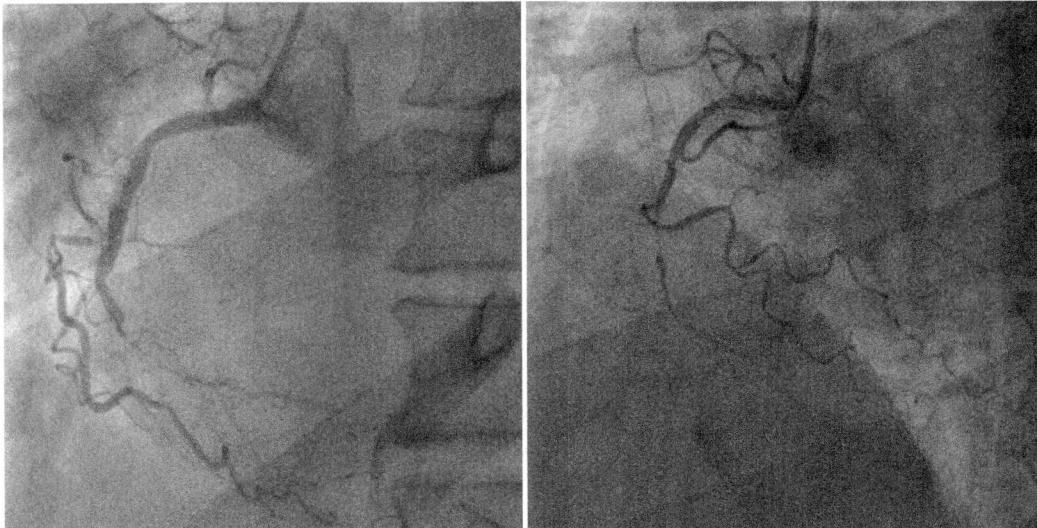

Fig. 3.4 The recanalization channel (microchannel) can be seen in RCA

main coronary arteries and is rarely seen in the branches. In order to determine the presence of calcification, it is helpful to slow the injection of the contrast medium slightly. If calcification is present, it is considered to be mostly in the main limb, but it is difficult to judge the location of the calcification site. Therefore, although calcification may be helpful in predicting travel path, it may cause confusion sometimes, so caution is needed.

3.1.4.4 Distal End Shape
It is also important to know the distal end shape as well as the CTO proximal end. Therefore, during coronary angiography, the angiogram should be taken longer than usual to ensure that the contrast agent is sufficiently pooled to the distal end. This is also important for accurately grasping the length of occluded lesions. The CTO distal tip is divided into tapered type and convex type. Usually the convex type, lesions are stiff, and the peripheral fibrous capsule is thick and rigid. On the contrary, it seems to be relatively easy to penetrate in the tapered type. However, if a false lumen is formed by the guide wire around the distal end, the true lumen easily changes in shape and is clogged. Careful handling of guide wires should be done at the distal end. A studious attention should also be taken,

when the courses are flexed immediately after distal CTO end, especially in the presence of sizable side branch around there.

3.1.4.5 Contrast "Island"
If the blood flow forms a complex network, we can see the island-shaped contrast filling inside the CTO lesion. This finding is a milestone in showing preferential cautions when manipulating guide wire, especially in long CTO lesions, and must be determined in advance (Fig. 3.5).

3.1.4.6 Branching Contrast Image
Side branching contrasts may be effective when predicting main branch route. In CTO lesions, contrast media may be seen up to the initial level, even if the contrast media are not clustered. This can also be a clue to the progression of guide wire, as is the case with contrast-island features.

3.1.4.7 "To and Fro" and "Negative Jet"
"To and fro" is the evidence that the contrast agent moves back and forth in the coronary artery, which is an indirect evidence that the blood enters the artery in a different way. "Negative jet" means that the contrast medium is partially thinned in the blood vessels, which means that the blood also comes in through the separate passage. In both cases, careful obser-

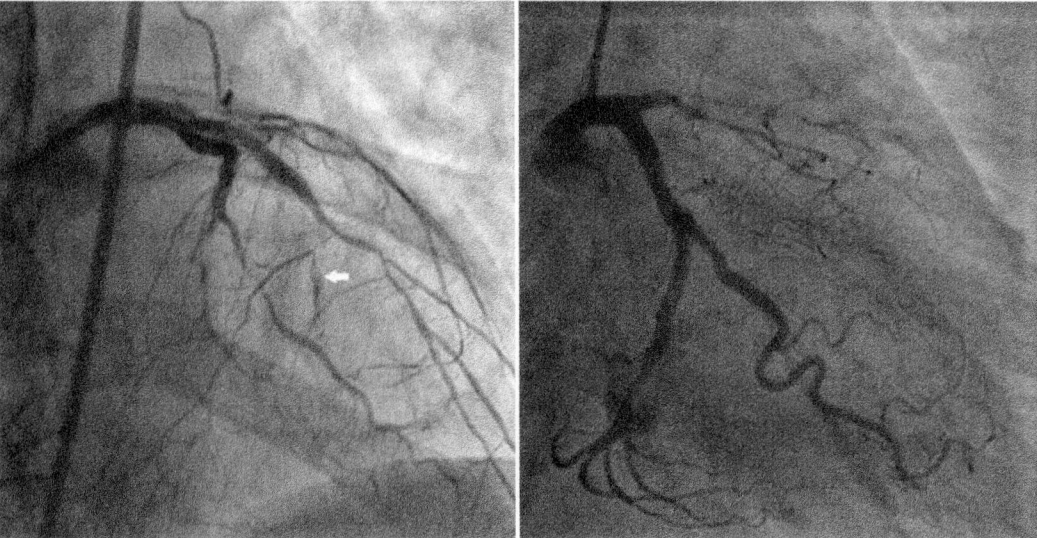

Fig. 3.5 In the late phase of image, contrast island is visible by the collateral blood flow

vation of the opposite side (contrast of right coronary artery, if the CTO is in the left coronary artery) should be observed. Particularly, in the right conus branch, segment 7 may be imaged in some cases, and there are cases where it is very effective in accurately determining the lesion length and grasping blood circulation. In order to accurately assess the CTO anatomy supplied by collateral circulation, bilateral simultaneous angiography is needed whenever possible.

3.1.5 Collateral Flow

In order to identify CTO lesions, it is important to observe the collateral blood flow in detail. In particular, if the donor artery comes out from the conus branch, the atrioventricular branch, or the right coronary artery origin (or independently from the aorta), the distal end of the CTO may not be fully visualized through the collateral flow. This phenomenon is often seen in the left anterior descending coronary artery because the distal end of the CTO is contrasted in the conus branch or in the right coronary artery or in the right ventricle.

Observation of CTO distal edge by collateral blood flow is also very important. Identification of the presence and shape of the branch at the distal end of the CTO is important when implementing the "side branch method." In addition, after the guide wire has passed the CTO lesion, it is necessary to grasp the distant vessel running in advance.

In the treatment of CTO by the retrograde approach, the course direction and morphology of the donor artery are important, so the operation through the collateral flow is one of the most important factors of success. Therefore, meticulous understanding of coronary angiogram must be necessary.

Grades of collateral filling:
- Grade 0—none
- Grade 1—filling of side branches of the artery via collateral channels without visualization of the epicardial segment
- Grade 2—partial filling of the epicardial segment via collateral channels
- Grade 3—complete filling of the epicardial segment of the artery via collateral channels

3.1.6 Image Projection

It is needless to say that CTO lesion coronary angiography requires multidirectional imaging. The bilateral injection angiogram is useful at exactly the same angle with the proximal end of the CTO lesion, and it plays an important role in understanding the CTO lesion length more accurately. In addition, rotational angiography or biplane angiograms, which also show three-dimensional positional relationships, can be effective tools in this regard.

3.1.7 Practical Tips of Diagnostic Coronary Angiography

3.1.7.1 Simultaneous Bilateral Angiography (Simultaneous Contrast)

Patients receiving collateral flow from the opposite coronary artery are basically required to undergo simultaneous imaging during PCI procedures. The goal is to (1) clarify the anatomical relationship around the occlusion site and (2) to pinpoint the status of the distal vessel occlusion, such as whether there is stenosis or occlusion. Simultaneous bilateral angiography should be performed when there is no clear occlusion route, and it cannot be grasped sufficiently. The best information obtained through coronary angiography before the procedure improves the success rate.

Looking at some of the basic things to keep in mind when performing this simultaneous angiography:

- Do not magnify the image too much.
- Donor artery should be contrasted first.
- CTO blood vessels should be visualized after 1–2 s.
- Avoid panning.
- Cine should be performed until all the contrast agent disappears.

3.1.7.2 Collateral Angiography (Contralateral Contrast)

While doing simultaneous angiography, the practitioner may judge the direction, in which the guide wire should proceed from the previous bilateral angiogram, or the frictional resistance felt during wire advance. If the microchannel is seen, even if the guiding wire is advanced to the microchannel and the net flow is lost, the contralateral puncture is performed to perform contralateral contrast. If the microchannel passes through the outer membrane layer and proceeds as it is, if the net flow is lost, the opposite side should be used to confirm that the direction is correct.

3.1.7.3 Biplane Cine Equipment

A bidirectional angiography equipment is another useful device for CTO PCI. Even if it seems that the wire goes in the right direction in one projection, while it is not in the other, the wire position is not correct. The ability to determine the guide wire position very precisely and instantly is the great advantage of the two-way angiography device. In the retrograde approach, a small amount of contrast agent is required after guide wire penetrates into the occlusion site in both the proximal and distal directions.

3.1.7.4 Selection of Projection Angle

The bidirectional angle to be selected by the bidirectional angiography device is firstly perpendicular (in the short-axis direction) from the entry point of the occlusion site to the long axis of the blood vessel and perpendicular to the core surface at that point (direction angle 1) (parallel to the core surface in the short-axis direction = direction angle 2) intersecting at a right angle with the direction angle 1 at the intersecting plane (within the short axis).

These directional angles are different depending on the occlusion region, and examples of the universal real direction angles are listed in Table 3.2. In RCA with long occlusion, the short axis changes significantly because the long-axis direction is very different from the proximal part and the distal part of occlusion. It is useful to change the direction angle, combined with guide wire advance. Changing the direction angle can also prevent skin injuries from radiation dose, by dispersing the skin surface dose.

3.1.8 Factors to Consider When Viewing the Preoperative Angiography

Recently, the CTO procedure considering the anatomical structure, namely, hybrid approach,

Table 3.2 Projection angle according to the CTO segment

Occlusion segment	Universal real direction angle	Universal perpendicular angle
#1, Ostium	LAO + CA	AP + CR
#1, RVB bifurcation	AP + CR, LAO + CA	LAO– LAO + CR
#4, AV, PD bifurcation	LAO + CR (LL)	AP + CR
#5, Ostium	AP + CR, AP + CA	Spider
#6, Ostium	RAO + CR	Spider
#6 and #7, Diagonal bifurcation	LAO + CR AP + CR	RAO + CR LL + CR
#11, Ostium	RAO (AP) + CA	Spider (LL + CA)
LCX, PL bifurcation	AP + CA	LL + CA

Abbreviation: *LAO* left anterior oblique, *CA* caudal, *AP* anteroposterior, *CR* cranial, *LL* left lateral, *RVB* right ventricle bifurcation, *AV* arteriovenous, *PD* posterior descending, *RAO* right anterior oblique, *LCX* left circumflex, *PL* posterolateral

has been proposed. Through four questions, we decide whether to use antegrade, retrograde, dissection, or reentry.

1. Is the proximal cap clearly visible on angiography or IVUS?
2. Is the lesion 20 mm or more in length?
3. Is the distal target clear?
4. Is collateral channel appropriate for the procedure?

Therefore, if you consider the answers to the above questions while thoroughly reviewing preoperative angiography, a more explicit approach strategy can be established.

3.2 Conclusion

Coronary angiography provides the most important information for the analysis and treatment of CTO lesions. All information that can be obtained from the contrast can be used to improve the success rate by performing the intervention under the best conditions. Although various interventional techniques are mentioned brilliantly, the best technique for treating CTO lesions is to observe coronary angiography images with considerable time and attention before the procedure. If the coronary angiographic projection is sufficiently observed, and the appropriate treatment policy is determined based on this, and the induction catheter and guide wire are selected as appropriate, the success rate will be further increased.

Suggested Reading

Brilakis ES. Manual of coronary chronic total occlusion interventions, A step-by-step approach. 1st ed. Waltham, MA: Elsevier; 2013.

Pershad A, Eddin M, Girotra S, Cotugno R, Daniels D, Lombardi W. Validation and incremental value of the hybrid algorithm for CTO PCI. Catheter Cardiovasc Interv. 2014;84:654–9.

Sianos G, Werner GS, Galassi AR, et al. Recanalisation of chronic total coronary occlusions: 2012 consensus document from the EuroCTO club. EuroIntervention. 2012;8:139–45.

Aris K, Barbara AD, Dimitri K, Khaldoon A, Minh V, Mauro C, Mitul PP, Stéphane R, Emmanouil SB. Approach to CTO intervention: overview of techniques. Curr Treat Options Cardiovasc Med. 2017;19:1.

Harding SA, Wu EB, Lo S, Lim ST, Ge L, Chen JY, Quan J, Lee SW, Kao HL, Tsuchikane E. A new algorithm for crossing chronic total occlusions from the Asia Pacific chronic total occlusion club. JACC Cardiovasc Interv. 2017;10(21):2135–43.

4

Pre- and Intraprocedure Computed Tomography-Based Assessment of CTO for the Successful CTO Intervention

Jin-Ho Choi, Byeong-Keuk Kim, and Sanghoon Shin

4.1 Introduction

Despite vast advances in the devices and interventional technique, the overall success rate of percutaneous coronary intervention for chronic total occlusion (CTO) is still an unsatisfactory 70–80%. Compared to successful opening of CTO, failed attempt for CTO has resulted in poor long-term outcome as well as higher contrast dye usage, radiation exposure, and complication rate [1–3]. The presence of CTO is one of the major causes of selecting surgical bypass surgery instead of percutaneous coronary intervention.

The most important component in the successful CTO procedure is selecting appropriate procedural candidate, which is preferably guided by understanding accurate lesion morphology and vascular course. Unlike conventional coronary artery lesions, invasive coronary angiography is limited in the direct visualization of CTO lesion morphology or vascular course. Recently introduced coronary computed tomography (CT) angiography enables noninvasive visualization evaluation of the total vascular system including CTO lesion. Coronary CT visualizes comprehensive anatomic findings which cannot be directly enhanced by contrast dye such as occluded segment, distribution of calcifications, and distal vasculature. There is no limitation of visualization angle in reconstructed anatomical images. In addition, non-CTO vascular segment including the shape of ostium, curvature and size of vessel proximal to CTO, the extent of collateral vessel development, presence of significant disease in donor vessel, and myocardial viability subtended by CTO vessel needs to be evaluated before starting procedure [4–7]. Image-guided CTO intervention based on pre-procedural coronary CT may increase procedural success rate as well as clinical outcome.

4.2 Information Derived from Coronary CT Angiography

Information provided by coronary CT angiography can be summarized as [1] anatomical finding of vessel segment proximal to CTO lesion [2], anatomical finding of CTO segment [3], and anatomical finding and perfusion of vessel distal to CTO lesion by collateral vessel (Fig. 4.1).

J.-H. Choi (✉)
Samsung Medical Center, Sungkyunkwan University
School of Medicine, Seoul, South Korea
e-mail: choijinh@skku.edu

B.-K. Kim
Severance Cardiovascular Hospital,
Yonsei University College of Medicine,
Seoul, South Korea

S. Shin
National Health Insurance Service Ilsan Hospital,
Goyang-si, Gyeonggi-do, South Korea

© Springer Nature Singapore Pte Ltd. 2019
Y. Jang (ed.), *Percutaneous Coronary Interventions for Chronic Total Occlusion*,
https://doi.org/10.1007/978-981-10-6026-7_4

4.2.1 Vessel Proximal to CTO Lesion

Selecting the appropriate guiding catheter is crucial for successful CTO procedure. Sufficiently powerful support is required to back up guidewire and devices such as balloon or microcatheter penetrating CTO lesion. Many operators prefer larger 7 or 8 French-sized catheters to smaller 5 or 6 French-sized catheters. However, diseased or narrowed ostium cannot accept large bore-guiding catheter and may need smaller guiding catheter. For left coronary artery, extra backup-type catheter is preferred to Judkins-type catheters. Amplatz-type guiding catheter may be suitable for selected left circumflex artery and right coronary artery but carries higher risk of ostial injury. These guiding catheter selection strategies can be predicted by pre-procedural coronary CT angiography (Fig. 4.2). Aorto-ostial

1. Anatomy of ostium and proximal vessel

2. Anatomy of CTO lesion   Donor vessel

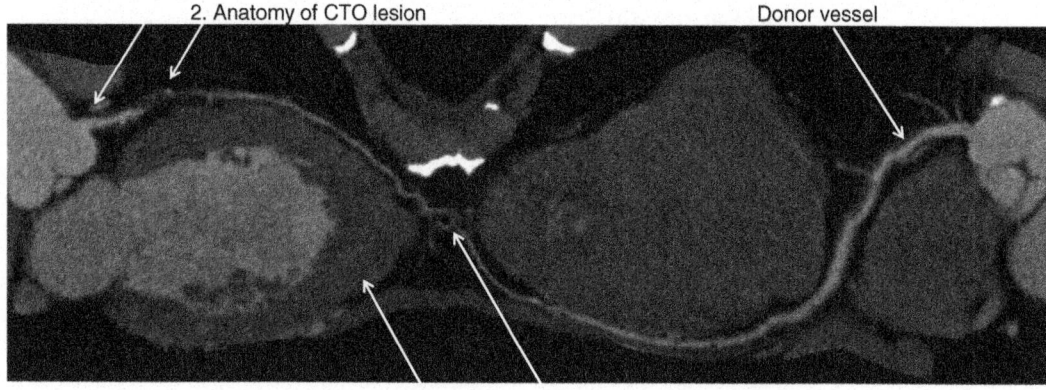

3. Physiology of myocardium   4. Physiology of collateral flow
(myocardial perfusion, viability)

Fig. 4.1 Anatomical and physiological information derived from coronary CT angiography

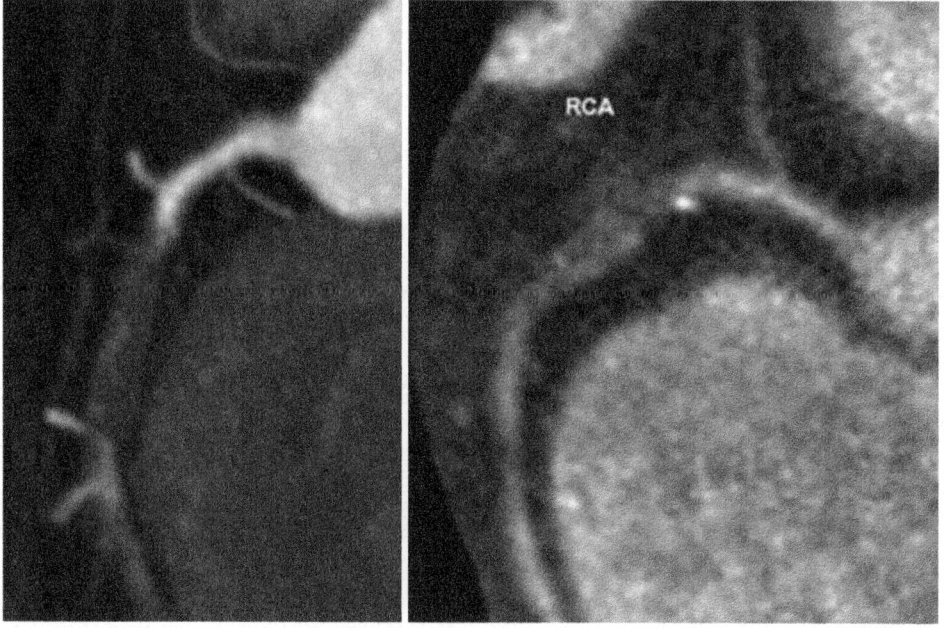

Fig. 4.2 Two cases of coronary CT angiography showing ostium of right coronary artery. Right coronary artery in the left panel shows large diameter without plaque and can accept large bore-guiding catheter. Right coronary artery in the right panel shows small luminal diameter with moderate to severe atherosclerotic plaque burden, for which large bore-guiding catheter cannot be cannulated

total occlusion is one of the most challenging CTO lesion and notorious for difficulty in finding and cannulating guiding catheter. Preprocedural coronary CT can visualize exact location of entry and guide CTO procedure (Figs. 4.3 and 4.4).

4.2.2 CTO Segment

4.2.2.1 Anatomical Findings of CTO

The pathogenesis of CTO is presumed to be the sequelae of symptomatic or asymptomatic non-fatal myocardial infarction, rather than progressive atherosclerotic occlusion [8]. Unresolved thrombotic occlusion is followed by organization and accumulation of proteoglycan. Proteoglycan is slowly replaced by collagen-rich plaque and calcified tissue, which is accompanied by shrinkage of positively remodeled vessel (Figs. 4.5, 4.6, and 4.7). The following clinical evidence supports this hypothetical age-dependent change of CTO plaque. The prevalence of symptomatic history or Q wave in electrocardiography is less than half in patients with CTO. However, cardiac magnetic

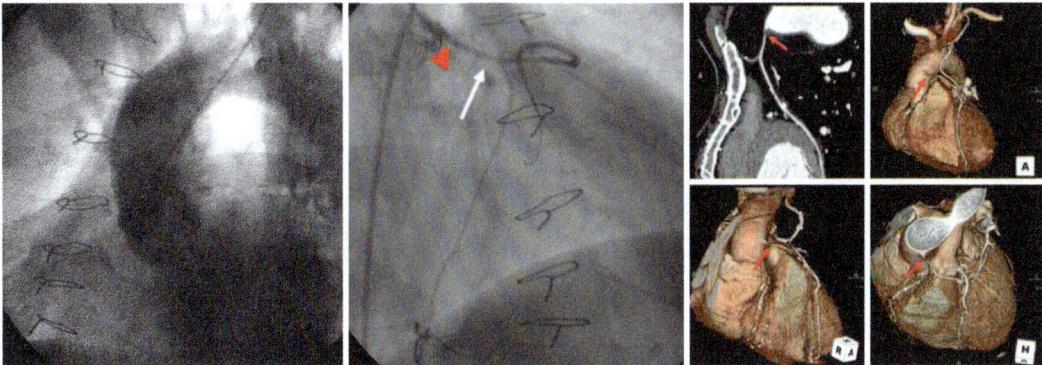

Fig. 4.3 A case of CT-guided PCI of invisible aorto-ostial graft occlusion lesion. Despite numerous attempts of guiding catheter cannulation and aortography, entry of graft ostial occlusion could not be identified. Following coronary CT angiography showed exact graft insertion site in ascending aorta. With this guidance, second attempt was successfully performed [27]

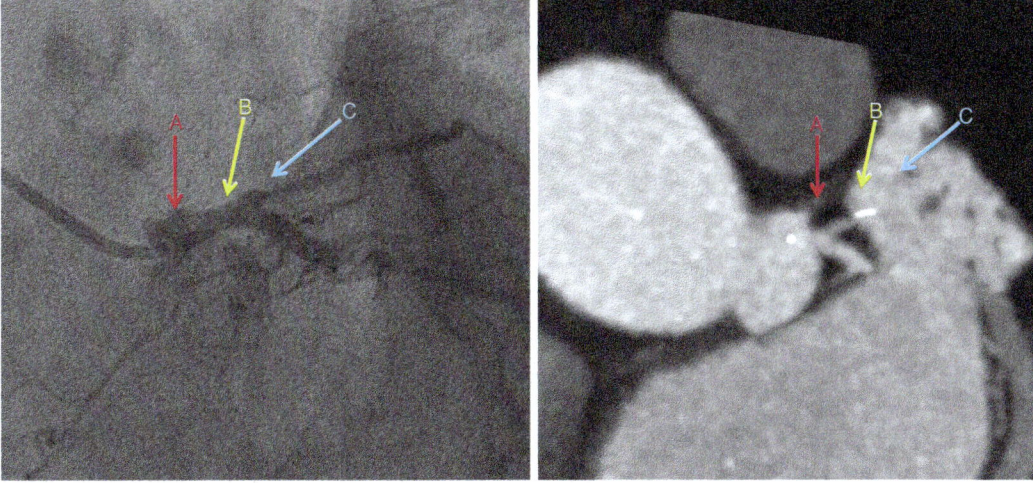

Fig. 4.4 CT-guided PCI of ostial occlusion of separated left anterior descending artery. Aorto-ostial total occlusion of separated left anterior descending artery. Comparison of angiographic finding (left panel) and coronary CT angiography finding (right panel) revealed that point A, not point B or C, is the actual entry of left anterior descending artery occlusion

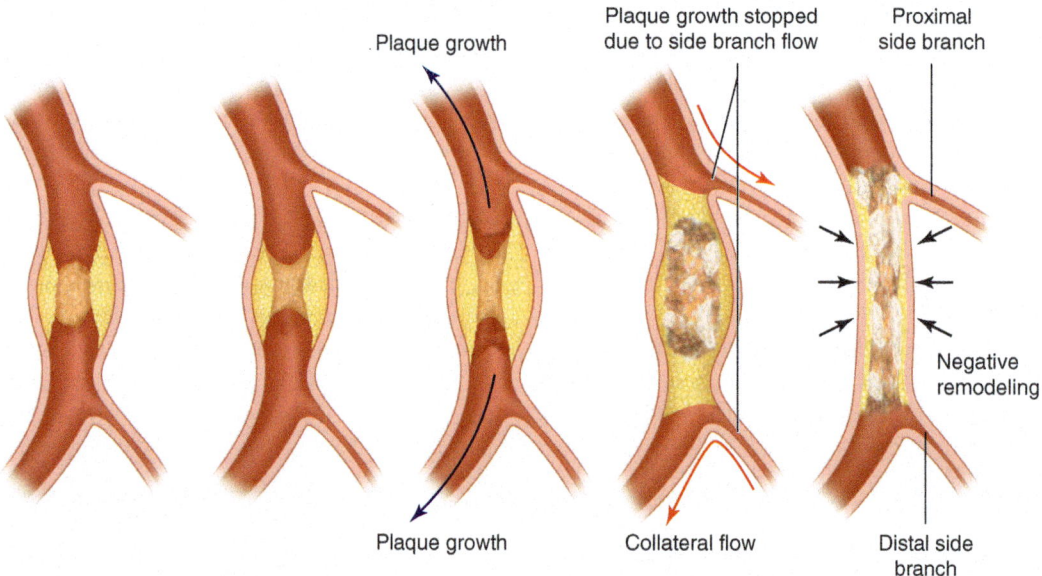

Fig. 4.5 Development of chronic total occlusion

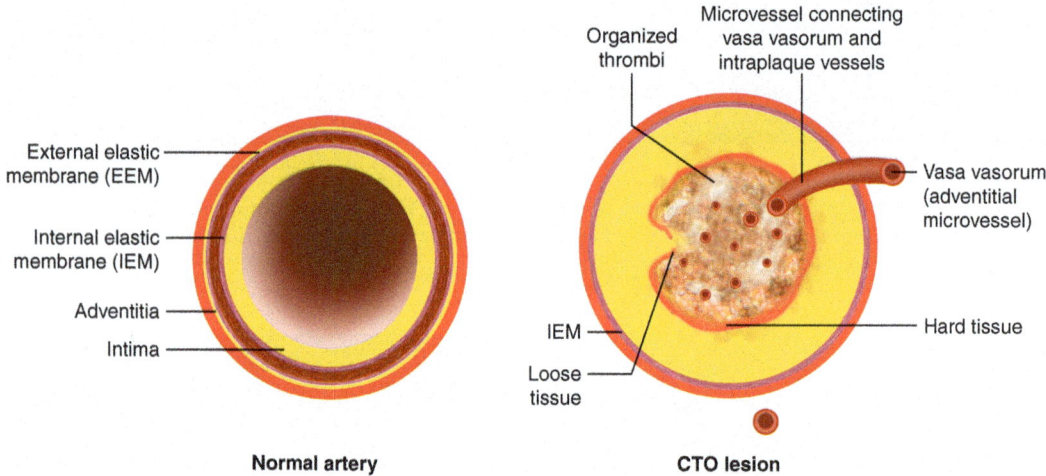

Fig. 4.6 Cross-sectional schematic illustration showing normal artery and CTO artery

resonance imaging revealed that most patients with CTO showed late gadolinium enhancement, which is an evidence of prior myocardial infarction [8]. Therefore, CTO is the sequelae of non-reperfused thrombotic acute coronary syndrome. Compared to patients without bypass surgery, patients who underwent bypass surgery have lower CTO procedural success rate. There was more negative remodeling, higher calcification, and less thrombotic materials in these patients which suggest longer duration of occlusion [9]. Coronary CT angiography showed shorter occlusion length and less adjacent side branches in CTO compared to subtotal occlusion. Therefore, most CTO is imaged as "inter-bifurcation disease." Subtotal occlusion can be regarded as the prequel of matured CTO and typically shows tapered stump, absence of adjacent side branch, and relatively short occlusion length. These findings can be imaged

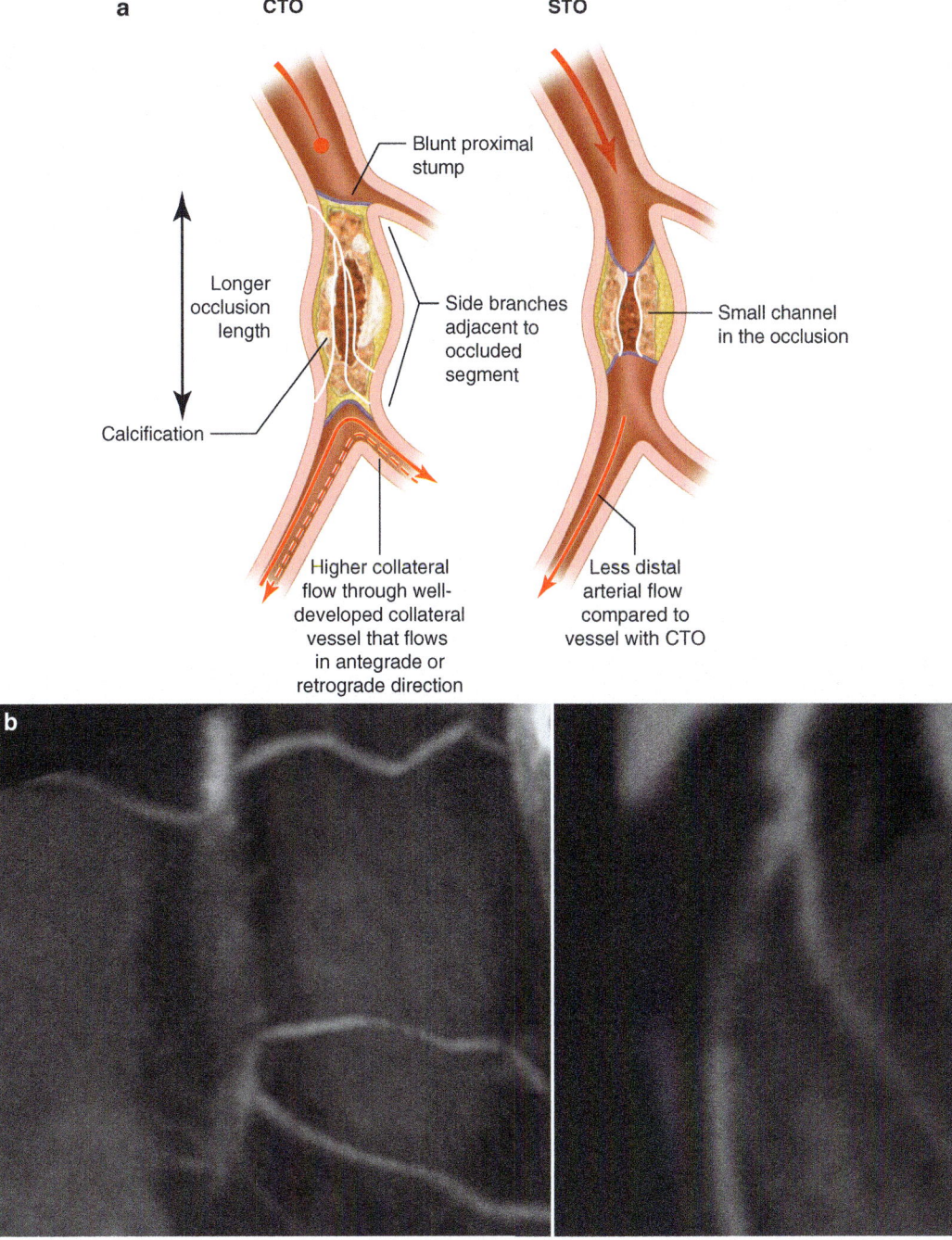

Fig. 4.7 Schematic illustration and cases of CTO and subtotal occlusion. Panel **a**: CTO lesion shown in the left panel shows adjacent side branches, blunt entry stump, and longer occlusion length. Panel **b**: Representative coronary CT images of CTO (left) and subtotal occlusion (right)

before procedure by noninvasive coronary CT angiography (Fig. 4.8) [10].

Due to the limited spatial resolution, sophisticated investigation of plaque characteristics is still challenging. Unsuccessful CTO procedure is frequently caused by failed penetration of hard fibrous tissue or calcified tissue, guidewire entrance into subintimal course, or extravascular

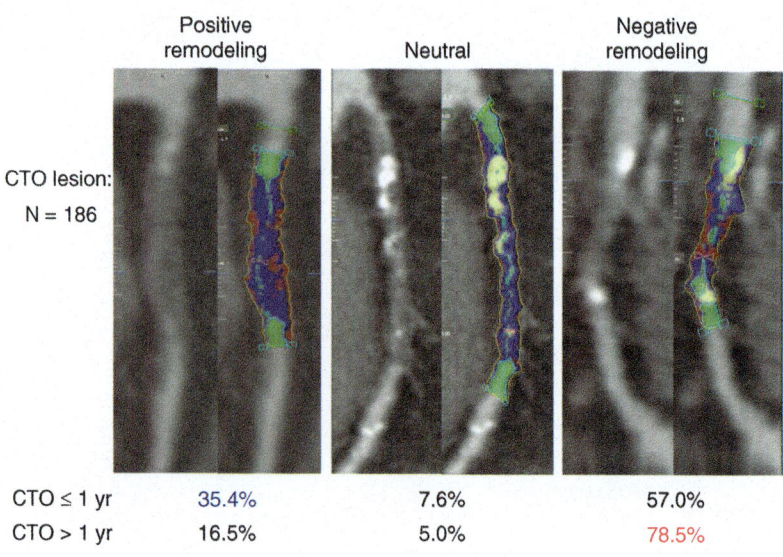

Fig. 4.8 Plaque characteristics according to the age of CTO. CTO lesion shown in the left panel shows adjacent side branches, blunt entry stump, and longer occlusion length

	Positive remodeling	Neutral	Negative remodeling
CTO ≤ 1 yr	35.4%	7.6%	57.0%
CTO > 1 yr	16.5%	5.0%	78.5%

space. Understanding of these pre-procedural characteristics would improve the procedural success rate and avoid wire entrance into false lumen or procedural failure. Recently introduced imaging fusion of invasive angiography and CT would help to understand the exact situation of wire penetration and to guide the device into the right direction, which would result in higher procedural success rate (Figs. 4.9 and 4.10).

Calcification is frequent in CTO plaque and causes blurring imaging artifact. Automatic or manual adjustment of the Hounsfield unit window and thin image slice is crucial for best image interpretation (Fig. 4.11). The extent of calcification is one of the major factors for successful CTO procedure. The extent of cross-sectional calcification is various, but most calcification is located in the vessel wall and "full-moon"-type complete occupation of vascular lumen is rare. Adjustment of the Hounsfield unit usually reveals calcium-free central tissue, which can be penetrated by a guidewire (Fig. 4.12).

The vascular course of long CTO is not easy to be grasped even after retrograde angiography due to hidden angulation or of CTO segment. Reconstructed coronary CT angiography projected with viewing angle same to catheterization frequently helps to understand the exact vascular course and advance guidewire into right pathway

or avoid potential extravascular advancement (Figs. 4.13 and 4.14).

4.2.3 Distal Vessel and Collateral Flow

The collateral vessel is imaged by injection of contrast dye into the donor artery in coronary angiography. The extent of collateral flow or vessel size is semiquantitatively assessed by Rentrop score or collateral connection score. Presence of well-developed collateral suggests higher chance of viable myocardium and higher chance of successful retrograde approach in CTO procedure. Coronary CT angiography is a snapshot of whole intracoronary contrast dye kinetics and enables evaluation of the extent of flow and direction of collateral flow based on the principle of transluminal attenuation gradient (Fig. 4.14) [6, 8, 11–16].

Coronary CT angiography visualizes collateral vessel having a diameter of more than 1.0 mm. Also, coronary CT angiography can visualize multiple collateral vessels simultaneously and even collaterals encircling large left or right atrium. Visualized collateral vessels can be a valuable pathway for retrograde approach unless very tortuous (Fig. 4.15).

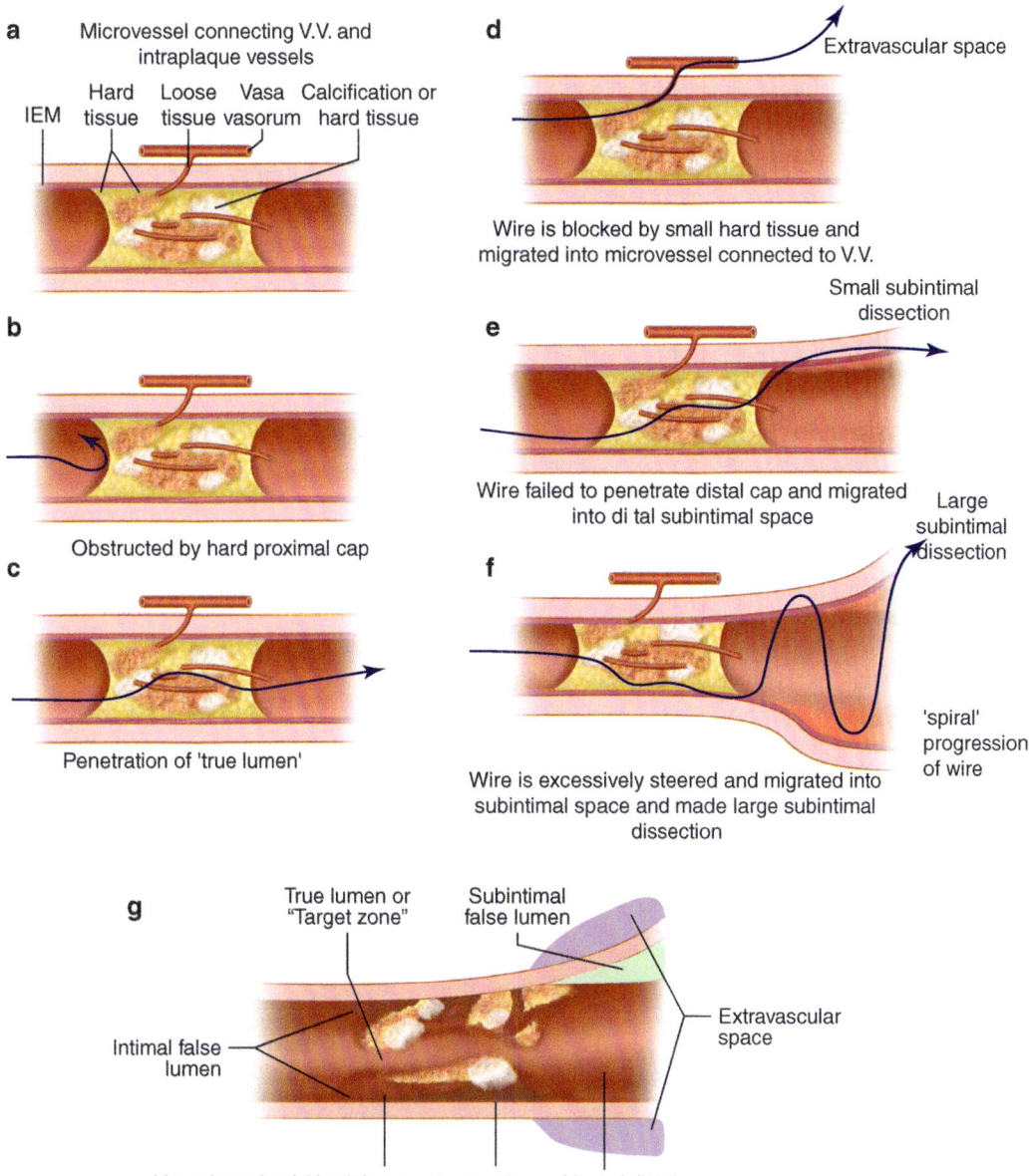

a Microvessel connecting V.V. and intraplaque vessels

IEM | Hard tissue | Loose tissue | Vasa vasorum | Calcification or hard tissue

b Obstructed by hard proximal cap

c Penetration of 'true lumen'

d Extravascular space

Wire is blocked by small hard tissue and migrated into microvessel connected to V.V.

e Small subintimal dissection

Wire failed to penetrate distal cap and migrated into di tal subintimal space

f Large subintimal dissection

Wire is excessively steered and migrated into subintimal space and made large subintimal dissection

'spiral' progression of wire

g True lumen or "Target zone"   Subintimal false lumen

Intimal false lumen

Extravascular space

Vessel proximal to CTO | Hard tissue penetration | Loose tissue tracking | Vessel distal to CTO

Fig. 4.9 Representative illustration of failed wire penetration situations. Panel **a**: Schematic drawing of CTO consisting fibrous hard tissue, soft or loose tissue, and calcification. Microvessels within CTO plaque may be connected into vasa vasorum (VV) in adventitial tissue or penetrate into distal vessel. Panel **b**: Guidewire (blue-colored curved arrow) cannot be penetrated into CTO plaque due to hard proximal cap. Panel **c**: Penetration of true lumen. Panel **d**: Guidewire penetrated the proximal cap but migrated into a microvessel which is connected into vasa vasorum and extravascular space. Panel **e**: Guidewire penetrates the proximal cap and mid-CTO body but fails to penetrate distal cap and migrates into distal subintimal space. Panel **f**: Excessive guidewire manipulation leads into entrance to subintimal space within CTO segment. Continuous aggressive guidewire steering and spiral progression of guidewire may result in large subintimal dissection in distal vessel. Panel **g**: Concept of "right intraplaque pathway into distal vessel"

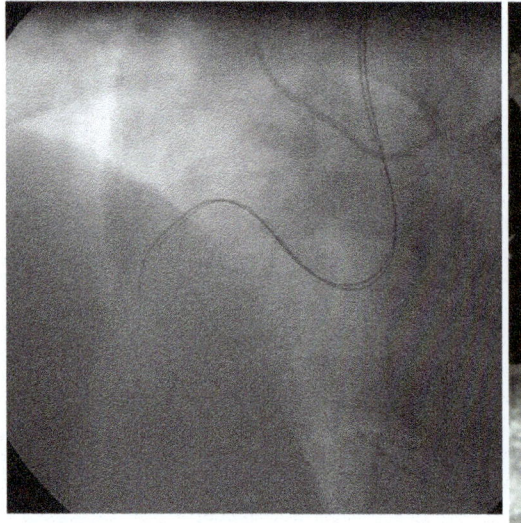

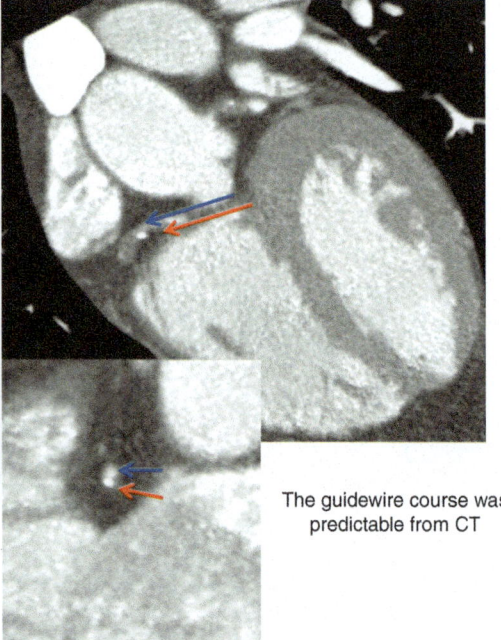

Guiding catheter: XB 2.0 6Fr.

Parallel wire technique - the outer
guidewire could enter distal true lumen

The guidewire course was
predictable from CT

Fig. 4.10 A case of CT-guided wire manipulation. Parallel wire technique was performed based on the preprocedural CT image. Progression of first guidewire was blocked by intra-CTO calcification in myocardial side and was blocked by calcification. Second guidewire was progressed into pericardial side of CTO plaque and successfully penetrated CTO lesion

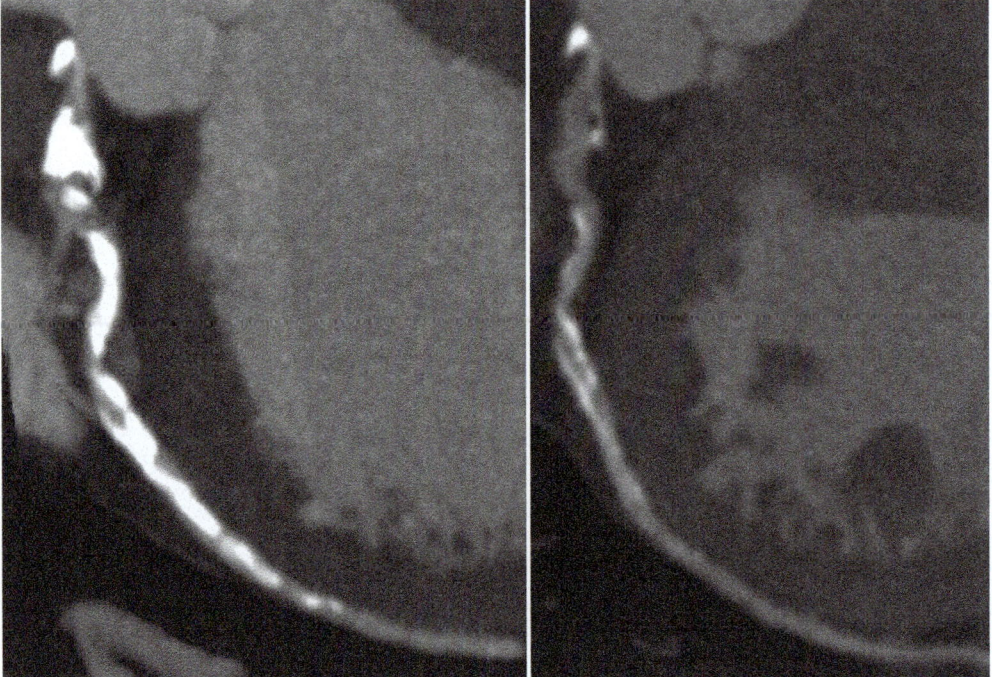

Fig. 4.11 Hounsfield window adjustment for adequate image analysis. Left panel shows extensive calcification along the vessel course and suggests significant stenosis. Adjustment of Hounsfield unit window and slice thickness reveals vascular wall calcification without significant luminal narrowing

Cross-sectional calcium

| 0% | < 50% | > 50% | 100% (full moon) |

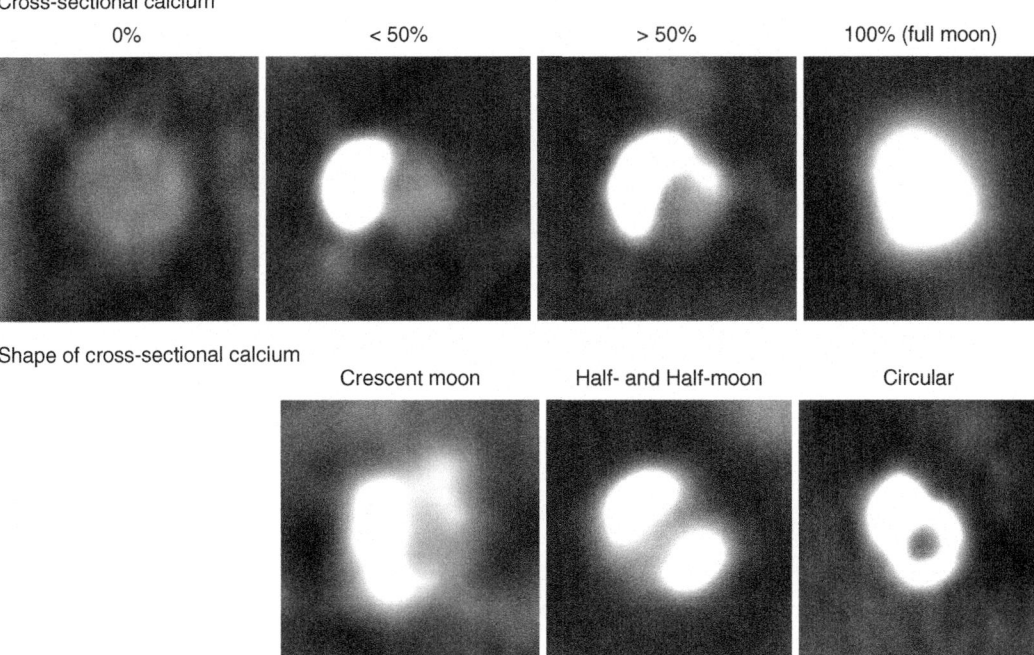

Shape of cross-sectional calcium

| Crescent moon | Half- and Half-moon | Circular |

Fig. 4.12 Cross-sectional calcifications in CTO segment

4.3 Prediction of CTO Procedure Success by Pre-procedural Coronary CT Angiography

PCI has been attempted less frequently for CTO compared to non-CTO lesion due to higher risk of procedural failure, higher risk of complication, and higher use of resources. Therefore, grading the procedural difficulty or predicting the probability of procedural success might help to select patients appropriate for PCI and improve procedural success rate. Currently, several angiographic scoring systems that predict successful CTO PCI based on anatomic and clinical parameters have been developed [14, 15, 17–23]. Most studies include blunt entry, long occlusion segment, the presence of side branch, and calcification as major anatomic predictors. Coronary CT angiography has a potential advantage over invasive angiography for direct visualization of CTO vessel trajectory from any arbitrary angle and precise extent of calcification [5, 6, 22]. Two CT-based scoring systems, CT-RECTOR and KCCT, showed better predictive performance compared to J-CTO angiographic score (Fig. 4.16) [24]. KCCT score also includes duration of occlusion and reattempt of previously failed procedure, which are two major clinical parameters that have been consistently reported as predictors of CTO PCI failure [19, 21, 22]. Incorporation of these widely validated anatomic and clinical parameters may explain the higher predictive performance of KCCT score compared with the other scoring systems (Fig. 4.17).

4.4 Intraprocedural Coronary CT Angiography for the Successful CTO Intervention

For the successful CTO recanalization, guidewire crossing of the CTO lesion would be the key, and the identification of the location of guidewire tip is the most essential. Recently, a coronary CT angiography system in the catheterization room allowing for the coronary CT scan and the coronary angiogram to be performed without relocation of the patients at any time during the

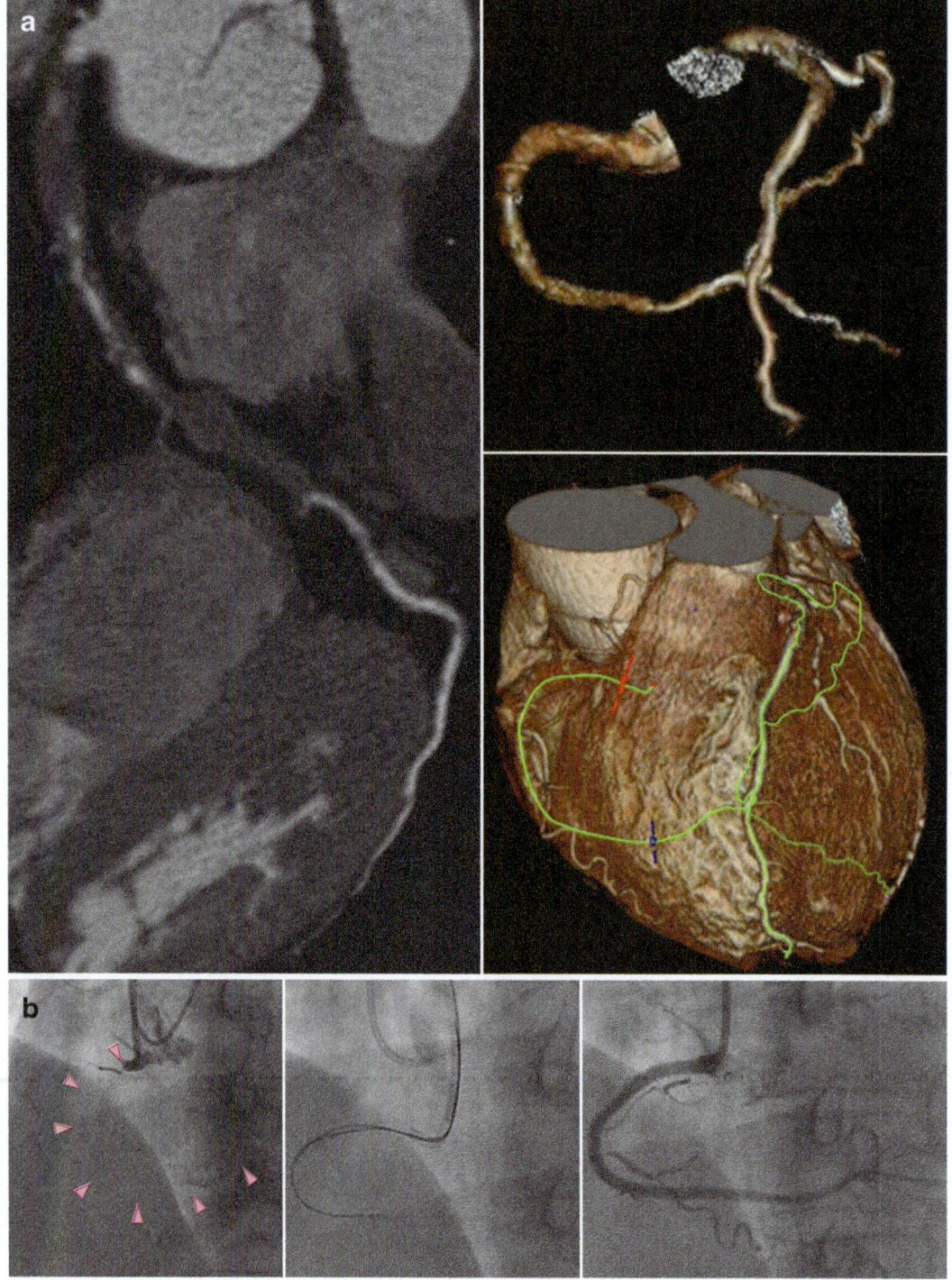

Fig. 4.13 Coronary CT angiography for visualization of long CTO segment. A case of very long CTO in right coronary artery. Panel **a**: Three-dimensional coronary CT angiography revealed two-tandem CTO segment with intervening contrast dye-filled non-CTO segment and distal vessel. Panel **b**: Successful CTO procedure was accomplished by retrograde approach from left circumflex into posterolateral artery

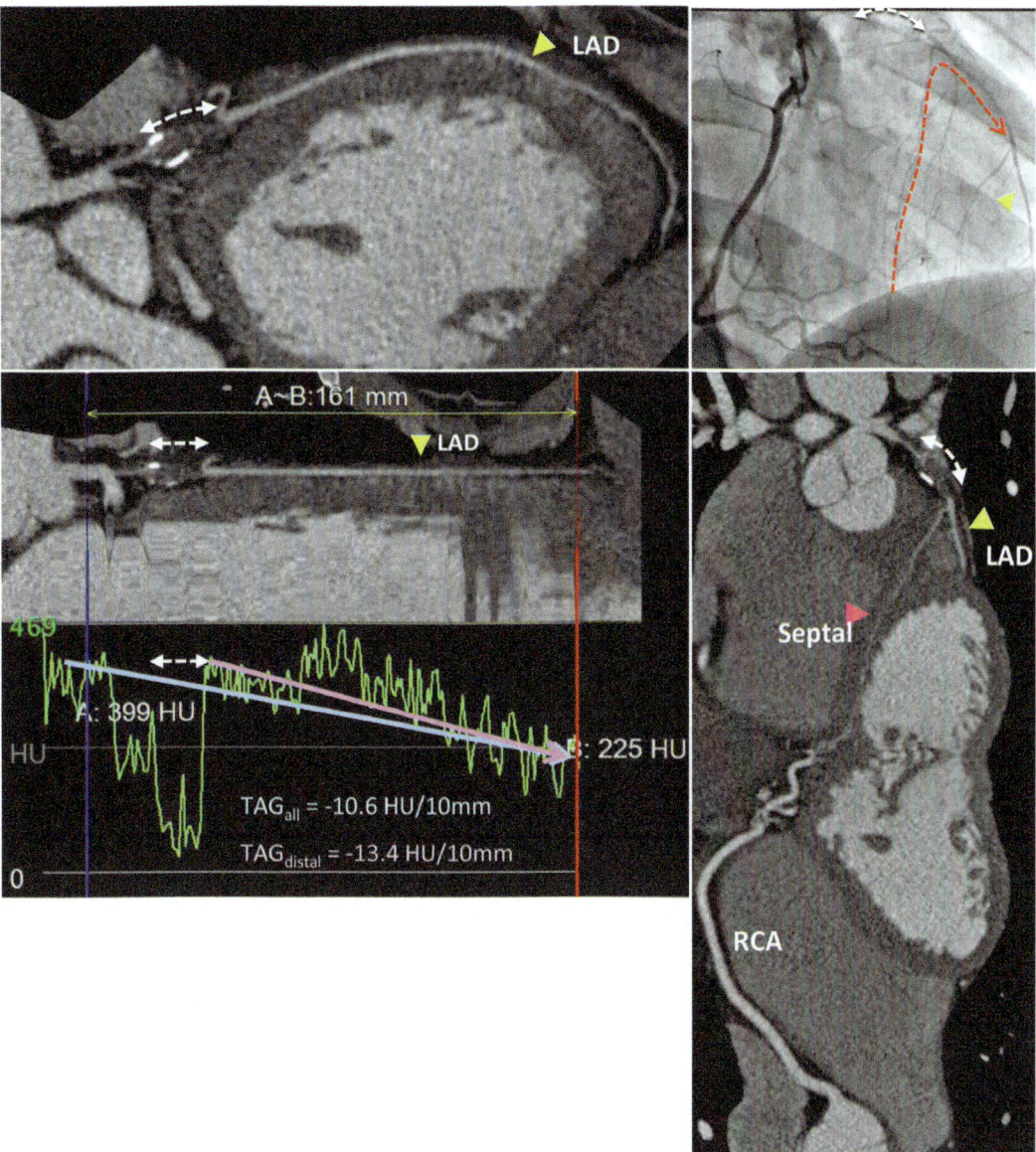

Fig. 4.14 Semiquantitative evaluation of collateral flow based on coronary CT angiography. TAG (transluminal attenuation gradient) is used to predict the extent and direction of coronary collateral flow

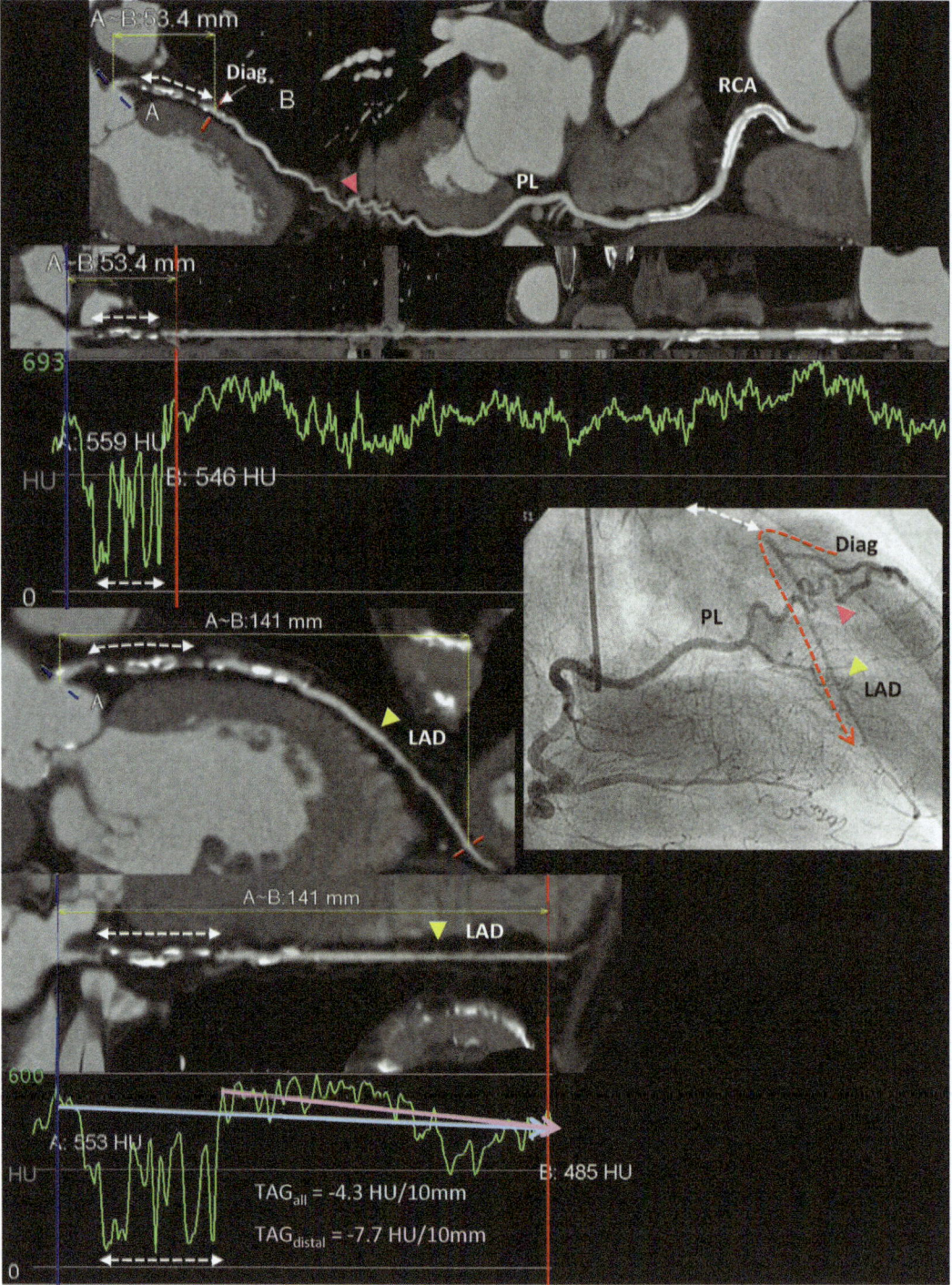

Fig. 4.14 (continued)

Fig. 4.15 Noninvasive visualization of coronary collateral artery. Panel **a**: Proximal LAD CTO. Septal collateral vessel supplying distal LAD. Panel **b**: Mid RCA CTO. Apical collateral vessel supplying distal RCA

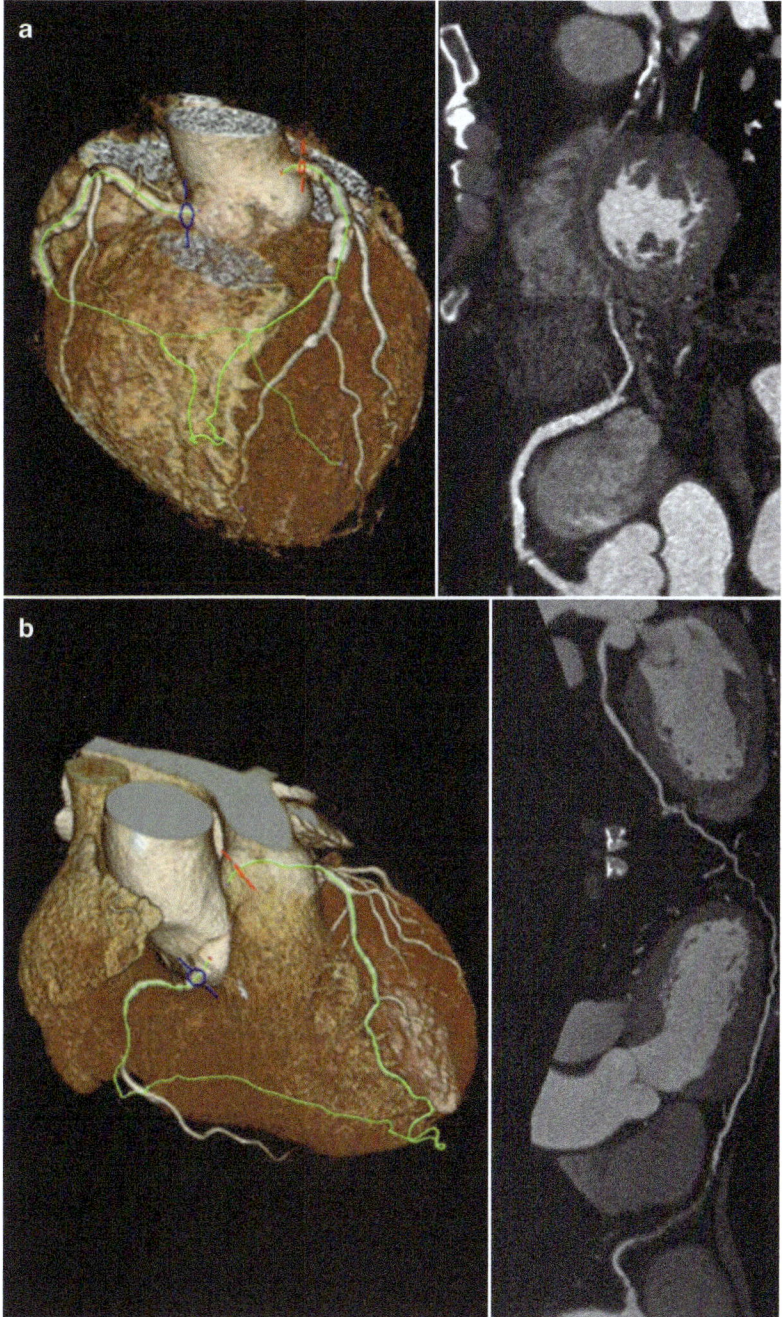

intervention was developed [25]. This system could identify the locations of guidewires during CTO procedures, without the need of invasive intravascular imaging, and revealed the location of the tip of a guidewire and the path during CTO intervention with a lesser contrast and radiation [25, 26]. Especially the intracoronary catheter-based contrast injection and combined assessment of axial and C-MPR images at different angles could enhance the role for determination of guidewire location (Fig. 4.18). Intraprocedural coronary CT angiography system would be helpful in case of the long or tortuous CTO and ambiguous guidewire position during CTO procedures.

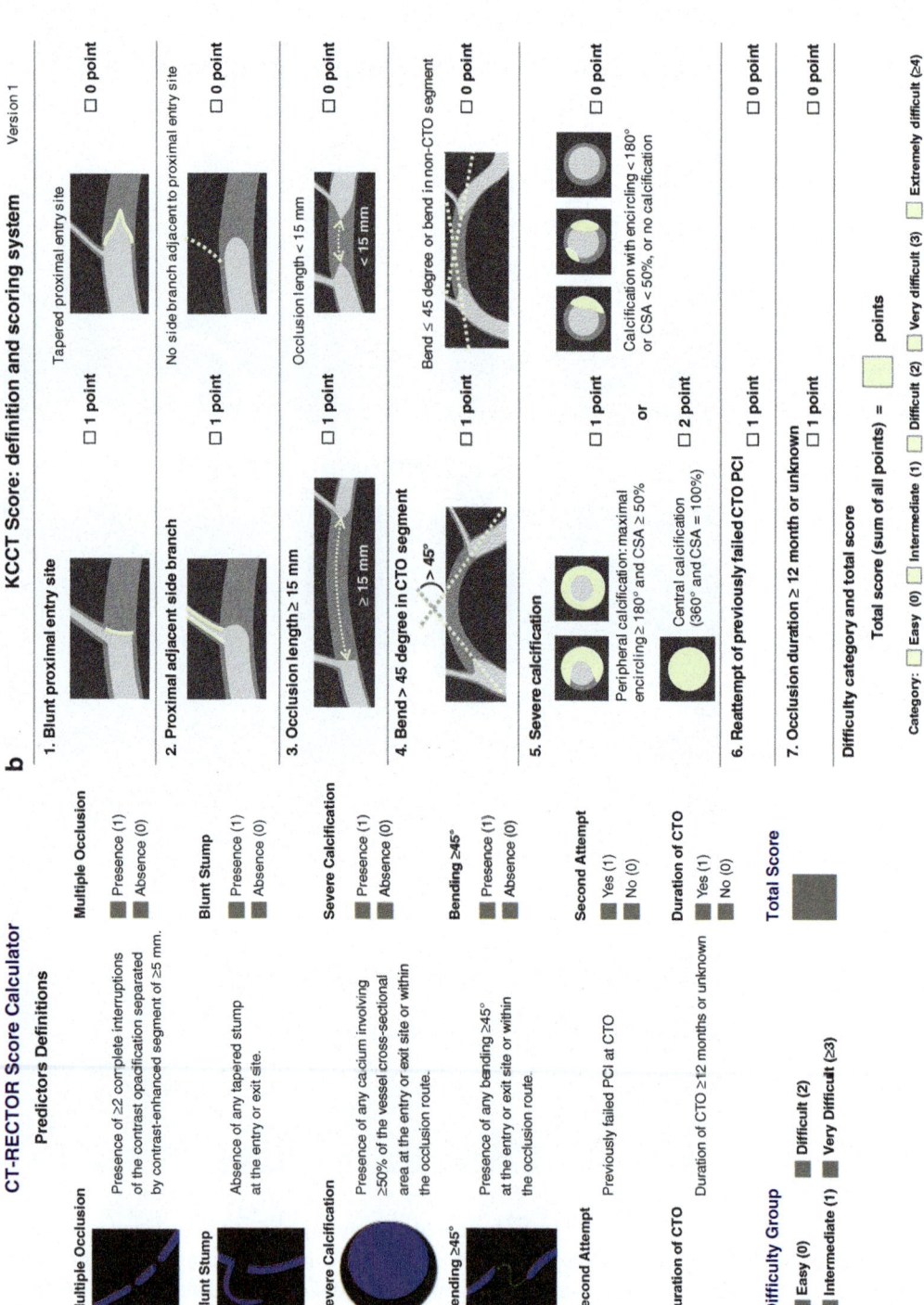

Fig. 4.16 Coronary CT angiography-based scoring system for CTO PCI. Panel **a**: CT-RECTOR score [22]. Panel **b**: KCCT score [16]

			CTO PCI success prediction scores				
			J-CTO (20)	PROGRESS-CTO (14)	CL-SCORE (15)	CT-RECTOR (21)	KCCT (16)
Anatomical predictors	CTO plaque	Proximal entry	Non-tapered stump	No tapered stump or poor cap visualization	Non-tapered stump	Non-tapered stump	Non-tapered stump
		Tortuosity	Bend > 45°	2 bends >70° or 1 bend >90°	-	Bend > 45°	Bend > 45°
		Occlusion length	≥ 20mm	-	≥ 20mm	-	≥ 15mm
		Side branch	-	-	-	-	Proximal side branch
		Calcification	Visualized calcification	-	Visualized calcification	Calcium CSA ≥ 50%	Calcium CSA ≥ 50%, worse if CSA =100%***
		Functional occlusion	-	-	-	-**	-**
	CTO vessel location		-	Worse in LCX	Worse in non-LAD	-	-
	Collateral		-	Non-interventional collateral	-	-	-
Clinical predictors	Previous MI		-	-	Previous MI	-	-
	CTO duration		-	-	-	≥ 12 mo or unknown	≥ 12 mo or unknown
	Reattempt		Reattempt	-	-	Reattempt	Reattempt
Primary endpoint			Wire cross ≤ 30 min	Procedural success	Procedural success	Wire cross ≤ 30 min	Wire cross ≤ 30 min
Number of predicting variables			5	4	5	5	7

Fig. 4.17 Comparison of scoring system for CTO PCI

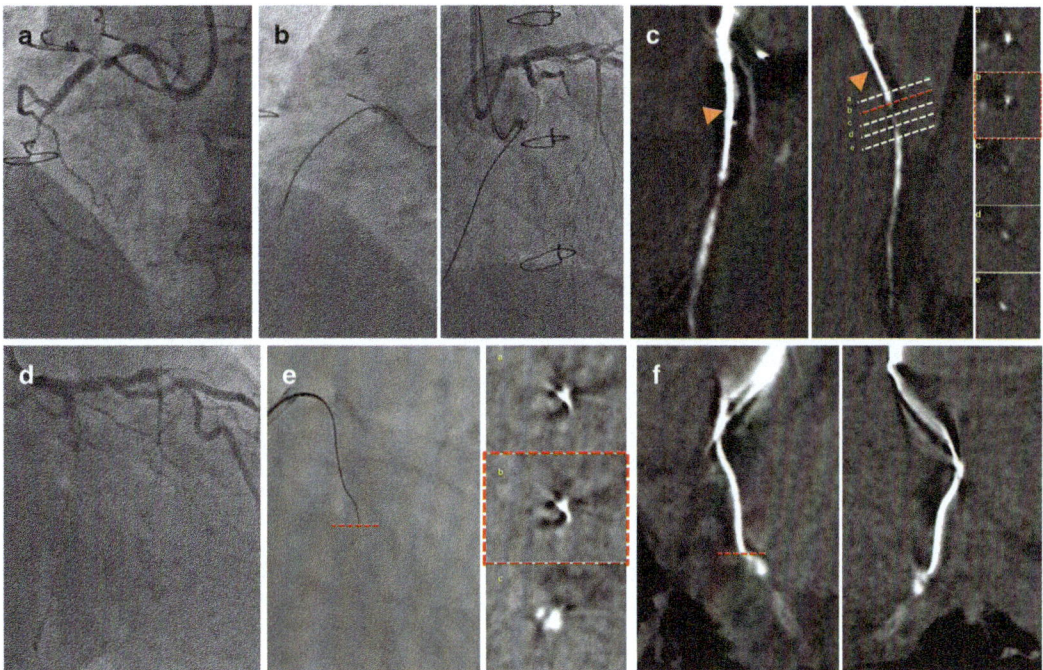

Fig. 4.18 Images of coronary CT angiography during CTO intervention. Scanning with contralateral intracoronary contrast injection (**A–C**); the distal portion of the guidewire-tip was enhanced by contrast filling of collateral channels. The artery course was clearly visible, and the tip location of a guidewire was more easily recognizable (b–d in **C**). Identification of guidewire location by using C-MPR images (**D–I**). Transverse axial images did not reveal the guidewire location (a–c in **E** and **I**); however, the C-MPR images at the different angles clearly indicated the location of a guidewire within the coronary artery (**F** and **I**). Especially, in retrograde CTO intervention, intraprocedural CT scan clearly visualized that two guidewires did not meet at the plane (**I**). Angiographic findings (**A–B, D–E, G–H**) indicating the guidewire location, C-MPR images (**C, F,** and **I**), and the matched cross-sectional images (a–e). The red broken lines and boxes indicate the wire-tip level and the corresponding axial images, respectively

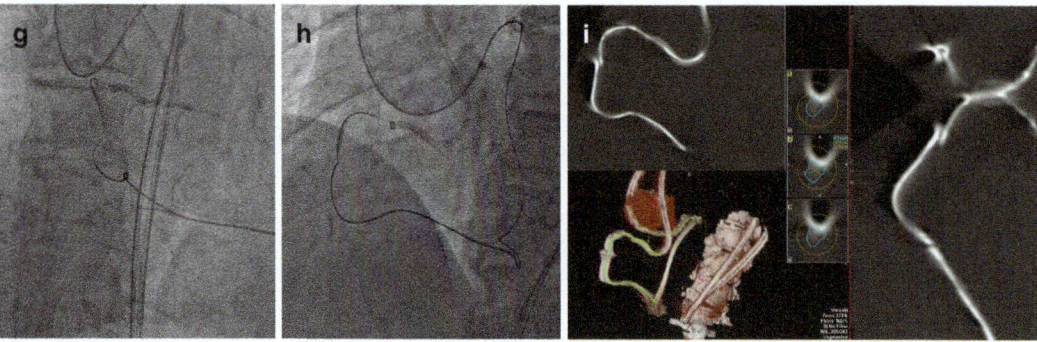

Fig. 4.18 (continued)

References

1. George S, Cockburn J, Clayton TC, Ludman P, Cotton J, Spratt J, Redwood S, de Belder M, de Belder A, Hill J, Hoye A, Palmer N, Rathore S, Gershlick A, Di Mario C, Hildick-Smith D, British Cardiovascular Intervention Society, National Institute for Cardiovascular Outcomes Research. Long-term follow-up of elective chronic total coronary occlusion angioplasty: analysis from the U.K. Central Cardiac Audit Database. J Am Coll Cardiol. 2014;64:235–43.
2. Patel VG, Brayton KM, Tamayo A, Mogabgab O, Michael TT, Lo N, Alomar M, Shorrock D, Cipher D, Abdullah S, Banerjee S, Brilakis ES. Angiographic success and procedural complications in patients undergoing percutaneous coronary chronic total occlusion interventions: a weighted meta-analysis of 18,061 patients from 65 studies. JACC Cardiovasc Interv. 2013;6:128–36.
3. Brilakis ES, Banerjee S, Karmpaliotis D, Lombardi WL, Tsai TT, Shunk KA, Kennedy KF, Spertus JA, Holmes DR Jr, Grantham JA. Procedural outcomes of chronic total occlusion percutaneous coronary intervention: a report from the NCDR (National Cardiovascular Data Registry). JACC Cardiovasc Interv. 2015;8:245–53.
4. Choi JH, Kim EK, Kim SM, Kim H, Song YB, Hahn JY, Choi SH, Gwon HC, Lee SH, Choe YH, Oh JK. Noninvasive discrimination of coronary chronic total occlusion and subtotal occlusion by coronary computed tomography angiography. JACC Cardiovasc Interv. 2015;8:1143–53.
5. Choi JH, Song YB, Hahn JY, Choi SH, Gwon HC, Cho JR, Jang Y, Choe Y. Three-dimensional quantitative volumetry of chronic total occlusion plaque using coronary multidetector computed tomography. Circ J. 2011;75:366–75.
6. Choi JH, Kim EK, Kim SM, Song YB, Hahn JY, Choi SH, Gwon HC, Lee SH, Choe YH, Oh JK. Noninvasive evaluation of coronary collateral arterial flow by coronary computed tomographic angiography. Circ Cardiovasc Imaging. 2014;7:482–90.

7. Choi JH, Koo BK, Yoon YE, Min JK, Song YB, Hahn JY, Choi SH, Gwon HC, Choe YH. Diagnostic performance of intracoronary gradient-based methods by coronary computed tomography angiography for the evaluation of physiologically significant coronary artery stenoses: a validation study with fractional flow reserve. Eur Heart J Cardiovasc Imaging. 2012;13:1001–7.
8. Choi JH, Chang SA, Choi JO, Song YB, Hahn JY, Choi SH, Lee SC, Lee SH, Oh JK, Choe Y, Gwon HC. Frequency of myocardial infarction and its relationship to angiographic collateral flow in territories supplied by chronically occluded coronary arteries. Circulation. 2013;127:703–9.
9. Sakakura K, Nakano M, Otsuka F, Yahagi K, Kutys R, Ladich E, Finn AV, Kolodgie FD, Virmani R. Comparison of pathology of chronic total occlusion with and without coronary artery bypass graft. Eur Heart J. 2014;35:1683–93.
10. Choi JH, Kim EK, Kim SM, Song YB, Hahn JY, Choi SH, Gwon HC, Lee SH, Choe YH, Oh JK. Noninvasive discrimination of coronary chronic total occlusion and subtotal occlusion by coronary computed tomography angiography. JACC Cardiovasc Interv. 2015;8:1143–53.
11. Zhang J, Li Y, Li M, Pan J, Lu Z. Collateral vessel opacification with CT in patients with coronary total occlusion and its relationship with downstream myocardial infarction. Radiology. 2014;271:703–10.
12. Li M, Zhang J, Pan J, Lu Z. Obstructive coronary artery disease: reverse attenuation gradient sign at CT indicates distal retrograde flow—a useful sign for differentiating chronic total occlusion from subtotal occlusion. Radiology. 2013;266:766–72.
13. Choi JH, Min JK, Labounty TM, Lin FY, Mendoza DD, Shin DH, Ariaratnam NS, Koduru S, Granada JF, Gerber TC, Oh JK, Gwon HC, Choe YH. Intracoronary transluminal attenuation gradient in coronary CT angiography for determining coronary artery stenosis. JACC Cardiovasc Imaging. 2011;4:1149–57.
14. Christopoulos G, Kandzari DE, Yeh RW, Jaffer FA, Karmpaliotis D, Wyman MR, Alaswad K, Lombardi W, Grantham JA, Moses J, Christakopoulos G, Tarar

MN, Rangan BV, Lembo N, Garcia S, Cipher D, Thompson CA, Banerjee S, Brilakis ES. Development and validation of a novel scoring system for predicting technical success of chronic total occlusion percutaneous coronary interventions: the PROGRESS CTO (Prospective Global Registry for the Study of Chronic Total Occlusion Intervention) score. JACC Cardiovasc Interv. 2016;9:1–9.

15. Alessandrino G, Chevalier B, Lefevre T, Sanguineti F, Garot P, Unterseeh T, Hovasse T, Morice MC, Louvard Y. A clinical and angiographic scoring system to predict the probability of successful first-attempt percutaneous coronary intervention in patients with total chronic coronary occlusion. JACC Cardiovasc Interv. 2015;8:1540–8.

16. Yu CW, Lee HJ, Suh J, Lee NH, Park SM, Park TK, Yang JH, Song YB, Hahn JY, Choi SH, Gwon HC, Lee SH, Choe YH, Kim SM, Choi JH. Coronary computed tomography angiography predicts guidewire crossing and success of percutaneous intervention for chronic total occlusion: Korean Multicenter CTO CT Registry Score as a tool for assessing difficulty in chronic total occlusion percutaneous coronary intervention. Circ Cardiovasc Imaging. 2017;10:e005800.

17. Safian RD, Freed MS. The manual of interventional cardiology. 3rd ed. Royal Oak, MI: Physician's Press; 2001.

18. Tan KH, Sulke N, Taub NA, Watts E, Karani S, Sowton E. Determinants of success of coronary angioplasty in patients with a chronic total occlusion: a multiple logistic regression model to improve selection of patients. Br Heart J. 1993;70:126–31.

19. Olivari Z, Rubartelli P, Piscione F, Ettori F, Fontanelli A, Salemme L, Giachero C, Di Mario C, Gabrielli G, Spedicato L, Bedogni F. Immediate results and one-year clinical outcome after percutaneous coronary interventions in chronic total occlusions: data from a multicenter, prospective, observational study (TOAST-GISE). J Am Coll Cardiol. 2003;41:1672–8.

20. Noguchi T, Miyazaki MS, Morii I, Daikoku S, Goto Y, Nonogi H. Percutaneous transluminal coronary angioplasty of chronic total occlusions. Determinants of primary success and long-term clinical outcome. Catheter Cardiovasc Interv. 2000;49:258–64.

21. Morino Y, Abe M, Morimoto T, Kimura T, Hayashi Y, Muramatsu T, Ochiai M, Noguchi Y, Kato K, Shibata Y, Hiasa Y, Doi O, Yamashita T, Hinohara T, Tanaka H, Mitsudo K, Investigators JCR. Predicting successful guidewire crossing through chronic total occlusion of native coronary lesions within 30 minutes: the J-CTO (Multicenter CTO Registry in Japan) score as a difficulty grading and time assessment tool. JACC Cardiovasc Interv. 2011;4:213–21.

22. Opolski MP, Achenbach S, Schuhback A, Rolf A, Mollmann H, Nef H, Rixe J, Renker M, Witkowski A, Kepka C, Walther C, Schlundt C, Debski A, Jakubczyk M, Hamm CW. Coronary computed tomographic prediction rule for time-efficient guidewire crossing through chronic total occlusion: insights from the CT-RECTOR Multicenter Registry (computed tomography registry of chronic total occlusion revascularization). JACC Cardiovasc Interv. 2015;8:257–67.

23. Luo C, Huang M, Li J, Liang C, Zhang Q, Liu H, Liu Z, Qu Y, Jiang J, Zhuang J. Predictors of interventional success of antegrade PCI for CTO. JACC Cardiovasc Imaging. 2015;8:804–13.

24. Rolf A, Werner GS, Schuhback A, Rixe J, Mollmann H, Nef HM, Gundermann C, Liebetrau C, Krombach GA, Hamm CW, Achenbach S. Preprocedural coronary CT angiography significantly improves success rates of PCI for chronic total occlusion. Int J Cardiovasc Imaging. 2013;29:1819–27.

25. Kim BK, Sumitsuji S, Cho I, Hong MK, Kim JS, HJ C, Jang Y. Role of intraprocedural coronary computed tomographic angiography in percutaneous coronary intervention of chronic total occlusion. EuroIntervention. 2016;11:1400.

26. Kim BK, Cho I, Hong MK, Chang HJ, Shin DH, Kim JS, Shin S, Ko YG, Choi D, Jang Y. Usefulness of intraprocedural coronary computed tomographic angiography during intervention for chronic total coronary occlusion. Am J Cardiol. 2016;117:1868–76.

27. Song BG, Choi JH, Choi SM, Park JH, Park YH, Choe YH. Coronary artery graft dilatation aided by multidetector computed tomography. Asian Cardiovasc Thorac Ann. 2010;18:177–9.

Dong-Kie Kim and Doo-Il Kim

5.1 Vascular Access

A careful choice of route of percutaneous coronary intervention (PCI) is needed especially in CTO intervention. An operator must consider lesion characteristics, the severity of calcification, and the presence of interventional collateral vessels.

5.1.1 Transfemoral Approach

The femoral artery is the most commonly used approaching site for coronary intervention. The reason for this is that, especially in cases of chronic total obstructive (CTO) lesions, a large diameter guide catheter can be used easily, which can provide more powerful backup support for dealing with complex lesions and can allow delivering multiple devices such as buddy wires, microcatheter, and intravascular ultrasound catheter at the same time.

However, patients with CTO lesions may also have peripheral artery occlusive disease, or pulsation of the lower limbs may not be palpable. Therefore, the femoral artery approach should be carefully selected, and radial artery or brachial artery can be chosen as an alternative route.

Since the puncture of the femoral artery is not so difficult, it is important to determine the exact puncture site. The appropriate site can not only facilitate the entry of the sheath but also can effectively stop the bleeding after the procedure. If the puncture level is low, distal vascular complications or pseudoaneurysms are likely to occur. If the puncture level is high, the risk of retroperitoneal hemorrhage increases.

The mid level of the common femoral artery (CFA) is the highly recommended site, and for the convenience of the operator, the right femoral artery is often selected. The common femoral artery is located 2–3 cm below the inguinal ligament, but sometimes the ligament is not palpable. Therefore, it is reasonable to make a target point about 1 cm below the inguinal skin fold. However, in an obese patient, it is difficult to refer to the skin fold because the inguinal skin fold is far below the inguinal ligament.

It is recommended to identify a fluoroscopic landmark or ultrasound guidance when setting the exact puncture site. It is also very useful in an obese patient or when a femoral pulsation is not easily palpable (Fig. 5.1).

One thing to keep in mind is to puncture the anterior wall of the artery whenever possible. This is because of the risk of hematoma or hemorrhagic complications when penetrating the posterior wall.

D.-K. Kim · D.-I. Kim (✉)
Inje University Haeundae Paik Hospital,
Busan, South Korea
e-mail: jo1216@inje.ac.kr

© Springer Nature Singapore Pte Ltd. 2019
Y. Jang (ed.), *Percutaneous Coronary Interventions for Chronic Total Occlusion*,
https://doi.org/10.1007/978-981-10-6026-7_5

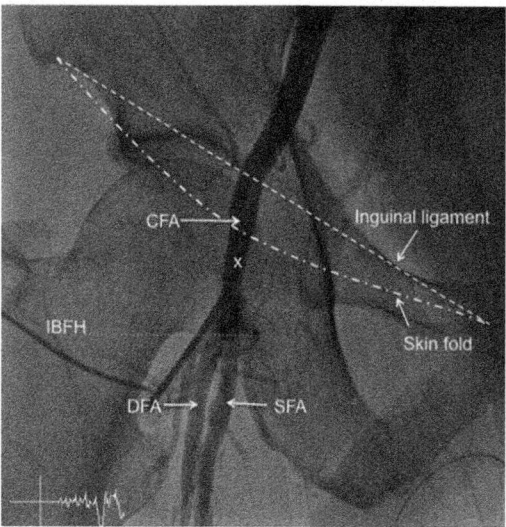

Fig. 5.1 Fluoroscopic landmarks of the common femoral artery. The adequate puncture site is marked as "x," which is located about 3 cm below the inguinal ligament, 1 cm below the inguinal skin fold, and medial 1/3 point of the femoral head. Abbreviations: *CFA* common femoral artery, *IBFH* inferior border of the femoral head, *DFA* deep formal artery, *SFA* superficial femoral artery. Courtesy by Dr. Dong-Kie Kim

5.1.2 Transradial Approach

The safety and efficacy of the transradial intervention have been known for over 10 years, and its indications are gradually expanding [1]. The transradial intervention has several advantages when compared with transfemoral intervention. Although the data on the transradial approach for CTO interventions is not sufficient yet, the transradial route needs less immobilization time for hemostasis, lower risk of bleeding complications of the puncture site, and shorter hospital stay. However, because of its poor backup support, transradial intervention has not been commonly performed especially in CTO intervention. This is mainly due to angulated course reaching from the radial artery to the subclavian artery that hampers tight sitting of the guide catheter on the opposite wall of the aorta [2]. It sometimes limits the use of guide catheters larger than 6 F which makes delivery of multiple devices impossible [2]. Also, it is disadvantageous compared to transfemoral intervention in terms of puncture time and a dose of radiation [3].

Recently introduced devices can overcome these limitations of transradial intervention. Hyperion® guide catheter (Asahi Intecc Co., Ltd., Burlington, MA, USA) has a bigger inner diameter than other guide catheters with same outer diameter and provides stronger backup support owing to its tertiary curve. Caravel microcatheter has a bigger inner diameter and smaller outer diameter than Corsair microcatheter. It is possible to use two Caravel microcatheters in 6 F guide catheter and to use an IVUS catheter and Caravel in 7 F guide catheter at the same time. The guide catheter extension devices such as the GuideLiner catheter (Vascular Solutions Inc., Maple Grove, MN, USA) or the GuideZilla catheter (Boston Scientific) can provide the extra support needed for balloon or stent delivery on the basis of the mother-child concept.

The radial artery approach is particularly advantageous in patients with coagulation disorders, prolonged INR due to warfarin, or severe obesity.

Most of short and straight CTO lesions are not difficult to perform on a 6 F catheter. If the radial artery in a young patient is big enough, a guiding catheter of 7 F or more can be inserted.

One thing to keep in mind when choosing the size of the guide catheter is that the larger the catheter, the greater the amount of contrast agent used. Because of the characteristics of the CTO lesions, a large amount of contrast media may be needed. Therefore, even if a large guide catheter is needed for the procedure, contralateral injection using a diagnostic catheter less than of 6 F via the transradial approach is helpful for reducing the amount of contrast agent.

5.2 Selection of Guide Catheter

Appropriate guide catheter selection is very important for a successful percutaneous coronary intervention (PCI) as the first step of the procedure. A proper choice of a right guide catheter makes the procedure simple, without exposing the patient to unnecessary risk.

A guide catheter provides two important functions which include a conduit function and a backup support function. The conduit function depends on the internal diameter of the guide. The backup support function depends on the shape of the catheter and its size also.

5.2.1 Size of Guide Catheter

Most uncomplicated coronary interventions are possibly performed using 6 F guide catheter and sometimes 5 F guide catheter. We can deliver single stents and single balloons together and also two balloons together using 6 F system [4]. Therefore, it is possible to perform anchoring balloon plus microcatheter or anchoring balloon plus monorail balloon technique with 6 F guide catheters in CTO intervention. However, it is difficult to use multiple guide wires, microcatheters, and IVUS catheters simultaneously (Table 5.1).

We need larger than 7 F guide catheters for successful CTO interventions. These systems will accommodate multiple wires and devices such as microcatheters and IVUS catheters. For retrograde CTO interventions, 8 F for the antegrade route and 7 F for the retrograde route are generally recommended.

Very tortuous, heavily calcified, or long CTO lesions may require the additional stiffness and backup support provided by larger diameter guide catheters. However, operators must manipulate carefully to avoid the trauma of the puncture site, aorta, and ostial coronary dissection. When compared with 6 F guide catheters, larger-sized guides are more related to increased risks of contrast-induced nephropathy and vascular site complications including bleeding, hematoma formation, pseudoaneurysm formation, and infection.

5.2.2 Shape of Guide Catheter

A good guide catheter may reduce damage to the coronary artery opening and ensures maximum support. As the first step of coronary intervention, operators select a suitable guide catheter according to the position of the coronary artery opening, the direction of the coronary artery, and the relation with the ascending aorta. The guide catheters that are often chosen are listed in Table 5.2.

5.2.2.1 Left Coronary Artery
Most commonly used catheters for left coronary interventions are extra backup catheters (EBU, Medtronic Inc., Minneapolis, MN, USA or XB,

Table 5.1 Comparisons of the size of guide catheters, IVUS catheters, and microcatheters

Device		Size	Manufacturer
Guide catheters	6 F	1.8 mm (ID)	
	7 F	2.0 mm (ID)	
	8 F	2.2 mm (ID)	
IVUS catheters	Eagle Eye®	1.17 mm (TD)	Volcano
	OptiCross®	1.03 mm (TD)	Boston Scientific
	Atlantis SR Pro®	1.07 mm (TD)	Boston Scientific
Microcatheters	FineCross®	0.60 mm (DOD)	Terumo
		0.87 mm (POD)	
	Corsair®	0.87 mm (DOD)	Asahi Intecc Co.
		0.93 mm (POD)	
	Caravel®	0.62 mm (DOD)	Asahi Intecc Co.
		0.85 mm (POD)	
	Crusade®	0.97 mm (DOD)	Kaneka Co.
		1.03 mm (POD)	

Abbreviations: *ID* inner diameter, *OD* outer diameter, *TD* transducer diameter, *DOD* distal outer diameter, *POD* proximal outer diameter

Table 5.2 Guide catheters chosen usually in coronary intervention

Target vessel	Guide catheters
LCA	XB, EBU, Judkins left, Amplatz left, Ikari left, Multipurpose
RCA	Judkins right, Hockey stick, Amplatz right, Amplatz left, LIMA, Multipurpose, Ikari right
LIMA	LIMA, modified LIMA, Judkins right
Saphenous graft	Amplatz left, Amplatz right, Multipurpose, Judkins right

Abbreviations: *LCA* left coronary artery, *RCA* right coronary artery, *LIMA* left internal mammary artery

Cordis Corporation, Bridgewater, NJ, USA). Their tip shape can make coaxial alignment easily and provide more passive support. However, a deep engagement with the target vessel sometimes produces vessel injury or dissection. Operators should pay attention to manipulate these catheters gently, especially dealing with the diseased left main stem.

Amplatz catheters can provide stronger backup support in the case of complex and difficult lesions such as severe tortuosity or heavy calcification.

5.2.2.2 Right Coronary Artery

A Judkins right catheter is one of the most popular guide catheters for right coronary interventions, but its backup support is too poor to choose for RCA CTO interventions. For stronger backup, Amplatz left catheters are generally recommended [5].

5.2.3 Support

5.2.3.1 Passive Support

Passive support of the guide catheter is dependent on its physical property and obtained by coaxial alignment with the coronary ostium against the aortic wall and the coronary sinus. Long-tipped and bigger-sized (7 F, 8 F) catheters have more passive support but the more increased risk of vessel injury or dissection.

5.2.3.2 Active Support

Active support is achieved by operators' skills, such as deep-seating technique or by molding the catheter in the coronary sinus. Active backup catheters have softer tips and a shape that can be easily altered by active guide catheter manipulation. Smaller-sized (5 F) guide catheters usually provide more active support than passive support. Intermediate-sized (6 F) catheters can provide both active and passive support.

5.2.3.3 Buddy Wire Technique

When stronger support is needed to perform complicated lesions, guide catheters can be stabilized by inserting additional one or two guide wires into the coronary arteries (Fig. 5.2a, b). That lessens the angle of the coronary artery and can hold guide catheters tightly by increasing friction resistance between wires and vessel wall.

5.2.3.4 Anchor Balloon Technique

A stronger support of guide catheter can be achieved by anchoring a side branch using balloon catheter (Fig. 5.2c). The recommended size of the balloon is equal to or larger than 0.25 mm in diameter compared to the side branch. Minimal inflation pressure that does not move the balloon catheter when pulled is needed for avoiding the side branch dissection or injury. It is sometimes helpful for the guide wire to pass through the CTO lesion by anchoring the over-the-wire balloon proximal to the lesion.

5.2.3.5 Mother-Child Catheter Technique

This is a way to enhance the backup support by engaging a large (mother) catheter for passive support in the target vessel and inserting a small (daughter) catheter into it for active support with less risk of complications such as dissections [6]. A 5 F mother-child system can generate strong backup support exceeding that of an 8 F guide catheter in a bench test. A 4 F system does not exceed that of a 7 F catheter [7].

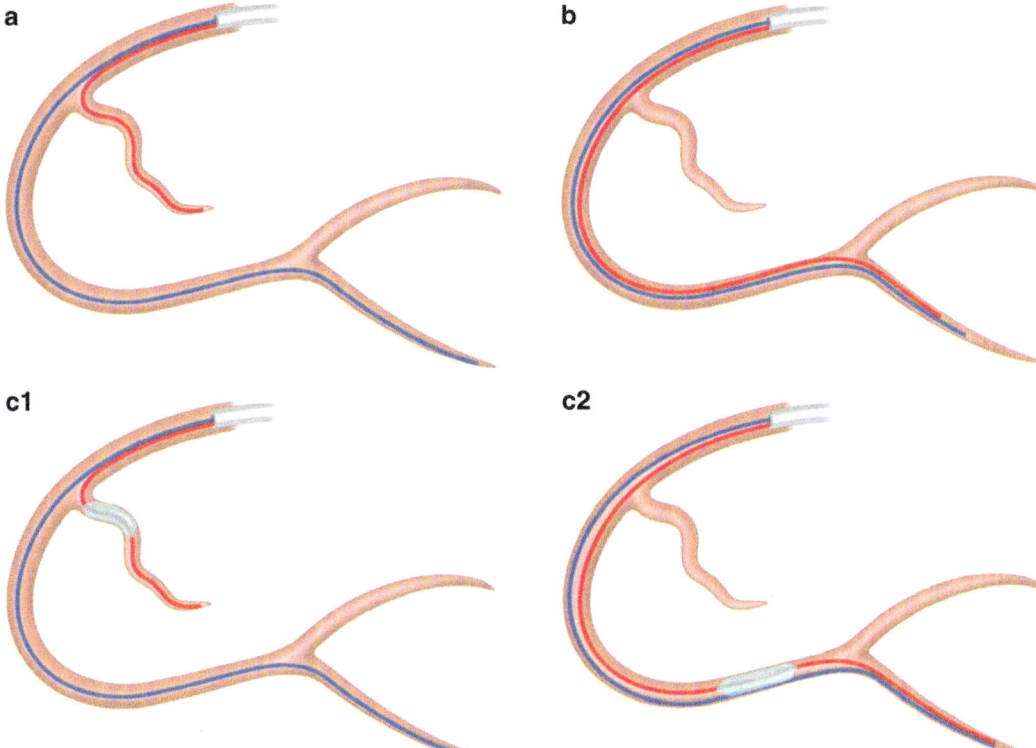

Fig. 5.2 Various techniques to increase backup support of guide catheter. Insertions of an additional wire into side branch (**a**) or distal to the main vessel (**b**) can help the guide catheter to stabilize. Balloon inflation at the side branch (**c1**) or at the distal segment of the main vessel (**c2**) also can provide stronger backup support

References

1. Rao SV, Ou F-S, Wang TY, Roe MT, Brindis R, Rumsfeld JS, Peterson ED. Trends in the prevalence and outcomes of radial and femoral approaches to percutaneous coronary intervention. JACC Cardiol Interv. 2008;1:379–86.
2. Patel T, Shah S, Pancholy S, Kwan T. Choosing catheter shapes for radial PCI. Cardiac Interventions Today. 2012;35–40.
3. Jolly SS, Amlani S, Hamon M, Yusuf S, Mehta SR. Radial versus femoral access for coronary angiography or intervention and the impact on major bleeding and ischemic events: a systematic review and meta-analysis of randomized trials. Am Heart J. 2009;157:132–40.
4. Prashant PU. Current and emerging catheter technologies for percutaneous transluminal coronary angioplasty. Res Rep Clin Cardiol. 2014;5:213–26.
5. Mishra S, Bahl VK. Curriculum in cath lab: coronary hardware—part I the choice of guiding catheter. Indian Heart J. 2009;61:80–8.
6. MacHaalany J, Abdelaal E, Bertrand OF. Guide catheter selection for transradial PCI. Cardiac Interventions Today. 2013;45–48.
7. Takeshita S, Shishido K, Sugitatsu K, Okamura N, Mizuno S, Yaginuma K, Suenaga H, Tanaka Y, Matsumi J, Takahashi S, Saito S. In vitro and human studies of a 4F double-coaxial technique ("mother-child" configuration) to facilitate stent implantation in resistant coronary vessels. Circ Cardiovasc Interv. 2011;4:155–61.

Basic CTO Guidewires and Tips for Proper Use

6

Cai De Jin and Moo Hyun Kim

6.1 Overview of CTO Guidewires

The conventional guidewire techniques for chronic total occlusion (CTO) lesions might not have been developed without the presence of various guidewires innovated and manufactured by dedicated Japanese company. Major guidewire techniques include "drilling," "penetrating," and "sliding" techniques. Asahi Intecc has developed several concepts which can define the performance of each guidewire, including tip load, shaping ability and memory, tip flexibility, shaft support, torque transmission, slipping ability, trackability, and trap resistance. Guidewires such as Miracle series focused on drilling concept by improving torque transmission, whereas Conquest series was optimized for the lesion where penetration technique is necessary. Fielder, Fielder FC, and Fielder XT were innovated for the facilitating retrograde approach by providing very lubriciousness and high torque controllability. Recently developed Gaia series (especially in Gaia third) wires focused on the concept of deflection and rotation (directional torque) which

is a unique feature as compared with contemporary GWs (e.g., Conquest Pro) for penetration. The milestones of CTO guidewire development are summarized in Table 6.1.

6.2 Guidewire Property Differences in Covers and Coatings

Polymer covers provide excellent lubricity and trackability with less tactile feedback. Hydrophilic coatings attract water to create a slippery "gel-like" surface and are therefore more lubricious with less tactile feedback resulting in easy advancement; hydrophobic coatings (Silicone- or Teflon-based) repel water to create a "wax-like" surface which enhances tactile feedback but decreases slipperiness and trackability (Fig. 6.1).

6.2.1 Spring-Type vs. Hydrophilic Wires

The differences in spring-type vs. hydrophilic wires are briefly summarized in Table 6.2.

1. Spring-type wires provide a better profile in terms of steerability, torquability, and tactile feedback from the tip compared with hydrophilic wires. Since they are less likely to cause

C. D. Jin
Department of Cardiology, The Affiliated Wuxi No. 2 People's Hospital of Nanjing Medical University, Wuxi, Jiangsu, China

M. H. Kim (✉)
Department of Cardiology, Dong-A University Hospital, Busan, South Korea
e-mail: kimmh@dau.ac.kr

© Springer Nature Singapore Pte Ltd. 2019
Y. Jang (ed.), *Percutaneous Coronary Interventions for Chronic Total Occlusion*,
https://doi.org/10.1007/978-981-10-6026-7_6

Table 6.1 Milestones of CTO guidewires

Year	Technological improvement of wires	Company	Product
1995	Polymeric coating	SciMED	Choice PT
1996	Hydrophilic coating	Terumo	Crosswire
1997	Incremental tip load (drilling concept)	Asahi	Miracle family
1998	Tapered-tip design	Guidant	HT CROSS-ITXT
1998	Combination of tapering without polymer jacket and hydrophilic coating in high tip stiffness (>9 g) (penetration concept)	Asahi	Conquest Pro
2008	Combination of tapering with polymer jacket and hydrophilic coating in low tip stiffness (<1 g) (sliding concept)	Asahi	Fielder XT
2010/2011	Composite core tip in low tip stiffness	Asahi	SION/Fielder XT-A/XT-R
2013	Combination of composite core tapering polymeric and hydrophilic coating in intermediate stiffness (>1.5, <5 g) (Deflection and rotation concept)	Asahi	Gaia family

Above data was obtained from Sianos et al. [1]

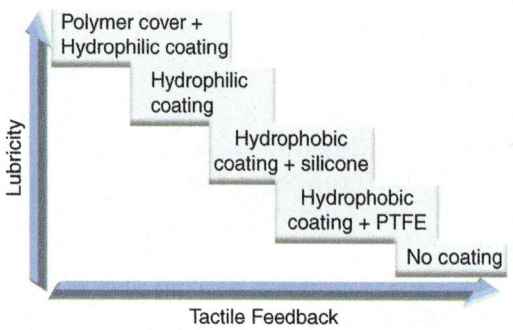

Fig. 6.1 Polymer covers and coatings in relationship between lubricity and tactile response. Figure modification is based on "Tools and Techniques – Clinical Update on Coronary Guidewires 2016: CTO" by Green et al. [2]

Table 6.2 Discrimination differences

Properties	Spring-type	Hydrophilic	Better
Torquability	+	−	Spring-type
Steerability	+	−	Spring-type
Tactile feedback	+	−	Spring-type
Trackability	−	+	Hydrophilic
Dissection/hematoma	Less	More	Spring-type
CTO lesion		Not used	

Even if we fail to cross it, we can feel the touch of the proximal cap and its rigidity. Spring-coil tapered-tip GWs like Conquest increase the risk of perforation, and thus they cannot be used as frontline wires for CTO.

2. By contrast, hydrophilic wires are not usually recommended as frontline guidewire, since they can easily drill into the subintimal space without tactile feedback resulting in expansion of it. They offer better manipulation in tortuous vessels, but don't respond well to the operator's attempt to make them follow a precise, predetermined path through hard plaque. However, after crossing the main part of the lesion, if there is a tortuous anatomy, you may take these GWs to negotiate the severe tortuosity. Thus, they are mainly used for retrograde approaches in modern techniques. The only exception is a hydrophilic soft wire such as Whisper wire in cases of CTO lesions with a straight microchannel [3] (Table 6.2).

6.3   Piercing the Proximal CTO Cap (Drilling, Penetrating, Sliding)

1. Drilling technique: The GW is rotated clockwise and counterclockwise, while the tip is pushed modestly against the CTO. The GW can be advanced like a "drill" going into its

dissection, they are safer and provide more control with some angulation when entering into the occlusion site. Even if an event occurs, it would be a minimal dissection or hematoma. Spring-coil non-tapered guidewires like Miracle 3 are the first choice for CTO lesions.

target. The drilling strategy implies stepping up gradually to stiffer wires according to visual and tactile feedback information from the wire tip. Straight-tip wires facilitate tactile feedback and steerability. The wire shaping should be done 1.0 mm from the distal tip with a shallow (15–20°) curve, and an additional secondary bend (10–15°) placed in the wire 5–8 mm proximal to the primary bend would be preferable to improve manipulation. The wire is rotated to and fro with the left hand, while the right hand is used for rotating 90–180° with rapid rotation and gentle probing and sometimes a full turn (the wire must be left to untorque to release the stored energy) with simultaneous moderated push and knocking. Non-tapered hydrophobic GWs like Miracle family were developed based on the drilling concept.

2. Penetrating technique implies applying direct pressure on an obstructive target by pushing a stiff wire slowly and gradually, with limited rotation movement (45–90°). The super stiff tapered-tip wires (like Conquest Pro 9-20) permit higher penetrating forces in blunt entry point, heavy calcific or resistant lesions, but have higher chance of perforation in tortuous angulated or bridging collateral lesions. After an initial attempt with a softer tip, progressively stiffer wires are the optimal choice in case of failure. Higher tip loads increased success rate but also raised the risk of wire perforation. Penetrability is dependent on tip stiffness (load), tip cross-sectional area, and the slipperiness of the coating. Therefore penetration power is more comprehensive than tip stiffness. The formula is tip load/area $[\pi(D/2)^2]$. Conquest Pro series behave like needles with high penetration power. To use the penetrating technique, the target has to be clearly identified by using multiangle projections with bilateral simultaneous contrast injection. Visual information is important as tactile feedback cannot be trusted. The Gaia Next series in development shows higher penetration power than the Gaia series (Fig. 6.2).

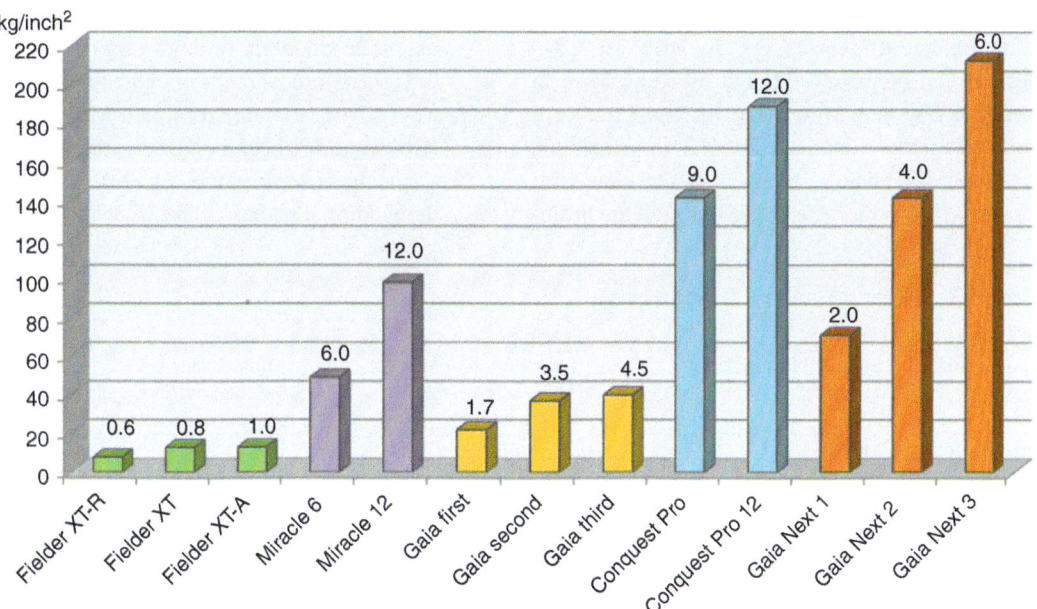

Fig. 6.2 Calculated penetration power. Special Gaia Next was obtained from "What is the GAIA Next" by Shigeru Nakamura, MD (Kyoto Katsura Hospital, CCT @ TCTAP 2017). The above data has been obtained by Asahi Intecc's permission

3. The sliding technique is performed by sliding a lubricious wire into the distal segment in the case of challenging microchannels, subtotal occlusion, and in-stent stenosis, which benefit from using hydrophilic coated and polymer jacket-type GWs (Fielder, Fielder FC, Fielder XTR/A, Gaia 1, Wizard 78, Whisper MS, PILOT 50, and Choice PT). These GWs should be carefully manipulated (minor rotations, shallow tip bend, gentle push) and not be forcefully pushed against resistance.

Overall (shown in Table 6.3), the above three techniques are appropriate for the short, focal, straight segment of non-calcified occlusions. In general, the drilling technique should be applied first, since the risk of perforation and intimal dissection is lower than the penetrating technique, as well as it works well even in tortuous vessels. Miracle series are better suited for the drilling technique than the Conquest series. When challenging complex CTOs (long, calcified, and tortuous lesion), a sprint-type wire is better, as having more torque is preferable. Subsequent step-up stiffness would be superior to an exchange to a different family of wires. If the proximal cap of the CTO is very hard, we need to penetrate it with tapered-tip GWs. The majority of CTO lesions can be passed through by using Miracle series GWs. However, some lesions need very stiff GWs like Conquest Pro 12, in which the penetrating technique is essential for successful crossing. Once the wire breaks through the proximal fibrous cap, it may be exchanged for a softer wire with a slightly greater primary tip bend if desired [4].

Tips

- *To make the wire tip stronger or stiffer*
  - The wire tip is deviated from the imaginary lumen/failed to engage into the intended direction in the proximal cap: (1) exchange for a stiffer wire alone and (2) additional advancement of a microcatheter close to the tip at this junction.
  - Guide catheter disengages with a wire tip pinpointed to the center of the occlusion: (1) exchange the guide for a stronger backup; (2) place another wire (anchoring); (3) inflate smaller balloon (anchoring) in SB proximal to CTO; (4) do deep seating with balloon; and (5) use microcatheter or daughter-and-mother technique [4].
  - Stiffer and more torquable wires are desirable, and spring-type wires are more preferable than the tapered ones, especially in curved and/or calcified portions.
  - The workhorse microcatheter is the Finecross (130, 150 cm, Terumo, Japan); the small tip and M-coating enable it to negotiate smoothly through a narrow space in CTO. Moreover, newer catheters such as MicroCross, CenterCross, and MultiCross (Roxwood Medical Inc., USA) are expected to further amplify the support for very demanding lesions. The Corsair (135,

Table 6.3 Piercing the proximal cap techniques

Concept	Drilling	Penetrating	Sliding
Application	Standard manipulation	Blunt entry point Heavy calcification Resistant lesion	Microchannels Subtotal occlusion In-stent restenosis
Guidewire	Miracle family	Conquest Pro	Fielder XT
Manipulation	90–180° rotation	45–90° rotation	Minor rotation to maintain tip freedom
Illustration			

The permission has been obtained by Asahi Intecc. Figure modification is based on "Guidewire Selection and Microcatheters" by Wasan Udayachalerm, MD. In NVCC HANOITEX 2016

150 cm, Asahi Intecc, Aichi, Japan) micro-catheter designed for collateral channel tracking can also be used in antegrade approach. It has more support, even beyond a calcified segment.

- Balloon inflation of the over the OTW system as coaxial anchor balloon technique is used to penetrate the proximal cap.
- If the wire still cannot cross the proximal cap, IVUS guidance may be required to accurately pinpoint the entry of occlusion.

6.4   Traversing the CTO Body

Once the wire has crossed the proximal cap, the operator should carefully advance the wire using the left hand while the right hand rotates the wire 180° back and forth. The wire, shaped (1 mm tip and <45° curved) to form an abrading tool, is used to grind through the lesion. If the wire buckles, it should never be forced into the lesion, rather retracted, reoriented, and rotated. Constant forward pressure is more successful than aggressive tapping against the occlusion ("jack hammering"), which does not transmit additional force [3]. Advancing with the wire rotated at a full angle may cause the wire tip to create a larger area of injury, which may result in dissection upon injecting contrast through the guide catheter. In contrast, if the angle of rotation is limited to a more favorable direction, the chance of creating a dissection would be minimal. If the wire tip repeatedly creates a false lumen, one is unlikely to get a better result with the same wire. Using the parallel wire technique [5] with a stiffer and tapered wire is a key component of successful strategy.

6.4.1   Tracking Loose Tissue

The tip of an intermediate GW is bent by 45–90° at the distal 2–5 mm so that it can be controlled and lead the wire through loose fibrous tissues without penetrating hard plaque. However, it is not clear which tip strength wire should be

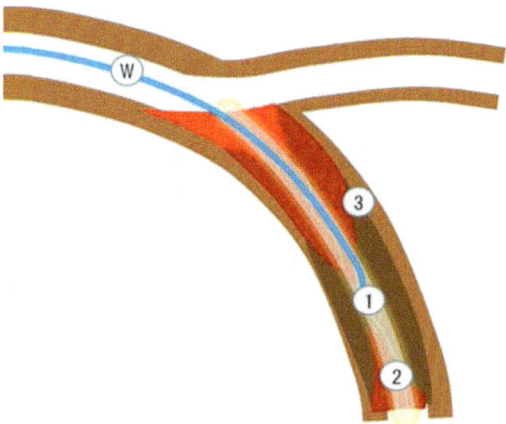

Fig. 6.3 Principle of "antegrade loose tissue tracking" (Figure is obtained from Sumitsuji et al. [6]). ① Wire tip force. ② Resistance in loose tissue. ③ Resistance in plaque. If we can control ①, between ② and ③, ② < ① < ③, wire might easily pass the CTO

selected for this technique due to different degrees of tissue rigidity. Usually, a 1.0 g tip-load hydrocoated wire is initially used. Wire handling and movement in loose tissue tracking are similar to that of those used in the case of acute myocardial infarction, in that the wire is advanced easily, smoothly with minimal rotations [6]. It will automatically advance with tracking in the loose tissue segments (Fig. 6.3).

- In each type of occluded lesion, there are small vascular channels (ranges from 160 to 230 μm) coursing from the proximal lumen, which cannot be visualized using coronary angiograms. The tapered-tip wire, like Cross-It (254 μm), which has a diameter close to that of those channels, and hydrophilic wires, with its lower friction, can advance more easily through these small channels [7].
- If the intermediate GW cannot penetrate the border between the loose and dense fibrous tissues, the wire can be exchanged for a stiffer one with tapered-tip (Conquest Pro) following OTW support system advancement. This has a greater possibility of penetrating through the dense connective tissues into the distal true lumen [3] (Fig. 6.4).

Fig. 6.4 The intermediate GW crossed the loose connective tissue but failed to penetrate into the dense fibrous tissue (**a**); tapered-tip stiff GWs could penetrate through the dense connective tissue into the distal true lumen using the OTW support system assistant (**b**) [3]

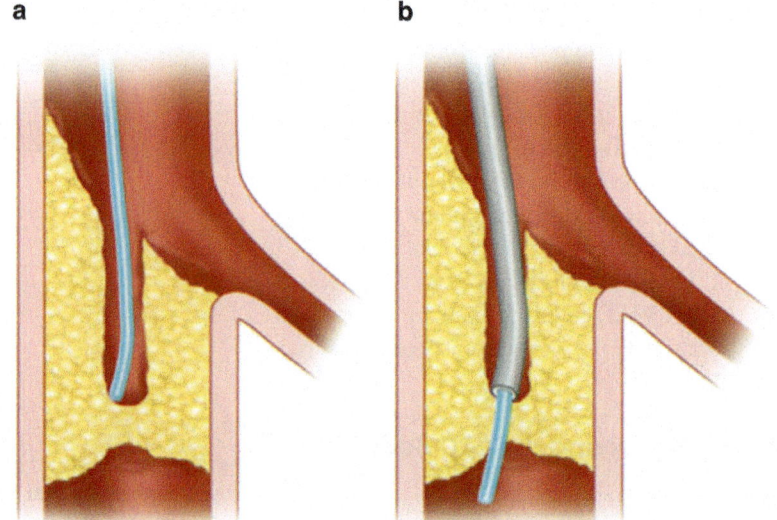

Tips

- *Tips for selecting the optimal wires are summarized in Tables 6.4 and 6.5 and Fig. 6.5.*
  - For a focal, tapered CTO lesion, start with a soft tapered polymer jacket wire for initial microchannel tracking. Fielder XT and Gaia 1 are currently the initial choice.
  - When failing to attempt tortuous artery or microchannel tracking, step up to intermediate GWs like Miracle 3, 4.5, and 6, Ultimate Bro 3, and Gaia 2.
  - In the case of hard, dense, and blunt occlusions, stiffer wires such as Conquest Pro 12 and 20 g, Gaia 2/3, and Miracle 12 should be attempted.
  - No consensus exists over the best initial antegrade GW. However, the author prefers a step-up approach with the moderate escalation of wire stiffness and switching to stiff-tapered ones with penetration ability [8]. Normally, ≥3 g tip-load GWs are used for CTO lesions.
- *Contemporary GWs limitation.*
  - Soft polymeric tapered GWs (Fielder XT family) are excellent for soft tissue tracking. They do have the capacity to deflect due to limited penetration efficacy within the occluded segment, resulting in *lack* of directional control (active wire control).

Table 6.4 GW selection (table generation is based on "Guidewire Crossing Techniques in CTO Intervention: A to Z" by Dash [8])

Indication	Wire type	Guidewire
Focal, tapered CTO	Soft	Fielder XT, Gaia 1
Tortuous or microchannel Tracking failure	Intermediate	Miracle 3, 4.5, and 6, Ultimate Bro 3, Gaia 2
Hard, dense, blunt	Stiff	Conquest Pro 12/20 g, Gaia 2/3, Miracle 12

Table 6.5 Sequence of GW selection in contemporary CTO techniques

CTO lesion type	Wire type (load)	Guidewire
Soft tissue tracking	Soft (<1 g)	Fielder XT-A/XT-R
Hard tissue tracking	Intermediate (2–6 g)	Gaia family
Calcified tissue penetration	Stiff (>9 g)	Conquest Pro

  - By contrast, stiff spring-coil GWs due to their high penetration efficacy are excellent for hard tissue penetration, but they have limited capacity to deflect and have *limited* directional control (*inadequate* active wire control).
  - Whereas there are two mechanisms of active wire control for tracking, including

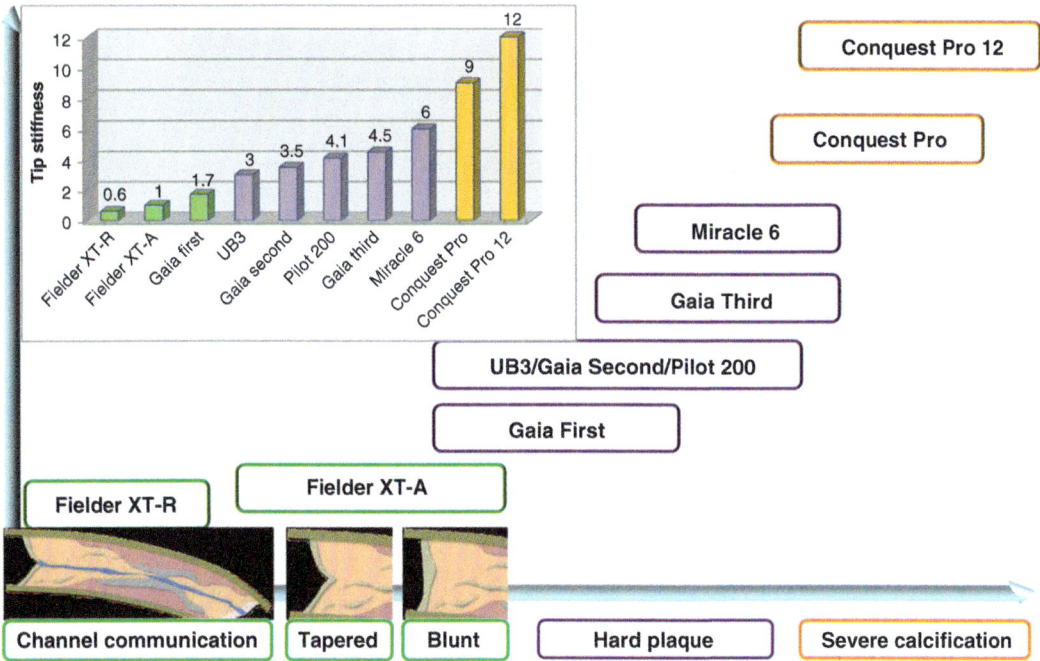

Fig. 6.5 Current algorithm for wire selection: figure modification is based on "An Overview About Dedicated CTO Wires" by Prof. Georgios Sianos, MD, in JIM, Milan, Italy, 2017. The above data has been obtained by Asahi Intecc's permission

(1) deflection control by longitudinal advancement and (2) direction (torque) control by rotation. The different concepts of contemporary GWs (e.g., Conquest Pro, Gaia third) for penetration are shown in Fig. 6.6.

- *Wire manipulation.*
  - *Both-hand maneuver*: left hand is used for to-and-fro movement and right hand for rotation, in cases where the wire tip direction needs to be changed or the wire presents the fingers with high resistance.
  - *Right-hand maneuver*: right hand does both movements. In this manipulation, the wire is advanced by dissecting the tissue with the wire tip (controlled drill). The wire tip is then advanced toward the intended direction with a sector swing.
  - Either manipulation is appropriate for CTO-PCI; in some cases, operators use both methods and alter their approach according to the situation. Do remember

the differences of wire tip movements with both maneuvers.

- *Hydrophilic GWs use in CTO.*
  Hydrophilic GWs are rarely used because they can easily go into the subintimal space without tactile feedback. The only exception is hydrophilic soft wires (like Whisper) in the case of CTOs with a straight microchannel. A faint channel, consistent with an intracoronary microchannel, is visible that may allow easy access to the distal lumen. Care must be taken in this circumstance not to create a false lumen. The operator converts a simple case into a big failure [3]. Conquest Pro is a hybrid wire (0.009 in. taper, hydrophilic coated except at the tip), thus reducing the friction as the wire shaft passes down the vessel and through the body of the occlusion while retaining tactile response at the distal tip end. Powerful wires with a combination of stiffness, hydrophilic coating, and tapered tip (Conquest Pro 9/12 g) should be reserved for experienced operators [3].

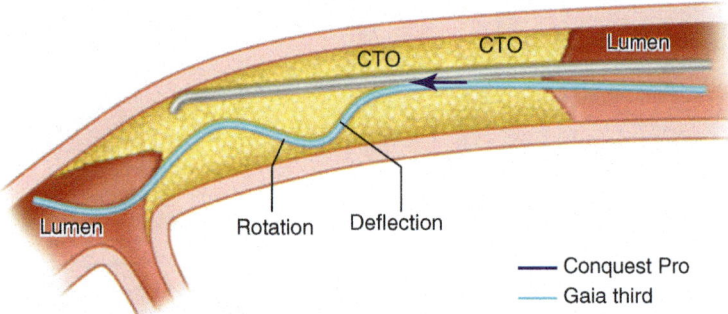

Fig. 6.6 Conquest Pro vs. Gaia third concept. Figure modification is based on "An Overview About Dedicated CTO Wires" by Prof. Georgios Sianos in JIM, Milan, Italy, 2017. The above information has been obtained by Asahi Intecc's permission. *Conquest Pro*, penetration force; *Gaia third*, deflection and rotation (directional torque) control

- *Where is the wire?*

  The interventional cardiologist should focus on these important feelings: (1) dimple feeling at the entry point, especially in the abrupt type, which is the key to success, but the dimple feeling does not always guarantee intimal plaque tracking; (2) strong resistance feeling when pulling back the wire inside the CTO body. If the guide is drawn into it, the wire tip has most likely migrated into the subintima; (3) no resistance feeling: The wire tip is in either the true lumen or the extravascular space [6] (Table 6.6).

- *Best way to know if the wire is in the subintima.*

  - In the case of abrupt CTOs, the wire could go into the wrong path without any resistance. There is little tactile feeling when penetrating the proximal cap. The wire seems to advance smoothly if the wire is in true lumen. The only evidence of wire in the true lumen is relative resistance during withdrawal of the wire. Wire tip rotation with movement-free and further advancement resistance is evidence of wire positioned in subadventitia (the wire turns around the vessel lumen, giving the appearance of a longer tip curve).

  - Pulling the GW back 1–2 mm is the best way to know whether the wire is in the intima. The wire stuck feeling confirms the tip is in the intima. The following (Table 6.6) can confirm that the wire tip is in the intima [4, 9].

- *To avoid entering the subintima.*

Table 6.6 Feeling from the fingertip [4]

Body
• Grasp: false lumen tracking or high resistance lesion
• Stuck: in the subintima
• Resistance: in the false lumen
• Movement decrease: in the false lumen
Exit
• Movement-free: in the (1) true lumen; (2) extravascular space

When trying to cross curved segments, avoid positioning the wire at the outer curve of the bend. If a false channel has been created, pull the wire back to proximal entry of the false channel, and then attempt a new channel [4].

- *If the wire goes the wrong way.*

  - If during penetration strategy the wire tip points to an unintended direction, either modify tip-shaping or switch to a stiffer one, which is more favorable than trying to use wire rotation.

  - When a wire tip deviates from the imaginary line, goes into subintimal space, or has a sticking sensation, it is better to switch to the parallel wire (seesaw wiring) technique.

6.5 Piercing the Distal Cap

More than 3-year-old occlusion typically tapers at the end to form a convex structure, making penetration of the distal fibrous more problematic. The optimal point for the penetration of convex-shaped distal fibrous cap is its center, although the newly created proximal channel often leads laterally. In curved vessels, the optimal point to attempt to perforate the distal fibrous cap is usually on the mural myocardial side [4].

Tips
- *Wire selection*
  - Spring-type wires with greater tactile feedback (less create a false lumen) are optimal. Stiffer ones, offering increased torque response (less resistance), may contribute to entering a false channel easily. Thus, lower-force ones are used initially (e.g., Miracle Brothers 3 g). If penetration is challenging, using a more stiff wire is optimal.
  - The optimal tip-shaping: angulation 15–30° with a 1.5–2.0 mm bend depending on the lumen size as part of either the parallel wire technique or IVUS-guided wiring (Conquest Pro 9/12 g is most suitable) [4].
- *Piercing distal cap feeling*
  - When wiring to the exit point, manipulation should be gentle and careful while controlling the tip in the direction of the distal true lumen for wire-crossing success. It is important to visualize the distal true

lumen on the angiographic examination assistant on different angles.
- Once the wire breaks through the distal cap to the true lumen, the resistance from the tip suddenly becomes lighter. It is very important to confirm that the tip has advanced to the distal vessel without any resistance by taking an angiogram [6].

6.6   Caveat

- Terminate the procedure to stabilize the dissection for a couple of weeks when:
  - There is suboptimal distal flow post-POBA due to long subintimal wiring.
  - Patient is hemodynamically unstable.

6.7   Recommendations of Preferred Wires for Each CTO Technique

Table 6.7 summarized the guidewire recommendations according to different wire techniques. For a successful outcome, the operator needs to be familiar with all of these techniques and needs to diversify whenever necessary.

Supplement table data is from "Tools and techniques—clinical update on coronary guidewires 2016: CTO" by Green et al. [2].

Table 6.7 Recommendations of preferred wires for each CTO technique

Use	Wire	Load (g)	Coating	Cover	Diameter	Tip composition
Access	SION blue	0.5	Hydrophilic Hydrophobic tip	None	0.014″	20 cm spring coil
	BMW Universal	0.6	Hydrophilic	Intermediate polymer	0.014″	Shaping ribbon
	Run through NS Intermediate	3.6	Hydrophilic	None	0.014″	25 cm spring coil
Microchannel crossing	Fielder XT	0.8	Hydrophilic	Polymer	0.014″ 0.009″ tip	16 cm spring coil
	Fielder XT-A	1.0	Hydrophilic	Polymer	0.014″ 0.010″ tip	16 cm spring coil

(continued)

Table 6.7 (continued)

Use	Wire	Load (g)	Coating	Cover	Diameter	Tip composition
Direct penetration	Confianza Pro	9 12	Hydrophilic Hydrophobic tip	None	0.014″ 0.009″ tip	20 cm spring coil
	PROGRESS 200T	13.0	Hydrophilic uncoated tip	Intermediate polymer	0.014″ 0.009″ tip	
	Gaia family (first, second, third)	1.7 3.5 4.5	Hydrophilic	None	0.014″ 0.010″ tip 0.011″ tip 0.012″ tip	15 cm spring coil
	PILOT 200	4.1	Hydrophilic	Full polymer	0.014″	15 cm spring coil
Collateral crossing	SION	0.7	Hydrophilic	None	0.014″	28 cm spring coil
	Fielder XT-R	0.6	Hydrophilic	Polymer	0.014″ 0.010″ tip	16 cm spring coil
	PILOT 50	1.5	Hydrophilic	Full polymer	0.014″	15 cm spring coil
	Fielder FC	0.8	Hydrophilic	Polymer	0.014″	11 cm spring coil
	SION black	0.8	Hydrophilic	Polymer	0.014″	12 cm spring coil
Knuckling	Fielder XT	0.8	Hydrophilic	Polymer	0.014″ 0.009″ tip	16 cm spring coil
	Fielder FC	0.8	Hydrophilic	Polymer	0.014″	11 cm spring coil
	PILOT 50	1.5	Hydrophilic	Full polymer	0.014″	15 cm spring coil
	PILOT 200	4.1	Hydrophilic	Full polymer	0.014″	15 cm spring coil
Reentering	Confianza	9	Hydrophobic	None	0.014″ 0.009″ tip	20 cm spring coil
	Stingray wire	12	Hydrophilic	None	0.014″ 0.0035″ tip	20 cm spring coil
Externalization	RG3	3	Hydrophilic	None	0.014″ 0.010″ tip	8 cm spring coil

References

1. Sianos G, Konstantinidis NV, Di Mario C, Karvounis H. Theory and practical based approach to chronic total occlusions. BMC Cardiovasc Disord. 2016;16:33.
2. Green P, Monga S, Ramcharitar S, Hanratty C. Tools and techniques—clinical update on coronary guidewires 2016: chronic total occlusions. EuroIntervention. 2016;11:1077–9.
3. Saito S, Tanaka S, Hiroe Y, Miyashita Y, Takahashi S, Satake S, et al. Angioplasty for chronic total occlusion by using tapered-tip guidewires. Catheter Cardiovasc Interv. 2003;59:305–11.
4. Nguyen TN, Hu D, Chen SL, Kim MH, Saito S, Grines C. Practical handbook of advanced interventional cardiology: tips and tricks. 4th ed: Wiley-

Blackwell: John Wiley & Sons, Ltd., 2013. ISBN: 978-0-470-67047-7.

5. Katoh O, Reifart N. New double wire technique to stent ostial lesions. Catheter Cardiovasc Diagn. 1997;40:400–2.

6. Sumitsuji S, Inoue K, Ochiai M, Tsuchikane E, Ikeno F. Fundamental wire technique and current standard strategy of percutaneous intervention for chronic total occlusion with histopathological insights. JACC Cardiovasc Interv. 2011;4:941–51.

7. Corcos T, Favereau X, Guerin Y, Toussaint M, Ouzan J, Zheng H, et al. Recanalization of chronic coronary occlusions using a new hydrophilic guidewire. Catheter Cardiovasc Diagn. 1998;44:83–90.

8. Dash D. Guidewire crossing techniques in coronary chronic total occlusion intervention: A to Z. Indian Heart J. 2016;68:410–20.

9. Basic OK. Wire-handling strategies for chronic total occlusions. In: King S, Yeung A, editors. Interventional cardiology. New York: McGraw-Hill; 2007. p. 367–83.

Guidewire Supporting Devices

7

Duck Hyun Jang and Cheol Woong Yu

7.1 Introduction

The role of microcatheter during CTO PCI is as follows:

1. Strong backup support during wiring
2. Reinforce torque transmission
3. Easy wire exchange
4. Selective angiography
5. Support double lumen for parallel wire technique
6. Septal channel dilator during retrograde approach

According to aim of use, optimal selection of microcatheter is very important for successful CTO PCI. Therefore, we should be familiar with characteristics of various microcatheters. This chapter introduces the profile and characteristics of microcatheters commonly used during CTO PCI.

7.2 Corsair

ASAHI Corsair (Asahi Intecc, Nagoya, Japan) was originally developed as a septal channel dilator, to ease retrograde approaches for CTO PCI. This is a unique device that can be used both

as a microcatheter and as a support catheter. 135 cm device was made for anterograde support, and 150 cm device was made for retrograde support. Tapered distal tip and ability to spin the device make the Corsair a very effective tool in CTO PCI. Different from other microcatheters, unique spiral structure (the so-called SHINKA-Shaft) effectively transmits rotational torque to the distal tip. This rotation gives ASAHI Corsair its high crossing performance through tortuous channels. Tapered soft tip provides superior tip flexibility which enables smooth advancement through narrow tortuous vessels, such as septal channels or other microchannels. Radiopaque marker is located closer to distal tip which enhances the visibility and safety of Corsair (Figs. 7.1, 7.2, and 7.3).

Using method:
1. When passing the catheter through the lesion, pushing with rotating the catheter reinforces the penetration ability.
2. When rotating the catheter, do not rotate over 10 times in the same direction which can cause catheter damage. After rotating 7–8 times in one direction, rotate in the opposite direction.
3. Do not use in a very severely calcified lesion (Corsair may be stuck in the lesion).

D. H. Jang · C. W. Yu (✉)
Korea University Anam Hospital, Seoul, South Korea
e-mail: iron0717@korea.ac.kr

© Springer Nature Singapore Pte Ltd. 2019
Y. Jang (ed.), *Percutaneous Coronary Interventions for Chronic Total Occlusion*,
https://doi.org/10.1007/978-981-10-6026-7_7

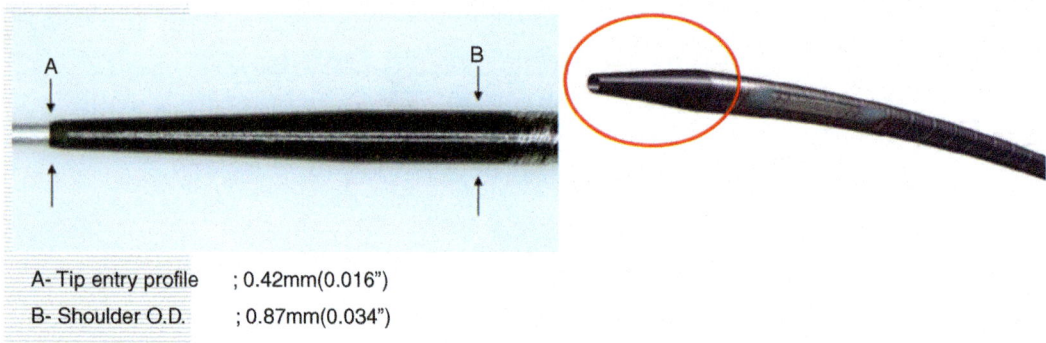

A- Tip entry profile ; 0.42mm(0.016")
B- Shoulder O.D. ; 0.87mm(0.034")

Fig. 7.1 Profile of distal tip in microcatheter Corsair

Φ0.12mm ×2pcs   Φ0.07mm ×8pcs

SHIKA-Shaft's unique spiral structure

Reinforced Tapered Shaft

A

B

C

Φ0.38mm

Φ0.45mm

Φ0.45mm

Φ0.42~0.82mm
(tapered)

Φ0.87mm

Φ0.95mm

1.3Fr

2.6Fr

2.8Fr

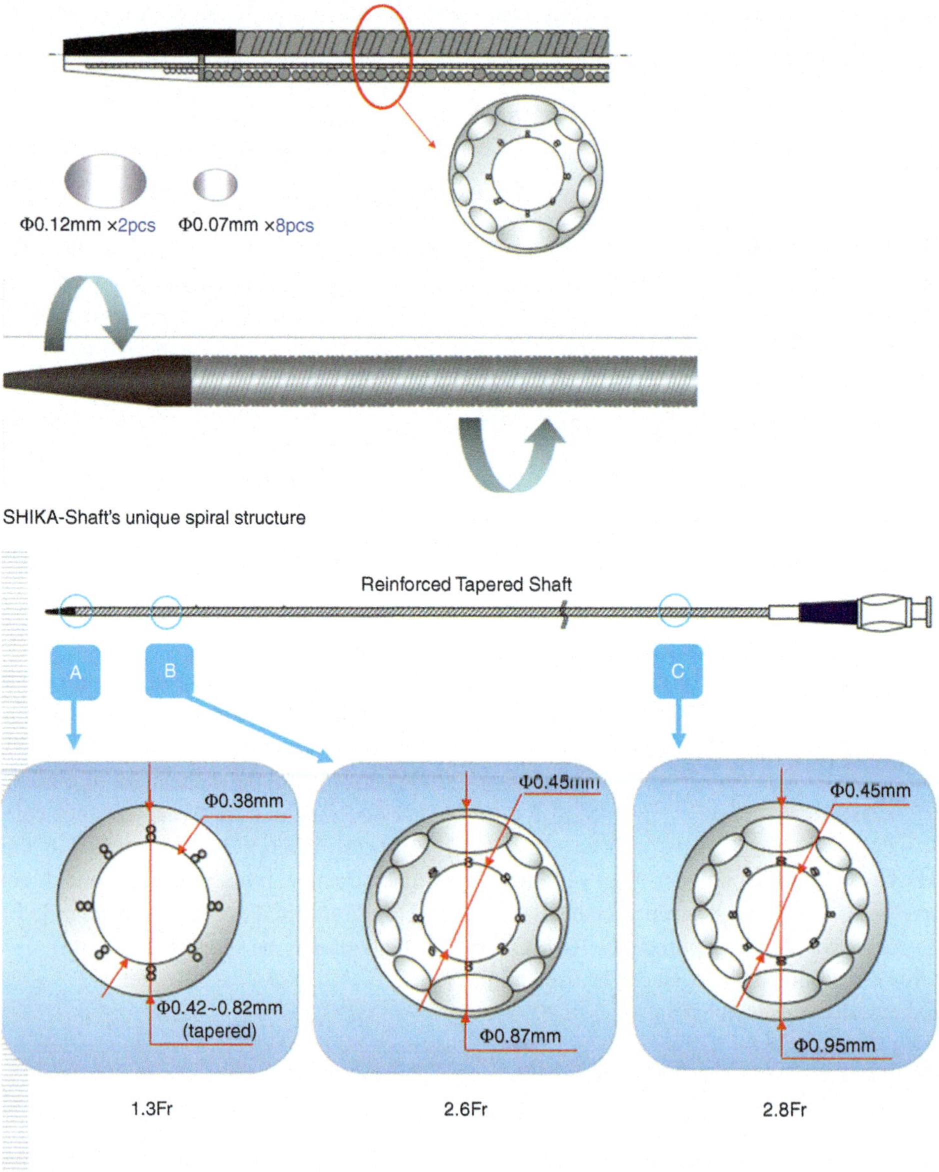

Fig. 7.2 Features and benefit of microcatheter Corsair

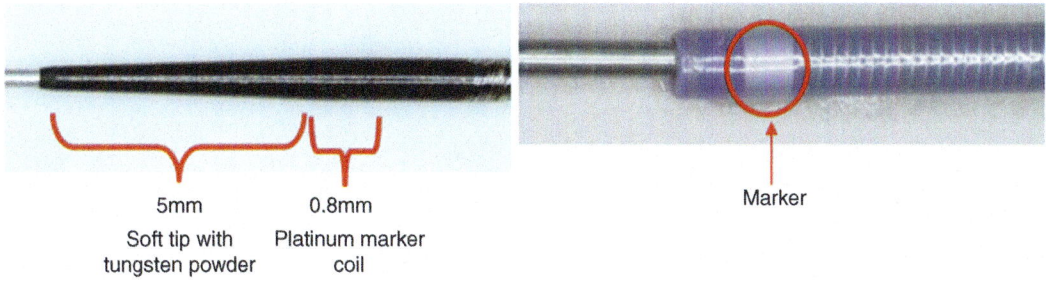

Fig. 7.3 Features of tip in microcatheter Corsair

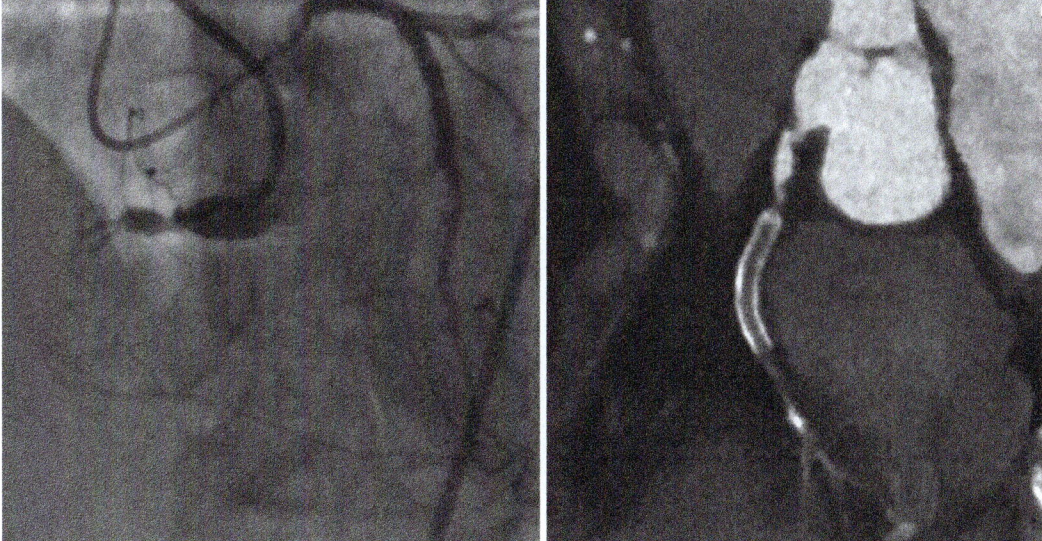

Fig. 7.4 Initial angiography and coronary CT

Example 1: CTO PCI Using Microcatheter (Corsair) for Retrograde Approach Via Septal Channel

Seventy-three-year-old female patient visited our hospital due to CCS II chest pain. Coronary angiography revealed that ostial right coronary artery (RCA) was severely stenosed, and mid RCA, which was treated with stent implantation using Endeavor (Medtronic Inc., Minneapolis, MN) 4.0 mm × 30 mm 6 years ago, was totally occluded with moderate calcification (Fig. 7.4). Coronary CT angiogram showed total occlusion with peripheral calcification at mid RCA (Fig. 7.4). Bilateral approach using Rt. radial and Rt. femoral artery was planned. Chronic total occlusion (CTO) lesion at m-RCA was attempted by anterograde approach at initial approach using guiding catheter 7 Fr short tip Amplatz Left 1 (SAL1) (Medtronic Inc., Minneapolis, MN) and several guidewires such as Floppy (Abbott Vascular, Santa Clara, CA, USA), Conquest Pro 12 (Asahi Intecc, Nagoya, Japan), and Gaia 2nd (Asahi Intecc, Nagoya, Japan) supported by microcatheter "Corsair." However, initial wiring attempt through anterograde approach failed, making false lumen. Thereafter, coronary angiogram was reviewed again, trying to find out optimal septal channel for retrograde approach, and finally second septal channel was selected for retrograde route. Finally Gaia 2nd (Asahi Intecc, Nagoya, Japan) supported by Corsair (Asahi Intecc, Nagoya, Japan) successfully passed the CTO

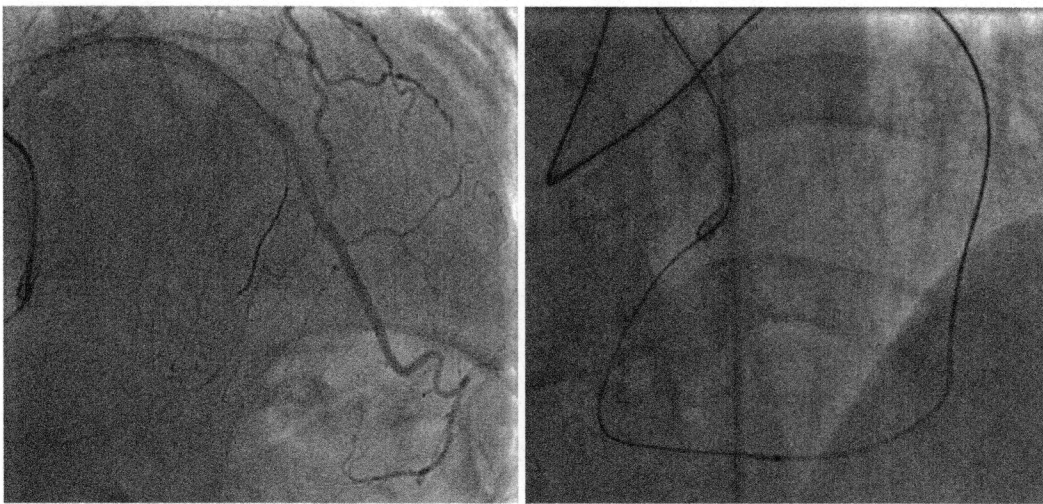

Fig. 7.5 Retrograde wiring (Gaia 2nd supported by Corsair)

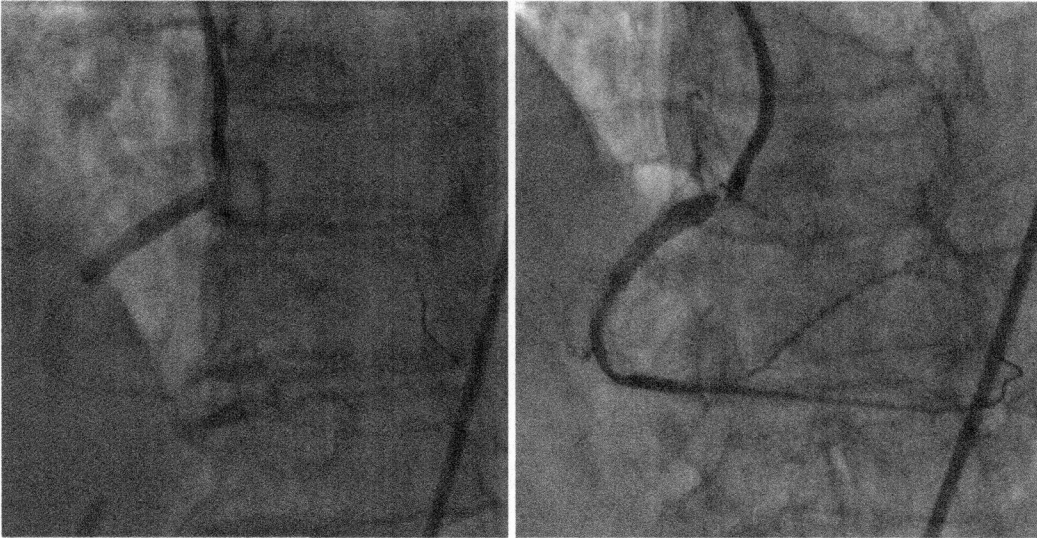

Fig. 7.6 Stent implantation and final angiography

lesion from the retrograde after successfully navigating septal channel with Fielder FC (Asahi Intecc, Nagoya, Japan) supported by Corsair (Asahi Intecc, Nagoya, Japan) (Fig. 7.5). After pre-dilatation with Lacrosse 2.5 mm × 15 mm (Goodman, Ireland), one stent (Xience Alpine 4.0 mm × 23 mm, Abbott Vascular, Santa Clara, CA, USA) was successfully implanted at the proximal RCA (Fig. 7.6).

7.3 FineCross

FineCross (Terumo Interventional Systems, Tokyo, Japan) has the smallest profile catheters and can be applied to pass the smaller-sized collaterals. They are composed of fully stainless steel braided shaft, which supports strong guidewire backup, and tapered inner and outer lumen, which supplies advanced crossability and provides a best guidewire support. Because the inner layer was coated by polytetrafluoroethylene (PTFE), optimal guidewire manipulation is possible. The proximal lumen's size (2.6 Fr/0.87 mm) is enough which facilitates buddy wire technique in 6 Fr guiding catheter, and distal lumen (1.8 Fr/0.60 mm) is enough for proper guidewire handling and contrast injection. This microcatheter has the lowest profile among microcatheters, but pushability is minimum. Because FineCross has the lowest profile, it can pass narrow CTO space smoothly. The distal 13 cm is consisted of ultra-flexible material to support optimal trackability at tight and tortuous anatomy. The floppy distal segment is manufactured to be atraumatic and offers a best balance between trackability and safety while navigating through the tortuous anatomy. FineCross GT has a more smaller tapering distal entry tip profile 1.7 Fr (0.57 mm) than FineCross. With such profile, the wire can be advanced into even smaller vascular lumens and tortuous lesions (Fig. 7.7).

Example 2: CTO PCI Using Microcatheter (FineCross) for Centrally Occupying Calcified Lesion

Fifty-five-year-old male patient visited the emergency department due to increasing dyspnea (NYHA IV). Echocardiography revealed that left ventricular function was severely depressed (EF 15%). Coronary angiography showed that proximal RCA was totally occluded with collateral flow Rentrop classification Grade II from left anterior descending artery (LAD). The decision was made to revascularize RCA. Coronary CT angiogram showed total occlusion of proximal RCA with centrally occupying calcification (Fig. 7.8). Because FineCross (Terumo Interventional Systems, Tokyo, Japan) microcatheter has the lowest profile and its distal outer diameter was smaller than other microcatheters, it has the benefit of passing the narrow and calcified CTO lesion. CTO lesion was attempted to cross by anterograde approach using guiding catheter 7 Fr SAL1 (Medtronic Inc., Minneapolis, MN) and guidewires such as Runthrough (Terumo Interventional Systems, Tokyo, Japan) and Gaia 1st (Asahi Intecc, Nagoya, Japan) supported by microcatheter "FineCross" (Fig. 7.9). Finally Gaia 1st supported by FineCross successfully crossed the CTO lesion. However, balloon could not be delivered through the CTO lesion. Therefore, after changing SAL1 guiding catheter to Amplatz Left 1 (AL1) (Medtronic Inc., Minneapolis,

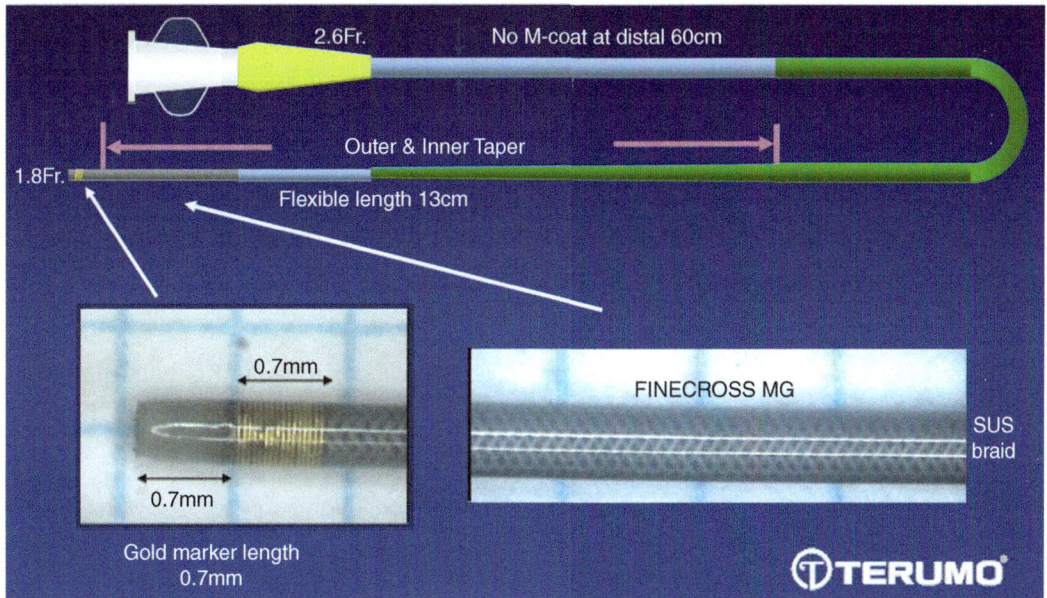

Fig. 7.7 Features of microcatheter FineCross

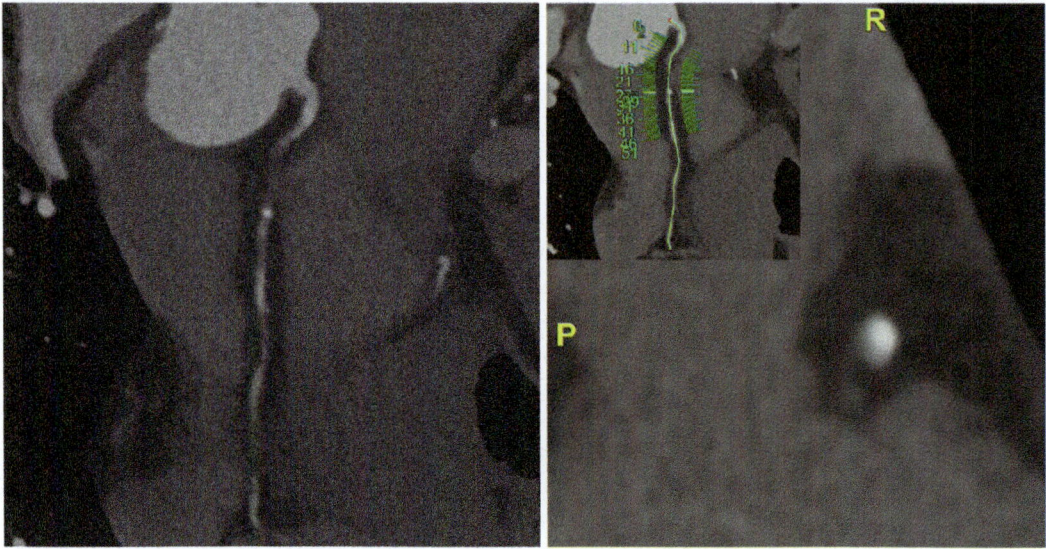

Fig. 7.8 Coronary CT angiogram showed total occlusion of proximal RCA with centrally occupying calcification

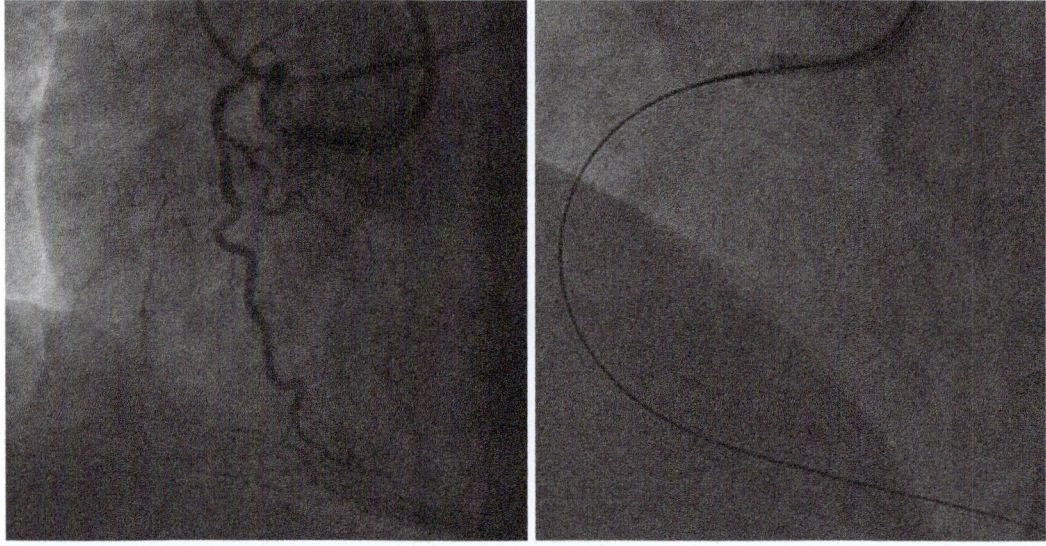

Fig. 7.9 Anterograde wiring with Gaia 1st supported by FineCross

MN), Gaia 1st guidewire was advanced again and changed to RotaWire for rotational atherectomy. After successful rotational atherectomy using 1.25-sized burr, Ikazuchi 1 mm × 6 mm (Cordis, Miami Lakes, FL, USA) was successfully delivered to the CTO lesion for pre-dilation. After multiple ballooning at lesion, Xience Alpine 2.5 mm × 38 mm (Abbott Vascular, Santa Clara, CA, USA) for mid RCA and BioMatrix 3.0 mm × 24 mm (Biosensors Europe SA, Morges, Switzerland) for proximal RCA were successfully implanted (Fig. 7.10). Three months later, follow-up echocardiograpy showed improved left ventricular systolic function (EF30~35%), and the patient's symptom has dramatically improved.

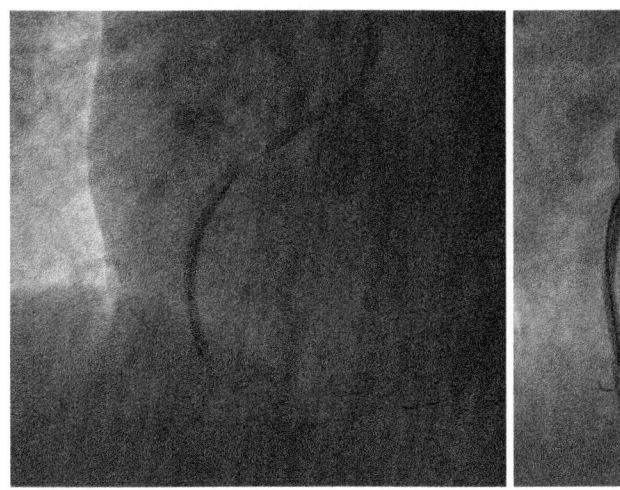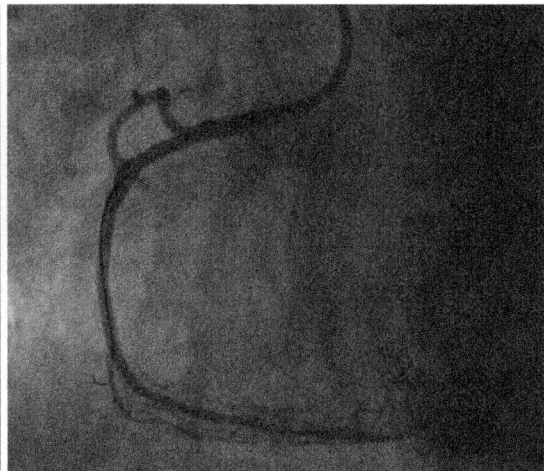

Fig. 7.10 Stent implantation and final angiography

7.4 Crusade

The most unique feature of the microcatheter Crusade (Kaneka Corp., Osaka, Japan) is that it consists of dual lumen. One is over the wire lumen, while other is rapid exchange lumen. This feature facilitated efficient wiring of difficult branches and wiring through stent struts. This microcatheter is also useful in antegrade parallel wire technique. The principle of parallel wire technique is to keep the first wire in place (subintimal space) and advance a second stiffer wire toward the distal true lumen using the first wire as a marker. Crusade has durable shaft and low profile tapered flexible tip (0.017 in.). Two radiopaque markers are located on the rapid exchange port 0.5 mm apart. These radiopaque markers make it easy to estimate the length of the lesion (Figs. 7.11 and 7.12).

Example 3: CTO PCI by Parallel Wire Technique Using Double-Lumen Microcatheter (Crusade) for Diffuse Long CTO Lesion
Fifty-seven-year-old man visited the hospital due to chest pain (CCS II). Angiography showed that proximal LAD was totally occluded with collateral flow (Rentrop classification Grade III) via very tortuous epicardial channel from RCA. Coronary CT angiogram showed diffuse long CTO lesion from proximal LAD to distal

LAD (Fig. 7.13). Because of no optimal retrograde channel, CTO PCI was decided using parallel wiring technique with double-lumen microcatheter "Crusade" through antegrade approach. With guiding catheter 7 Fr extra backup 3.75 (EBU 3.75) (Medtronic Inc., Minneapolis, MN), parallel wiring technique using Miracle 6g (Asahi Intecc, Nagoya, Japan) and Conquest Pro 12 (Asahi Intecc, Nagoya, Japan) supported by Crusade (Kaneka Corp., Osaka, Japan) was performed (Fig. 7.14). Finally, Conquest Pro 12 guidewire advanced distal true lumen. After multiple ballooning, two stents (Xience Prime 2.5 mm × 38 mm and 2.75 mm × 12 mm (Abbott Vascular, Santa Clara, CA, USA)) were successfully implanted

7.5 Caravel

A multipotent microcatheter that completes the simple lesion and simplifies the complex lesion.

Caravel (Asahi Intecc, Nagoya, Japan) is intended to provide support to facilitate the placement of guidewires in the coronary and peripheral vasculatures and can be used to exchange from one guidewire to another. It has an excellent crossing profile of 0.62 mm (1.9 Fr), and braided wires maintain lumen diameter and guidewire performance. In case when a lower profile support

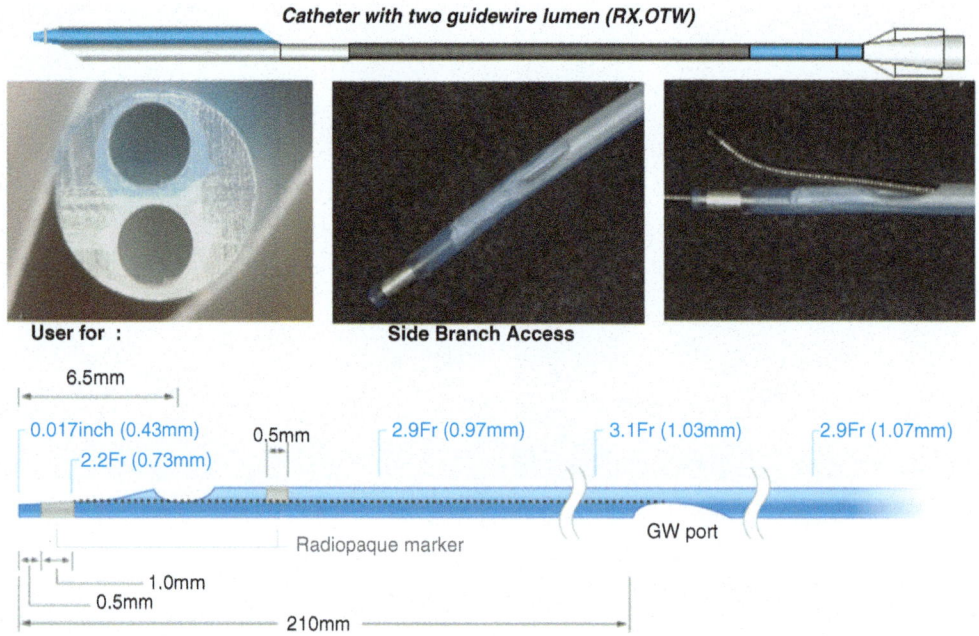

Fig. 7.11 Features of microcatheter Crusade

Fig. 7.12 Benefits of microcatheter Crusade

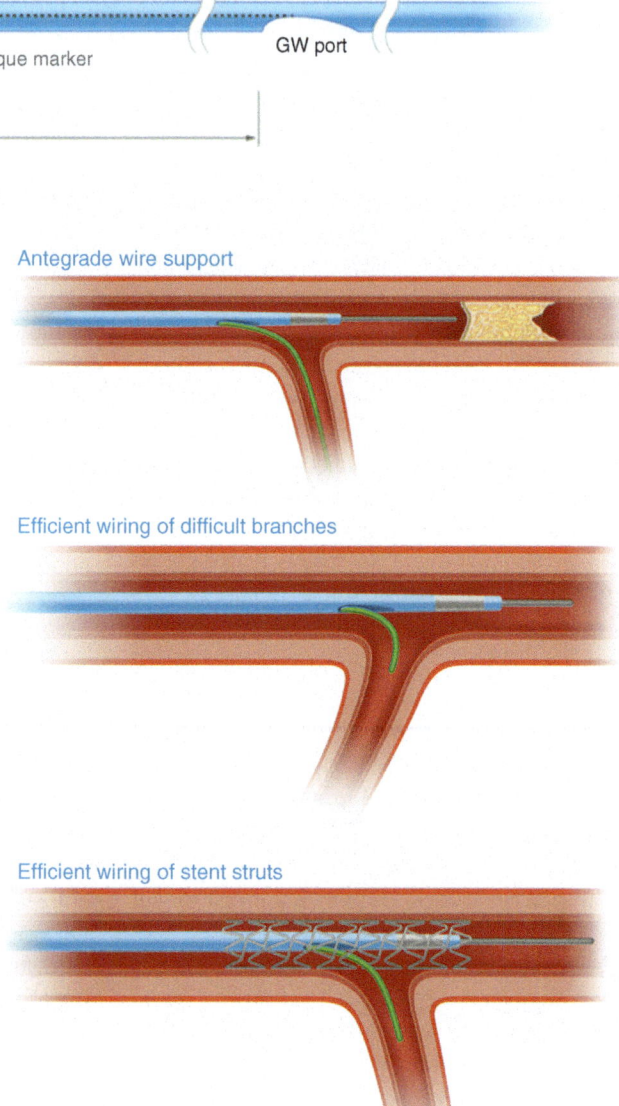

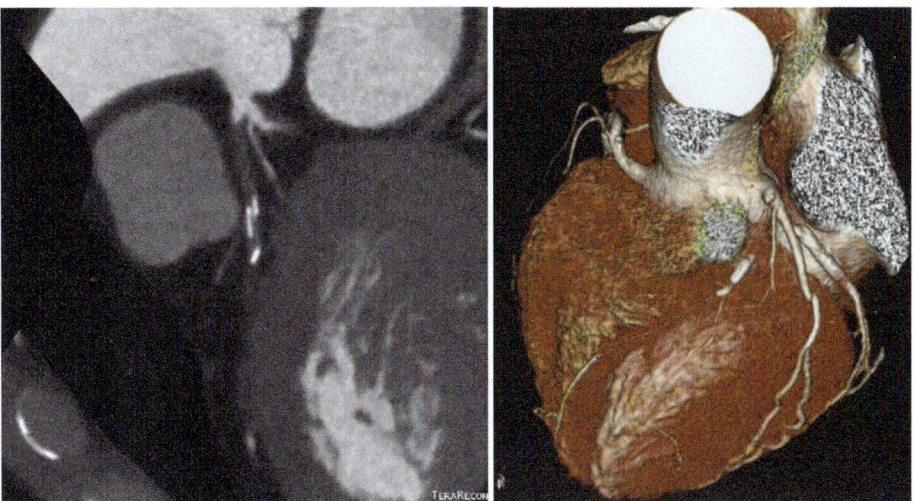

Fig. 7.13 Coronary CT angiogram showed diffuse long CTO lesion from proximal LAD to distal LAD

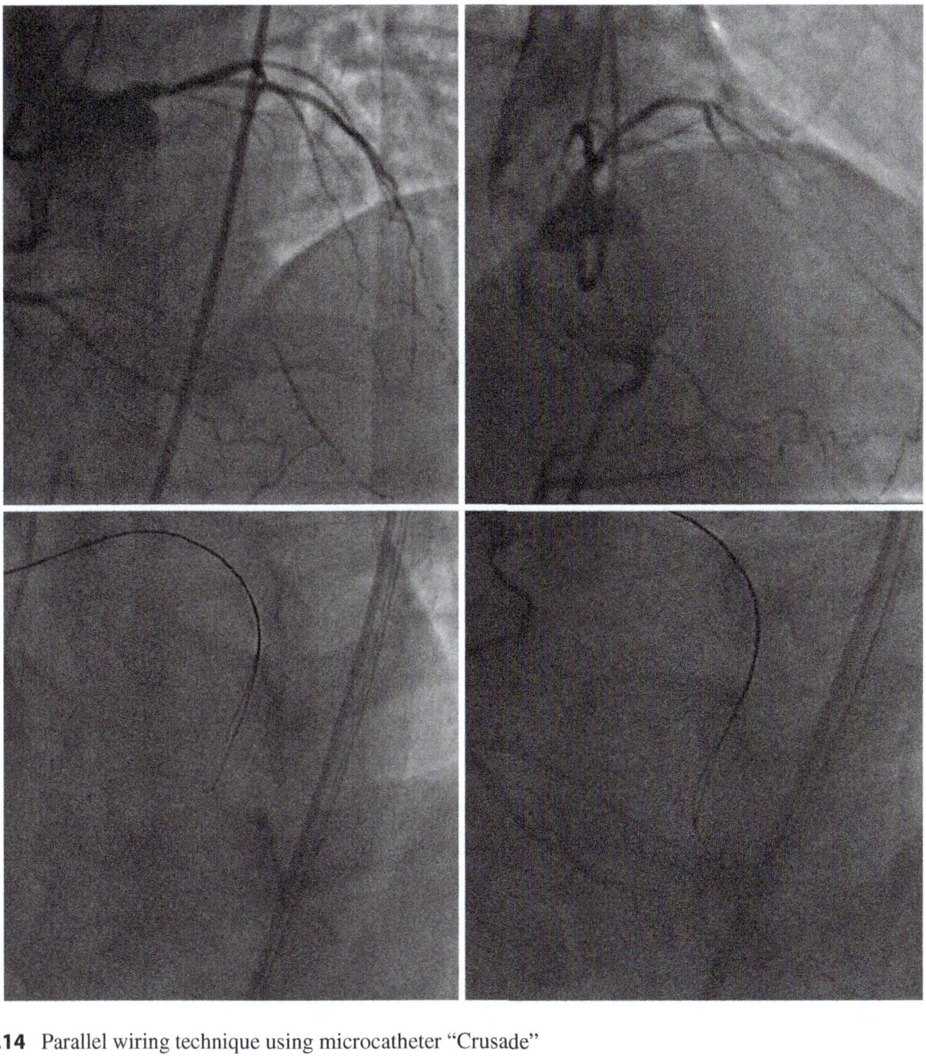

Fig. 7.14 Parallel wiring technique using microcatheter "Crusade"

catheter is needed in anterograde approach and when it navigates very narrow and tortuous lesion in retrograde approach, Caravel could be considered as the suitable microcatheter. Because of its lower outer profile, 6 Fr guiding catheter can house two Caravel microcatheters, as well as 7 Fr catheter with one Caravel and IVUS catheter (Fig. 7.15).

Smooth Transition

There is a smooth transition with subtle changes in the flexibility from the flexible tip to the shaft so the Caravel™ tracks well around an acute bend (Fig. 7.16).

7.6 Conclusion

There are several kinds of microcatheter with various profiles and characteristics for CTO PCI. The outer diameter of microcatheter at the level of distal, mid, and proximal portion, degree of hydrophilic coating, flexibility of tip, tapered tip, torque transition from shaft to tip, structure of inner shaft, etc. are important functional and structural characteristics of microcatheter. Appropriate selection of microcatheter with its unique individual characteristics is of utmost importance for the success in CTO PCI.

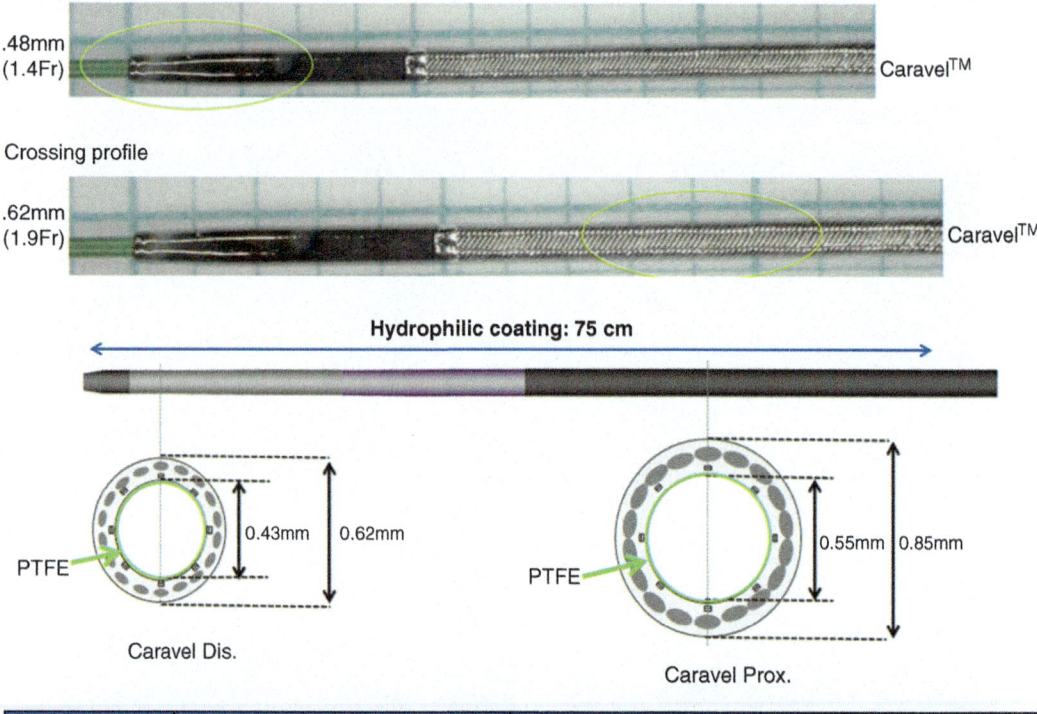

Products	O.D			I.D			Length	Coating Length
	Entry	Distal	Proximal	Entry	Distal	Proximal		
ASAHI Caravel	0.48 mm (1.4 Fr)	0.62 mm (1.9 Fr)	0.85 mm (2.6 Fr)	0.40 mm (0.016 inch)	0.43 mm (0.017 inch)	0.55 mm (0.022 inch)	135 cm	75 cm
ASAHI Corsair	0.42 mm (1.3 Fr)	0.87 mm (2.6 Fr)	0.93 mm (2.8 Fr)	0.38 mm (0.015 inch)	0.45 mm (0.018 inch)	0.45 mm (0.018 inch)	135 cm 150 cm	60 cm

Fig. 7.15 Profile of microcatheter Caravel

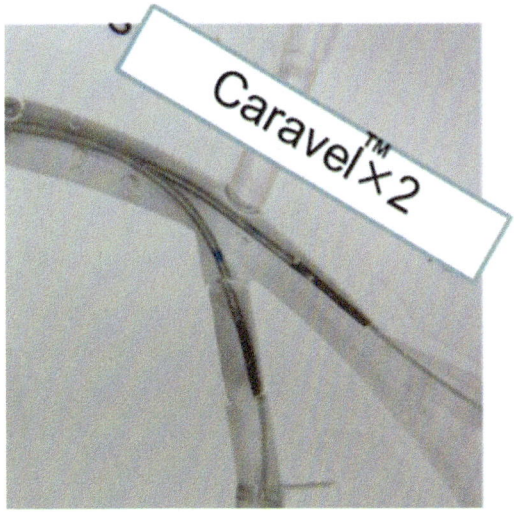

Guiding catheter: ASAHI Hyperion™ 7 Fr

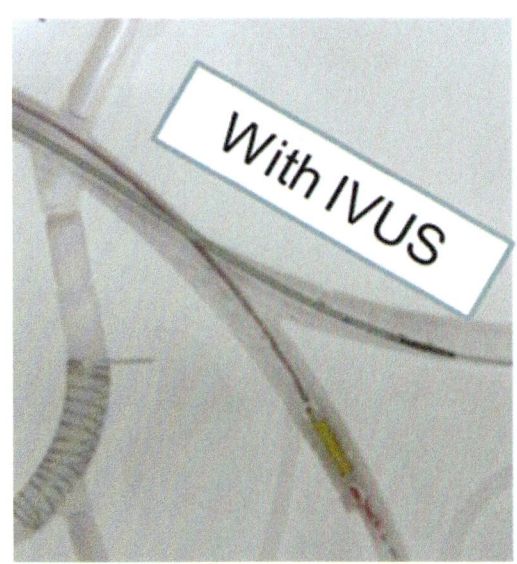

Guiding catheter :ASAHI Hyperion™ 6 Fr

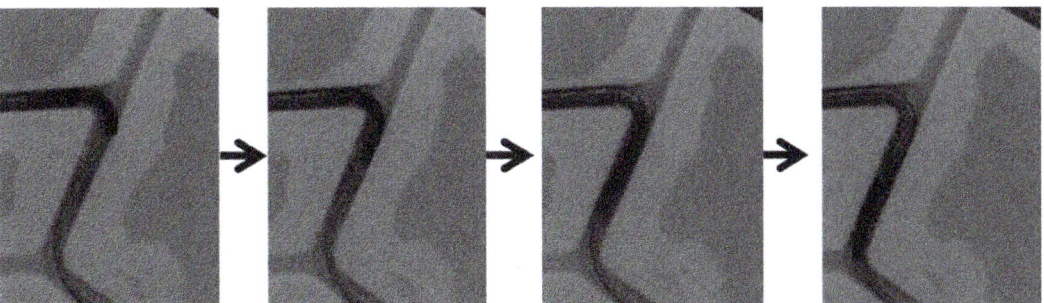

Fig. 7.16 Features of microcatheter Caravel

Bibliography

1. Aris K, Barbara AD, Dimitri K, et al. Approach to CTO intervention: overview of techniques. Curr Treat Options Cardiovasc Med. 2017;19:1.
2. Debabrata D. Guidewire crossing techniques in coronary chronic total occlusion intervention: A to Z. Indian Heart J. 2016;68:410–20.
3. Editorial. Language of CTO interventions—focus on hardware. Indian Heart J. 2016;68:450–63.
4. Georgios S, Nikolaos VK, Carlo DM, et al. Theory and practical based approach to chronic total occlusions. BMC Cardiovasc Disord. 2016;16:33.
5. Terumo-europe.com [Internet]. Coronary micro-guide catheter. http://www.terumo-europe.com.
6. Vascularperspectives.com [internet]. KANEKA Crusade Dual Lumen Microcatheter. http://www.vascularperspective.com.
7. ASAHI Corsair manual. ASAHI Corsair/ver2/01-09.
8. ASAHI Caravel manual. ASAHI Caravel/ver.1/AMC-K16211.

Antegrade Approach of CTO PCI

8

Seung-Hwan Lee, Bong-Ki Lee, and Jun-Won Lee

8.1 Planning of Antegrade Approach

The most important step for successful CTO intervention is to establish a pre-procedural strategy and prepare for every possible situations during procedure. Careful review of coronary angiography and coronary computed tomography angiography (CCTA), if available, provides crucial information for vessel direction and degree of calcification. Then, guiding catheter, supportive microcatheter, and guidewire should be considered appropriately case by case.

8.2 Device Selection and Handling

With development of PCI devices, success rate of CTO PCI has been raised together. CTO PCI is a representatively complex procedure, so highly dependent to operator's technique and device

S.-H. Lee (✉) · J.-W. Lee
Division of Cardiology, Department of Internal Medicine, Yonsei University Wonju College of Medicine, Wonju Severance Christian Hospital, Wonju, South Korea
e-mail: carshlee@yonsei.ac.kr

B.-K. Lee
Division of Cardiology, Department of Internal Medicine, Kangwon National University Hospital, Kangwon National University School of Medicine, Chuncheon, South Korea

selection. Adequate device selection is crucial for successful CTO PCI.

8.2.1 Choice of Guiding Catheter

For the selection of shape and size of guiding catheter, lesion location, lesion length, tortuosity, and degree of calcification should be considered. In general, larger guiding catheter enables various techniques such as anchor-balloon technique, IVUS-guided navigation of guidewire, and the use of double microcatheters.

8.2.2 Choice of Microcatheter

The next step is to select suitable microcatheter which can affect procedural performance in terms of location of occluded segment, vessel tortuosity, and trackability. For example, FineCross microcatheter (TERUMO, Tokyo, Japan) may be advantageous than Corsair microcatheter (Asahi Intecc, Aichi, Japan) when directional property of guidewire is required in the proximal right coronary artery (RCA) lesion or ostium of left anterior descending artery (LAD) or left circumflex artery (LCX).

After passage of CTO-dedicated guidewire followed by microcatheter, stiff guidewire should be exchanged to conventional soft guidewire to avoid vessel injury. Corsair microcatheter may be better than FineCross microcatheter to overcome resistant

© Springer Nature Singapore Pte Ltd. 2019
Y. Jang (ed.), *Percutaneous Coronary Interventions for Chronic Total Occlusion*,
https://doi.org/10.1007/978-981-10-6026-7_8

lesion. If microcatheter fails to pass the lesion, pre-dilation with small balloon (1.0mm size) can make a space for the passage of microcatheter.

8.2.3 Choice of Guidewire

Selection of guidewire is determined by two factors. The one is the lesion character of proximal cap to be punctured. The other is the presence of microchannel for the navigation of a guidewire. Guidewires should be exchanged, if necessary,

with "step-up" or "step-down" strategy for the purpose of puncture or navigation.

The rotation of tip of guidewire should be carefully performed between 45 and 90 degrees. Guidewire should be advanced with a feeling of "push and pull" or "drilling" keeping from bending the tip of guidewire over 90 degrees.

In case of stumpless CTO with side branch, IVUS-guided navigation of guidewire could be helpful. The guidewire of higher tip load with proper tip shape is better for penetrating the proximal cap of CTO lesion (Figs. 8.1 and 8.2).

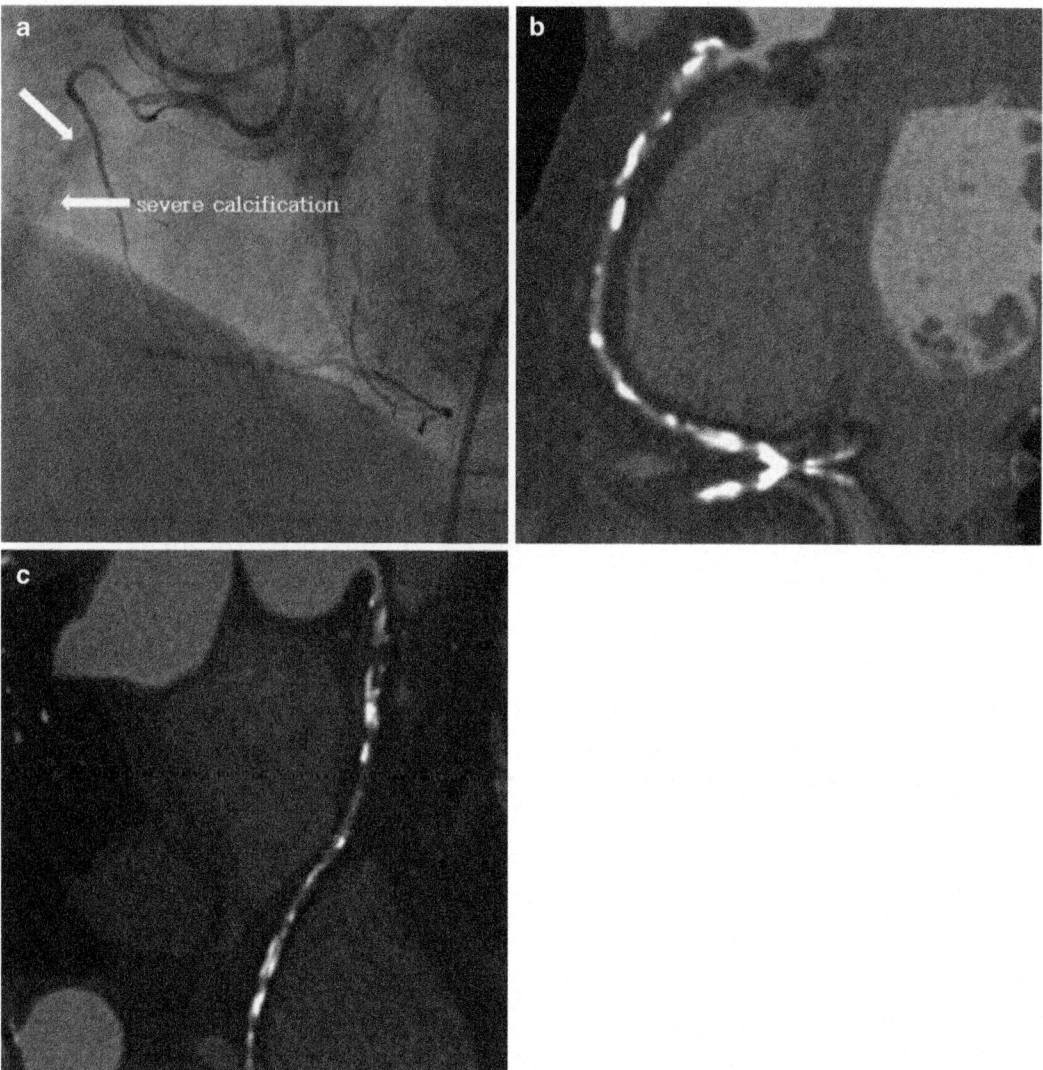

Fig. 8.1 Pre-procedural planning with baseline angiogram and coronary CT angiography. (**a**) Angiography shows stumpless chronic total occlusion with severe calcification at proximal RCA. Collateral flow comes from LAD; (**b, c**) multiplane reconstruction (MPR) image of

coronary CT angiography provides the direction of occluded segment and location of calcification which can be a milestone for introducing a guidewire. In this case, true lumen of mid-RCA is located between two calcifications (Case courtesy of Dr. Seung-Hwan Lee)

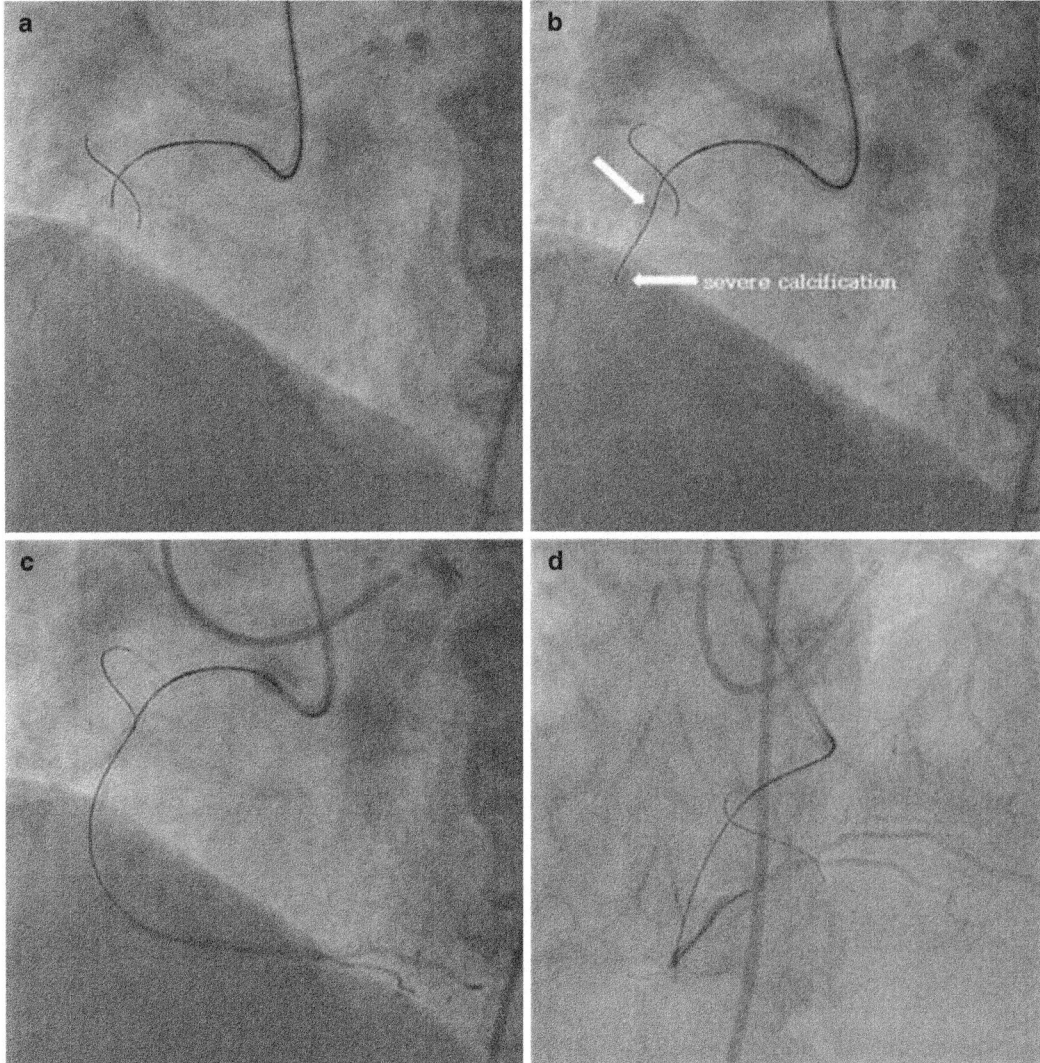

Fig. 8.2 Selection of guidewire and microcatheter. (**a**) Proximal fibrous cap was punctured using Gaia 2nd guidewire with a Corsair microcatheter; (**b**) "step-up" exchange of guidewire from a Gaia 2nd to a Miracle 6g which is better for navigation of the true lumen of calci-fied CTO lesion; (**c**) successful passage of a Miracle 6g guidewire into distal true lumen (LAO 45° view); (**d**) confirmation of guidewire into distal true lumen (LAO 10° and cranial 20° view) (Case courtesy of Dr. Seung-Hwan Lee)

8.3   Handling of Guidewire

Most failures in CTO PCI are associated with failure of guidewire crossing. Choosing the wire strategy is crucial for successful CTO PCI. In general there are four strategies to advance guide-wire [1, 2].

1. Sliding technique: If the closed channel is composed with softer tissue (loose fibrous tissue, proteoglycan, RBC, and inflammatory cells) with recanalized channels, this technique is preferred. Slightly higher tip load (1–2 g) and relatively high lubricity with lower friction (hydrophilic or polymer coated)

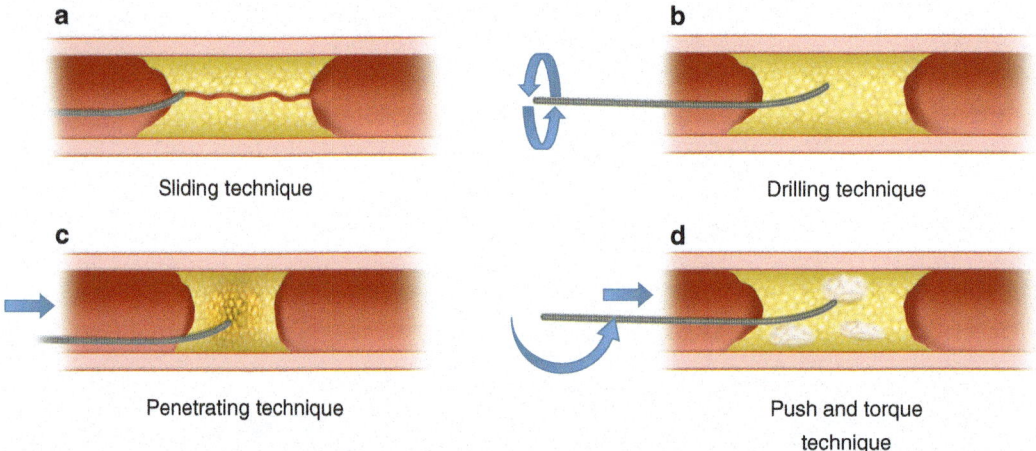

Fig. 8.3 Technique of guidewire handling (illustrated by Dr. Bong-Ki Lee)

are required such as Fielder XT-A, Fielder FC, Runthrough NS, Choice PT, or Pilot 50. If wire passing is unsatisfactory, wire escalation to a higher tip load and higher penetration power is recommended. This strategy has the lowest risk of subintimal tracking or perforation (Fig. 8.3a).

2. Drilling technique: when CTO segment is composed of a harder tissue (collagen, elastin, or calcium), this technique is useful. The wire is rotated fast but controlled through 360° with gentle advancement like drilling of a borewell. Proper wire property for this technique contains higher tip load (3–12 g) with/without taper, higher lubricity, and higher lateral support as Miracle or Conquest series of wires (Fig. 8.3b).

3. Penetrating technique: this technique is forcing the wire through the occluded lesion like a screw. The rotation movements are smaller (45°–90°), and the forward penetration force is higher. The wire is stiffer with/without a tip tapering as Miracle 12, Conquest Pro 9, 12, or 20 (Fig. 8.3c).

4. Push and torque technique: the wire is pushed with force, but only gentle rotation, and then the wire gets requisite position. The wire is negotiated through a soft tissue till it encounters a hard tissue. Then the wire is redirected into another plane of soft tissue and advanced longitudinally. If wire cannot be advanced, slightly move backward then forward again into different planes. Suitable wire has moderate tip load (1.5–4.5) with 1:1 torquability for precious steering as Gaia wires (Fig. 8.3d).

If these wiring techniques do not work to penetrate the tissue especially due to a lot of calcium, we should consider an alternate technique such as subintimal tracking or retrograde approach. Immoderate attempts of antegrade approach can cause extension of false lumen or vessel perforation. Appropriate collateral channel for retrograde approach should be verified from first planning strategy, if available.

8.4 Anchor-Balloon Technique

One of the major obstacles for passing guidewire or device is severe tortuosity of vessel or occlusion at proximal segment, especially proximal RCA CTO. If side branch is nearby proximal occluded lesion, balloon inflation with small-size balloon into the side branch, called as "anchor-balloon technique," can overcome lack of backup support of guiding catheter (Fig. 8.4).

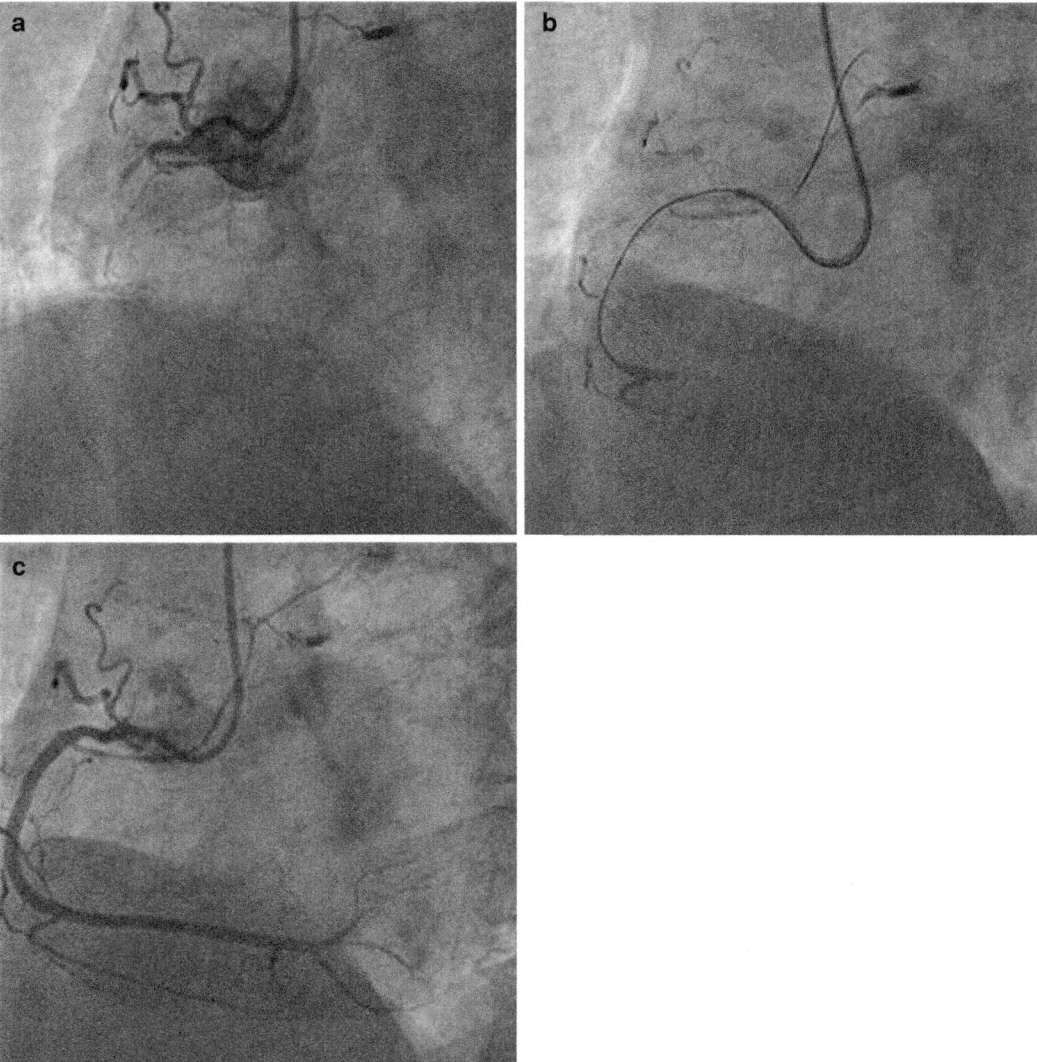

Fig. 8.4 A CTO PCI case used anchor-balloon technique. (**a**) Baseline angiography shows chronic total occlusion of proximal RCA; (**b**) balloon passes the CTO lesion with the help of anchor-balloon technique using 2.0 mm size balloon to the side branch; (**c**) final angiography showed successful result (Case courtesy of Dr. Seung-Hwan Lee)

8.5 Step-by-Step Approach

8.5.1 Parallel Wire Technique Using Dual Lumen Catheter

If first guidewire enters into the false lumen, careful manipulation of guidewire is required not to make a big deflection of tip of guidewire over 90 degrees which can make huge false lumen. Difficulty of reentrance into true lumen with first guidewire needs a switch treatment strategy. The choice of second guidewire is recommended to have better torquability and high tip load. Using dual lumen microcatheter is beneficial for parallel wire technique. The Crusade catheter (Kaneka, Osaka, Japan) is a double-lumen microcatheter that contains both a monorail and an over-the-wire (OTW) port (Fig. 8.5). It is ideally suited to parallel wiring by allowing the introduction of multiple wires without removal of the catheter from an optimal position. A second penetrating wire is therefore introduced using a microcatheter, and an attempt is made at redirection into the true lumen (Fig. 8.6).

8.5.2 Hairpin Wire (Reverse Wire) Technique

If first guidewire goes to side branch of CTO bifurcation with steep angulation, the use of dual

lumen microcatheter with second guidewire can be a next treatment option. Otherwise, "hairpin wire (reverse) technique" can be effective. U-shaped 014" soft guidewire is advanced into guiding catheter and passes the side branch. Then, slow pullback of guidewire can enter into distal main branch (Figs. 8.7 and 8.8).

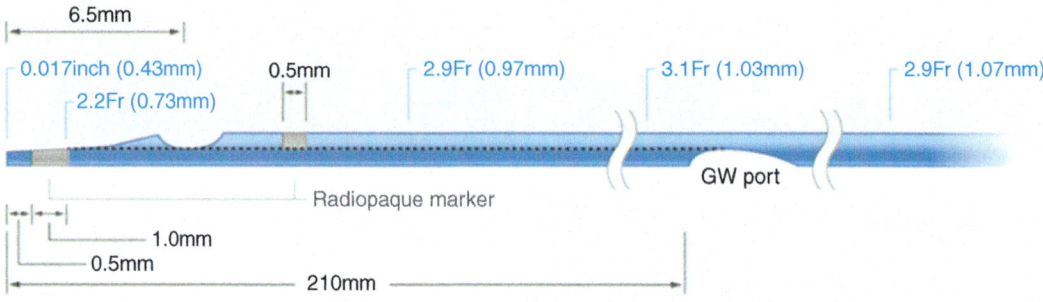

Fig. 8.5 The Crusade dual lumen microcatheter (illustrated by Dr. Bong-Ki Lee)

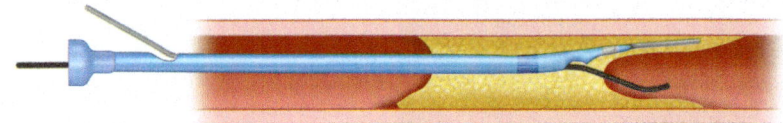

Fig. 8.6 Parallel wire technique using a dual lumen microcatheter (illustrated by Dr. Bong-Ki Lee)

Fig. 8.7 Hairpin (reverse) wire technique using a dual lumen microcatheter (illustrated by Dr. Bong-Ki Lee)

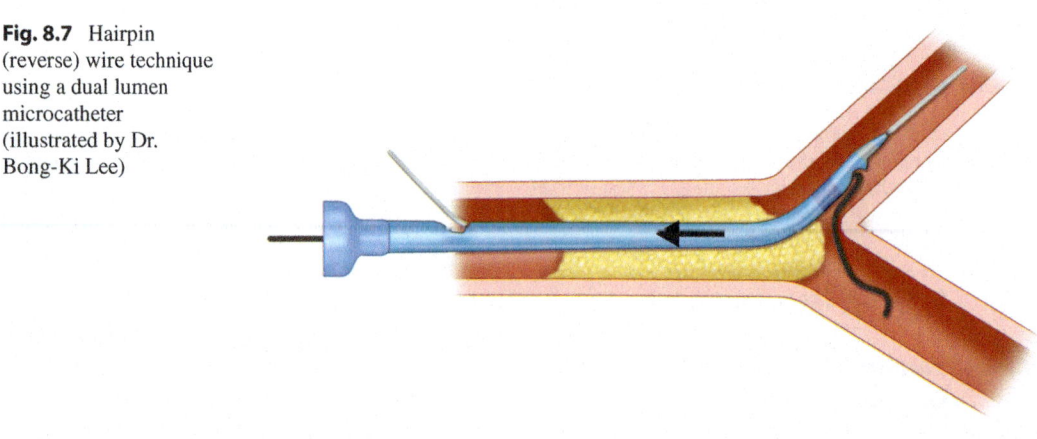

Fig. 8.8 A CTO PCI case used parallel wire technique with a dual lumen catheter and hairpin wire (reverse wire) technique. (**a**) CTO of just proximal portion of bifurcation md-LAD with severe calcification. Collateral flows are observed from RCA to LAD; (**b**) second guidewire (Gaia 2nd) failed to penetrate the true lumen of mid-LAD despite use of dual lumen microcatheter; (**c**) inflation with 1.5 × 15 mm balloon was performed at proximal CTO bifurcation lesion; (**d**) hairpin wire technique using a Runthrough® guidewire; (**e**) successful insertion of a Runthrough® guidewire into distal LAD; (**f**) final angiography (Case courtesy of Dr. Seung-Hwan Lee)

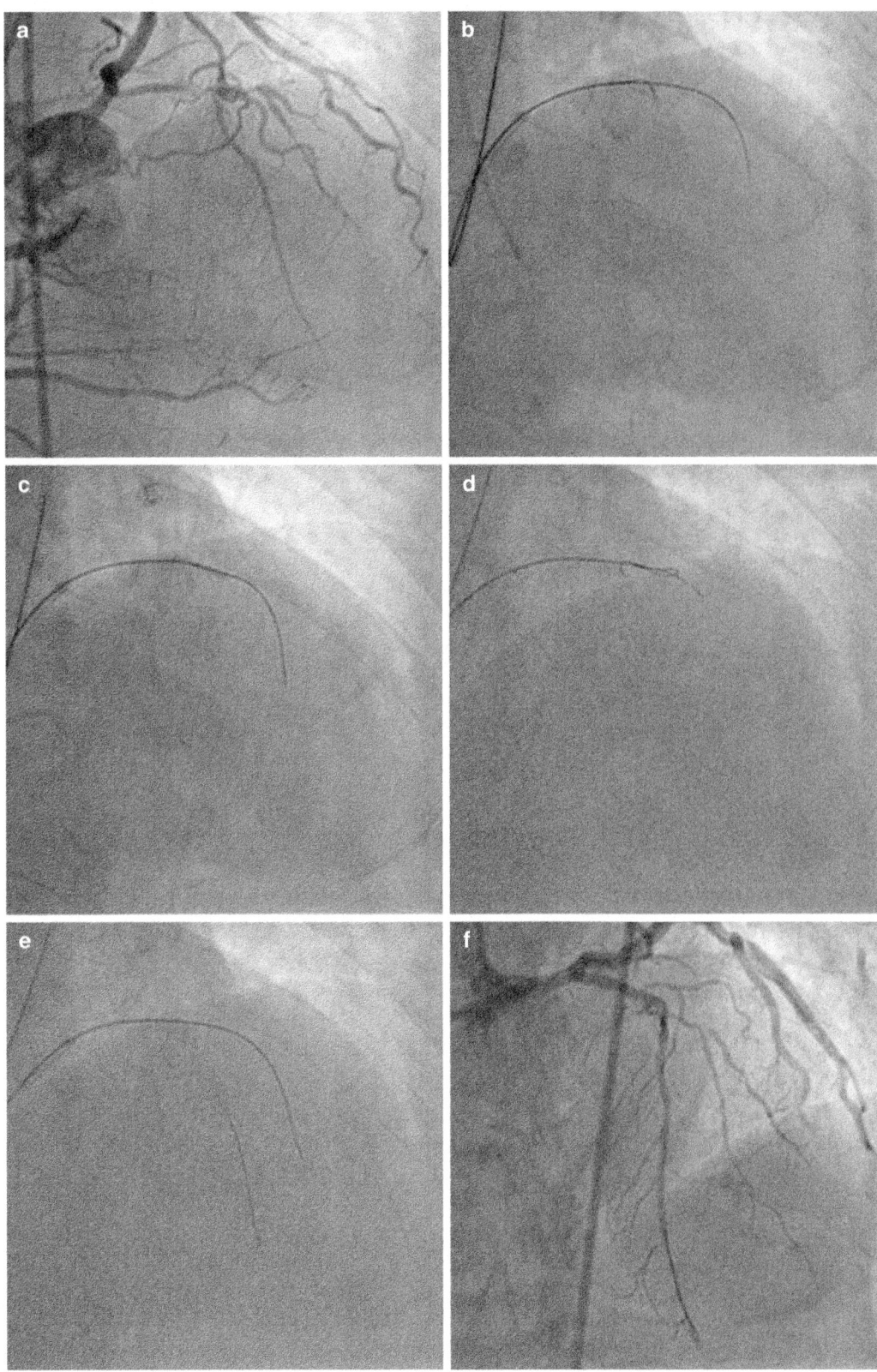

References

1. Sumitsuji S, Inoue K, Ochiai TE, Ikeno F. Fundamental wire technique and current standard strategy of percutaneous intervention for chronic total occlusion with histopathological insights. JACC Cardiovasc Interv. 2011;4(9):941–51.

2. Dave B. Recanalization of chronic total occlusion lesions: a critical appraisal of current devices and techniques. J Clin Diag Res. 2016;10(9):OE01–7.

Tips and Tricks of Antegrade CTO PCI

9

Kenya Nasu

Successful percutaneous coronary intervention (PCI) of chronic total occlusions (CTOs) has been associated with significant clinical benefits, but remains technically demanding [1–5]. Especially in antegrade approach, failure to cross the CTO with a guidewire is the most common cause of CTO PCI failure. Antegrade CTO crossing can be accomplished by not only maintaining true lumen position but also reentry from subintimal; however, antegrade reentry does not always work well [6]. Therefore, manipulation of CTO guidewire is one of the most important points to increase success rate in antegrade approach. For understanding the manipulation, we should assimilate the basic potential of guidewire for CTO recanalization and the effect of wire motion in CTO lesions.

9.1 The Necessary Potential of Guidewire for CTO Recanalization

In antegrade CTO PCI, penetration of the proximal cap is the first step. After penetrating the cap, the tip of guidewire is deflected by advancement of guidewire. The direction of the guidewire tip is controlled by rotating wire (Fig. 9.1). Thus, penetration efficiency, deflection control, and direction control are the basic potentials of guidewire during manipulation. We always try to recanalize CTO lesions by repeating these basic procedures. Therefore, it is very important to understand the fundamental of this mechanics.

1. Penetration efficiency
   (a) Factor 1: Tip profile; lower profile is associated with better penetration efficiency (e.g., Conquest Pro 12g has better penetration efficiency than Miracle12g).
   (b) Factor 2: Tip flexibility; less flexibility is associated with better penetration efficiency (e.g., Conquest Pro 12g has better penetration efficiency than Conquest Pro 9g).
   (c) Factor 3: Hydrophilic coating; hydrophilic coating accelerates penetration efficiency (SION Black > SION).
2. Direction control
   (a) Factor 1: Torque response; better torque response is associated with better direction control (e.g., Gaia family).
   (b) Factor 2: Torque power; better torque power is associated with better direction control; however, less torque power is associated with better flexibility (e.g., Miracle 12g is easier to change direction than Miracle 3g).

K. Nasu (✉)
Department of Cardiovascular Medicine,
Toyohashi Heart Center, Toyohashi, Aichi, Japan
e-mail: nasu@heart-center.or.jp

© Springer Nature Singapore Pte Ltd. 2019
Y. Jang (ed.), *Percutaneous Coronary Interventions for Chronic Total Occlusion*,
https://doi.org/10.1007/978-981-10-6026-7_9

Fig. 9.1 Basic step of
wire advancement in
CTO lesion

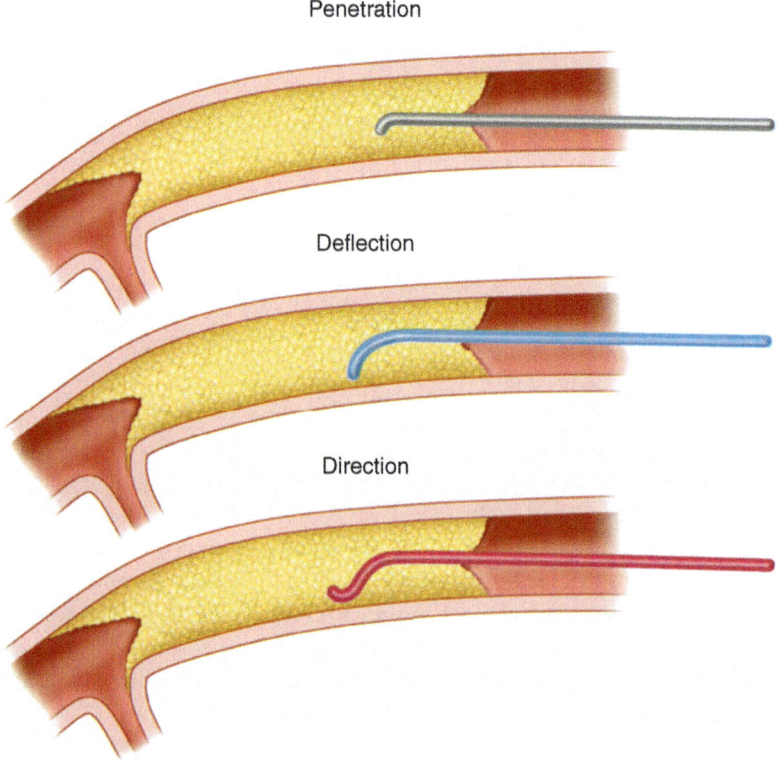

Penetration

Deflection

Direction

(c) Factor 3: Tip shape; smaller shape and acuter angle are associated with better direction control.

3. Deflection control
   (a) Factor 1: Tip profile; lower profile is easier to make deflection (e.g., XT-R is more easily deflected than Sion Black).
   (b) Factor 2: Tip flexibility; better flexibility is easier to make deflection (e.g., Miracle 3g is more easily deflected than Miracle 12g).
   (c) Factor 3: Tip shape; bigger shape and acuter angle are easier to make deflection.

These potentials are summarized in Fig. 9.2. Some factors are overlapped between the two potentials. (1) Lower profile is associated with better penetration efficiency and deflection control. (2) Acuter angle of guidewire tip is associated with both direction and deflection control. On the other hand, conventional CTO wire makes trade-off between the two poten-

tials as follows: (1) Less flexibility is needed for the better penetration efficiency. However, better flexibility is need for the better deflection control. (2) Smaller shape has an advantage for direction control, however, is limited in deflection control. (3) For better torque power, poor flexibility is better; however, poor flexibility is associated with poor deflection control.

To overcome these trade-off relations, Gaia family (Asahi Intecc, Japan) has been developed (Fig. 9.3). Micro-cone tip (Fig. 9.3a) of Gaia has better penetration efficiency and easier deflection control with keeping flexibility at proximal and distal cap (for trade-off point No. 1). Most appropriate pre-shaping (Fig. 9.3b) (length and angle) can keep direction and deflection control (for trade-off point No. 2). ACTONE (Fig. 9.3c) on the core wire (composite core wire system) can improve torque with keeping flexibility (for trade-off point No. 3).

Penetration efficiency	Direction control	Deflection control
<Tip profile> Lower profile ↓ Better penetration efficiency	<Torque response> Better torque response ↓ Better direction control	<Tip profile> Lower profile ↓ Better deflection control
<Tip flexibility> Less flexibility ↓ Better penetration efficiency	<Torque power> Better torque power ↓ Better direction control Less torque power ↓ Better flexibility	<Tip flexibility> Better flexibility ↓ Better deflection control
<Hydrophilic coating> Hydrophilic coating ↓ Better penetration efficiency	<Tip shape> Smaller shape and acuter angle ↓ Better direction control	<Tip shape> Bigger shape and acuter angle ↓ Better deflection control

Fig. 9.2   Summary of guidewire potentials

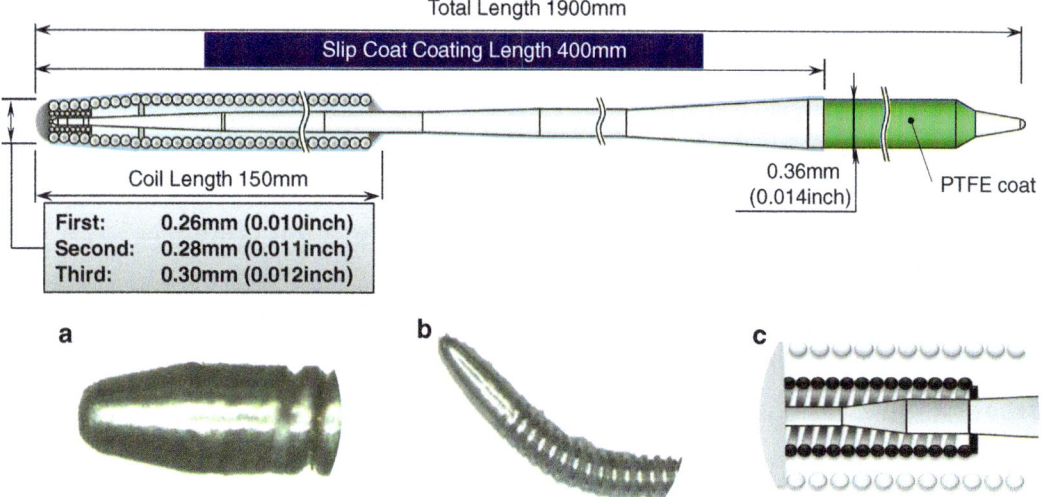

Fig. 9.3   Basic structure and characteristics of current Gaia (Courtesy by Asahi Intecc)

9.2   The Influence of Wire Rotation on Atherosclerotic Plaque in CTO Lesions

Although there has been a huge technical improvement with CTO guidewires, wire manipulation itself is performed by the human - the CTO operator. To learn the appropriate wire manipulation, we should consider the influence of wire movement on CTO lesion. In histopathological findings, layered structure of fibrous tissue is observed in CTO lesions (Fig. 9.4a). As a

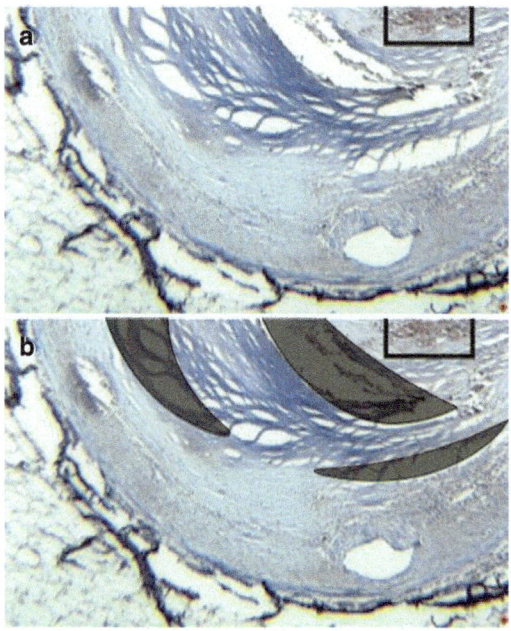

Fig. 9.4 Layer structure of CTO lesion in histopathological findings (Courtesy by Dr. Osamu Kato)

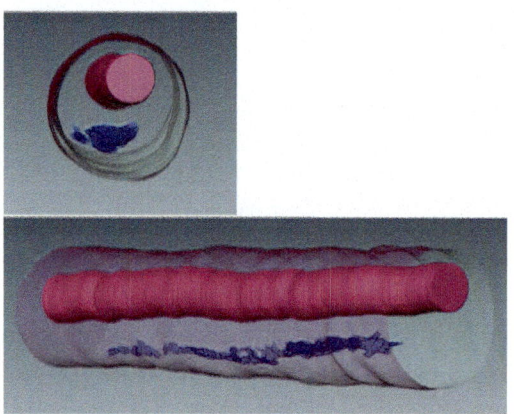

Fig. 9.5 Semilunar space in 3D IVUS image (Courtesy by Dr. Kenya Nasu)

response to the rotation of CTO wire, semilunar space is created easily in the layered structure of fibrous tissue (Fig. 9.4b). Figure 9.5 is 3D intravascular ultrasound (IVUS) image after recanalization of CTO lesion by parallel wire technique. Blue area is a space made by rotation of first wire and showed semilunar shape.

9.3 CTO Guidewire Control in CTO Lesions

After making some space around a guidewire tip by wire rotation, deflection of guidewire tip is reduced. To change the direction of guidewire tip, maximum flexure and wire deformation are needed. However, those phenomena cause the expansion of semilunar space and deflection control becomes more difficult. Thus, making space around guidewire tip induces the difficulty of guidewire control in CTO lesions. In other words, CTO guidewire can work well in the solid tissue (without any space around wire tip). In clinical setting, we can use deflection control at the distal cap of the CTO in case without any space around guidewire tip (Fig. 9.6a). However, after making some space around guidewire tip (Fig. 9.6b), deflection control to penetrate distal cap becomes difficult, and guidewire goes in to subintimal space easily (Fig. 9.6c). Thus, wire rotation is necessary for direction control; however, we can make space around the guidewire tip. On the other hand, better penetration force is one of the important factors to advance in CTO lesion without unnecessary space formation.

9.4 Next-Generation CTO Guidewire for Appropriate Wire Manipulation

For appropriate guidewire manipulation, Gaia family had been developed and is widely used in current CTO PCI field. Although Gaia has good penetration efficiency, it doesn't have good penetration force to keep flexibility. In some CTO cases with severe calcification, Gaia (especially Gaia first) can penetrate proximal cap, however, cannot advance in the calcified site. Finally, core wire and rope coil may be fractured (Fig. 9.7). For prevention of these complications, Gaia Next has been developed as a novel standard CTO wire. Basic structure of Gaia Next is completely same as current Gaia without the structure of rope coil. The rope coil of

Fig. 9.6 Influence of space around wire tip for distal cap penetration

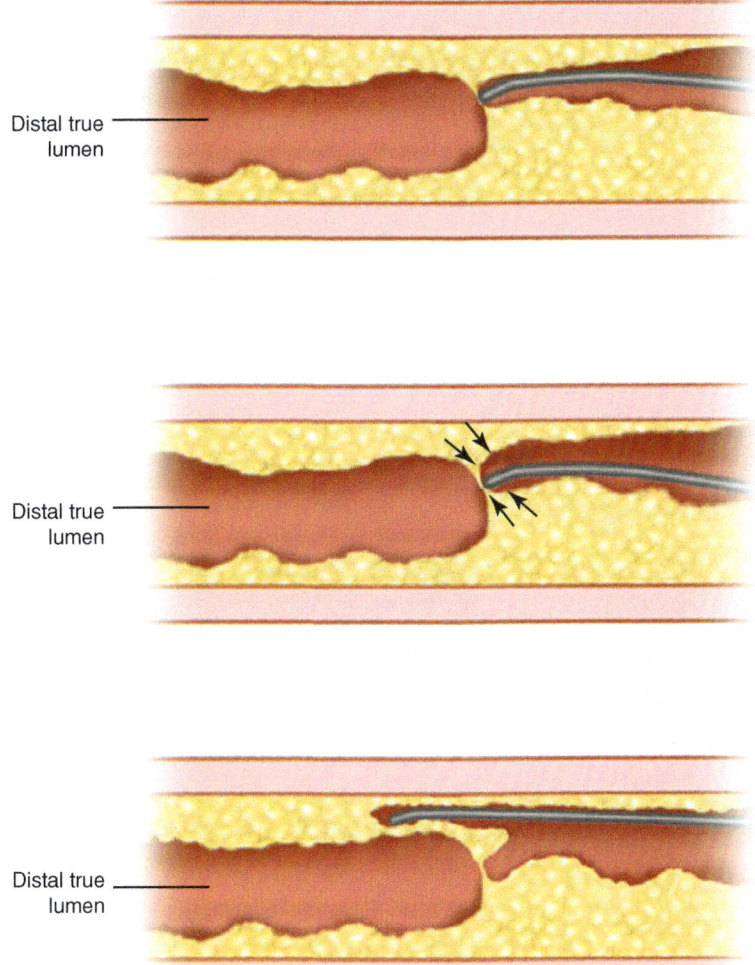

Distal true lumen

Distal true lumen

Distal true lumen

Gaia Next (XTRAND coil) consists of seven wires although only single wire is used for rope coil in conventional guidewires (Fig. 9.8). In addition, each wire is braided by seven thinner wires. XTRAND coil can tighten and support core wire by rotation of Gaia Next itself. The durability against wire tip trapping is doubled, and 90% torsion of coil is reduced compared with current Gaia family. Gaia Next has better linear torque response, thanks to the current Gaia, and hastens the rise of the torque (Fig. 9.9). Therefore, more delicate guidewire manipulation is possible in Gaia Next era.

9.5 Summary

Understanding the basic potential of guidewire for CTO recanalization and effect of wire motion in CTO lesions is very important in antegrade approach. However, the appropriate skill of the operator who actually performs the CTO PCI is also important. Delicate guidewire manipulation should be associated with not only prevention of unnecessary dissection but also successful wire recanalization without complications.

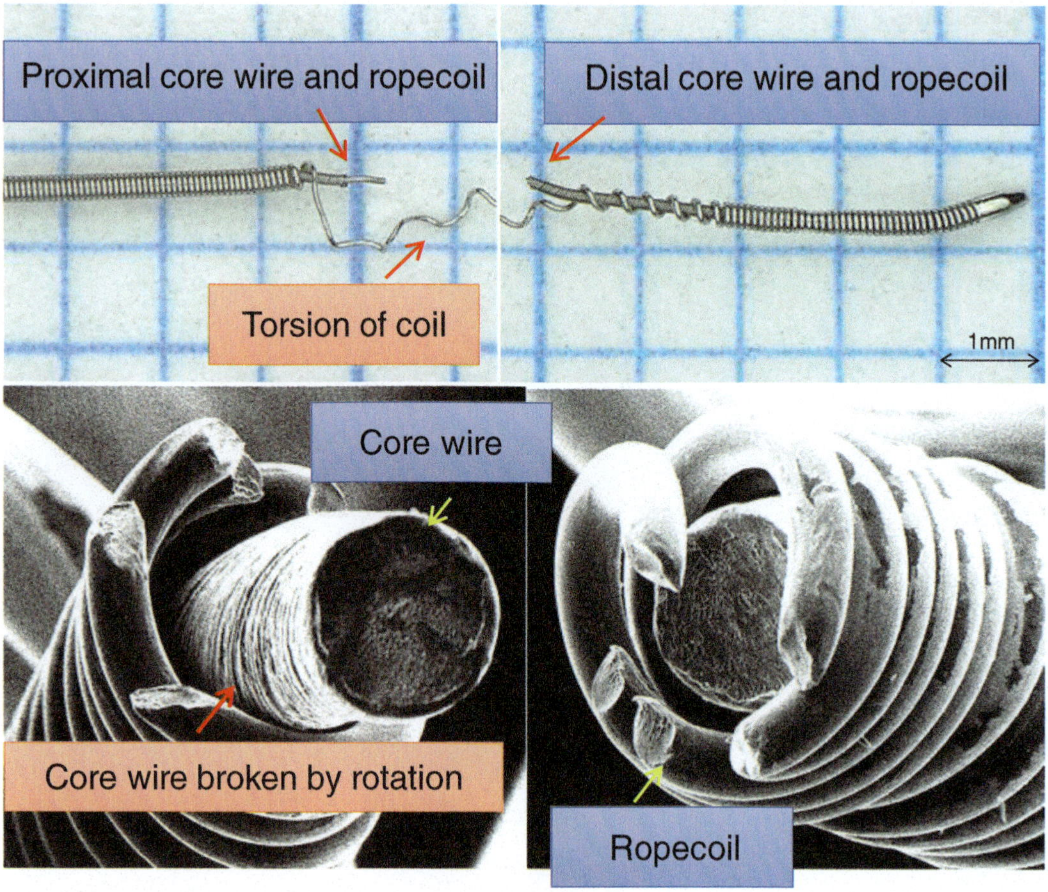

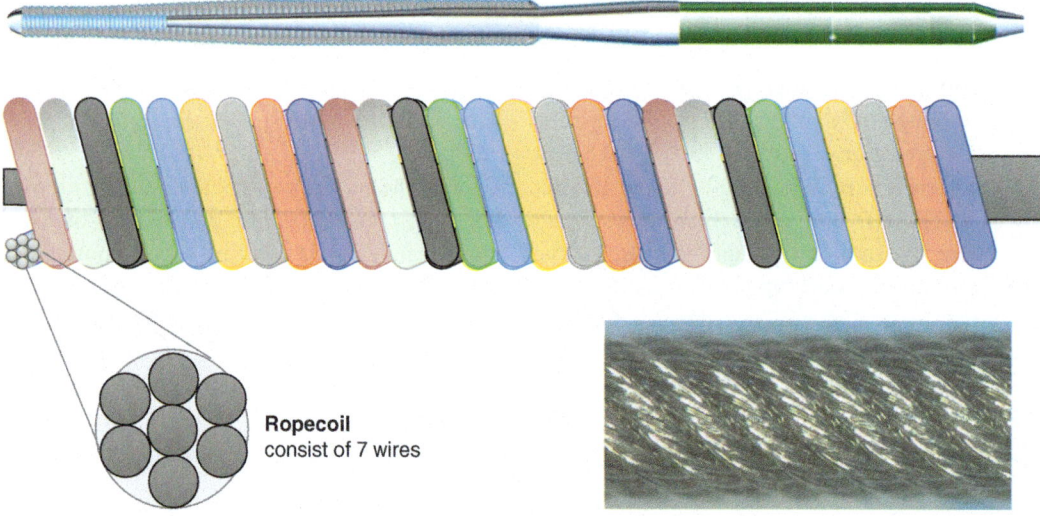

Fig. 9.7 Core wire and rope coil fracture of current Gaia (Courtesy by Asahi Intecc)

Ropecoil
consist of 7 wires

Fig. 9.8 Basic structure and characteristics of current Gaia Next (Courtesy by Asahi Intecc)

Fig. 9.9 Torque response of current Gaia and Gaia Next (Courtesy by Asahi Intecc)

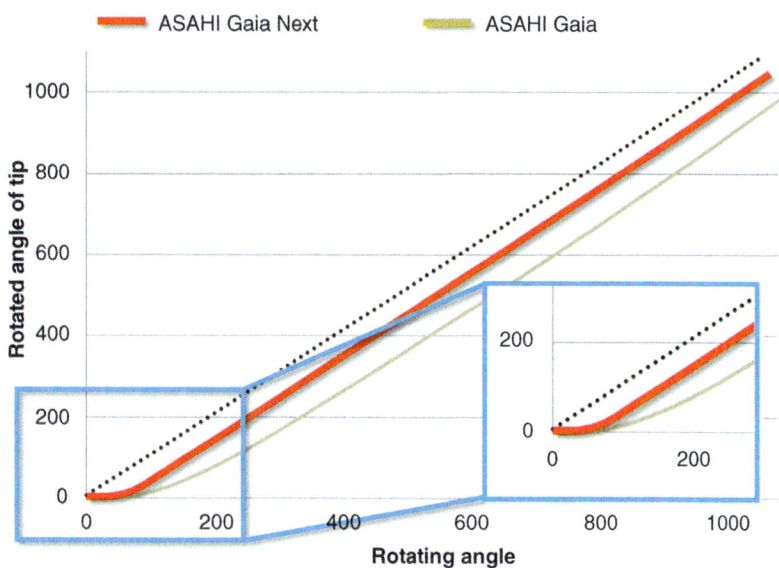

References

1. Cohen HA, Williams DO, Holmes DR Jr, et al. Impact of age on procedural and 1-year outcome in percutaneous transluminal coronary angioplasty: a report from the NHLBI Dynamic Registry. Am Heart J. 2003;146:513–9.
2. Anderson HV, Shaw RE, Brindis RG, et al. A contemporary overview of percutaneous coronary interventions. The American College of Cardiology-National Cardiovascular Data Registry (ACC-NCDR). J Am Coll Cardiol. 2002;39:1096–103.
3. Galassi AR, Tomasello SD, Reifart N, et al. In-hospital outcomes of percutaneous coronary intervention in patients with chronic total occlusion: insights from the ERCTO (European Registry of Chronic Total Occlusion) registry. EuroIntervention. 2011;7:472–9.
4. Morino Y, Kimura T, Hayashi Y, et al. In-hospital outcomes of contemporary percutaneous coronary intervention in patients with chronic total occlusion insights from the J-CTO Registry (Multicenter CTO Registry in Japan). J Am Coll Cardiol Intv. 2010;3:143–51.
5. Colmenarez HJ, Escaned J, Fernandez C, et al. Efficacy and safety of drug-eluting stents in chronic total coronary occlusion recanalization: a systematic review and meta-analysis. J Am Coll Cardiol. 2010;55:1854–66.
6. Wilson WM, Walsh SJ, Bagnall A, Yan AT, Hanratty CG, Egred M, Smith E, Oldroyd KG, McEntegart M, Irving J, Douglas H, Strange J, Spratt JC. One-year outcomes after successful chronic total occlusion percutaneous coronary intervention: the impact of dissection re-entry techniques. Catheter Cardiovasc Interv. 2017;90(5):703–12.

Intravascular Ultrasound Guidance for the Successful Wiring

10

Jang Hoon Lee and Hun Sik Park

10.1 Introduction

Intravascular ultrasound (IVUS) can provide useful information for vessel size and atherosclerotic plaque characteristics by cross-sectional imaging during percutaneous coronary intervention (PCI). In patients with chronic total occlusion (CTO) lesion, IVUS also can provide information about the lesion characteristics including atherosclerotic plaque morphology, vessel size, and lesion length and enable stent implantation properly. Moreover, using IVUS catheter, we can avoid PCI-related complications by appropriate sizing of the CTO lesion. In addition, IVUS is very helpful for wiring strategy for CTO intervention. In this chapter, we demonstrated the IVUS-guided wiring technique with the standard antegrade approach and with the more recent retrograde approach. IVUS could be used with each of these cases: (1) to find entrance of the CTO lesion, (2) guidewire penetration from subintimal space to true lumen, and (3) reverse CART technique with retrograde approach [1].

J. H. Lee · H. S. Park (✉)
Department of Internal Medicine,
Kyungpook National University Hospital, School of
Medicine, Kyungpook National University,
Daegu, South Korea
e-mail: hspark@knu.ac.kr

10.2 The Role of IVUS-Guided Wiring for CTO-PCI

1. To Find the Entrance of the CTO Lesion

   In the case of stumpless CTO (Fig. 10.1), guidewire should be crossed to the side branch just proximal to the CTO lesion before identifying the entrance of CTO. Then, an IVUS catheter should be placed at the side-branch distal portion if the branch is large enough to advance an IVUS catheter [2]. During the pullback, we can obtain images of CTO entry point. Based on the series of IVUS images, operators can identify CTO entry point by two methods. First, operators can obtain real-time IVUS image when the catheter is positioned just at the occlusion in the main vessel. Then, we can penetrate guidewire through the most suspected site under real-time IVUS guidance. However, if it is difficult to fix an IVUS catheter position at the occlusion because of beating heart or if the IVUS image is not clear to discriminate wire position, the success rate to enter the entrance of CTO will be low. Second, guidewire could get into the suspected entrance of CTO first, and then an IVUS examination could be performed to confirm wire position whether it is in the true lumen or not. If the wire is in the true lumen, it can be carefully advanced to the distal true lumen. However,

© Springer Nature Singapore Pte Ltd. 2019
Y. Jang (ed.), *Percutaneous Coronary Interventions for Chronic Total Occlusion*,
https://doi.org/10.1007/978-981-10-6026-7_10

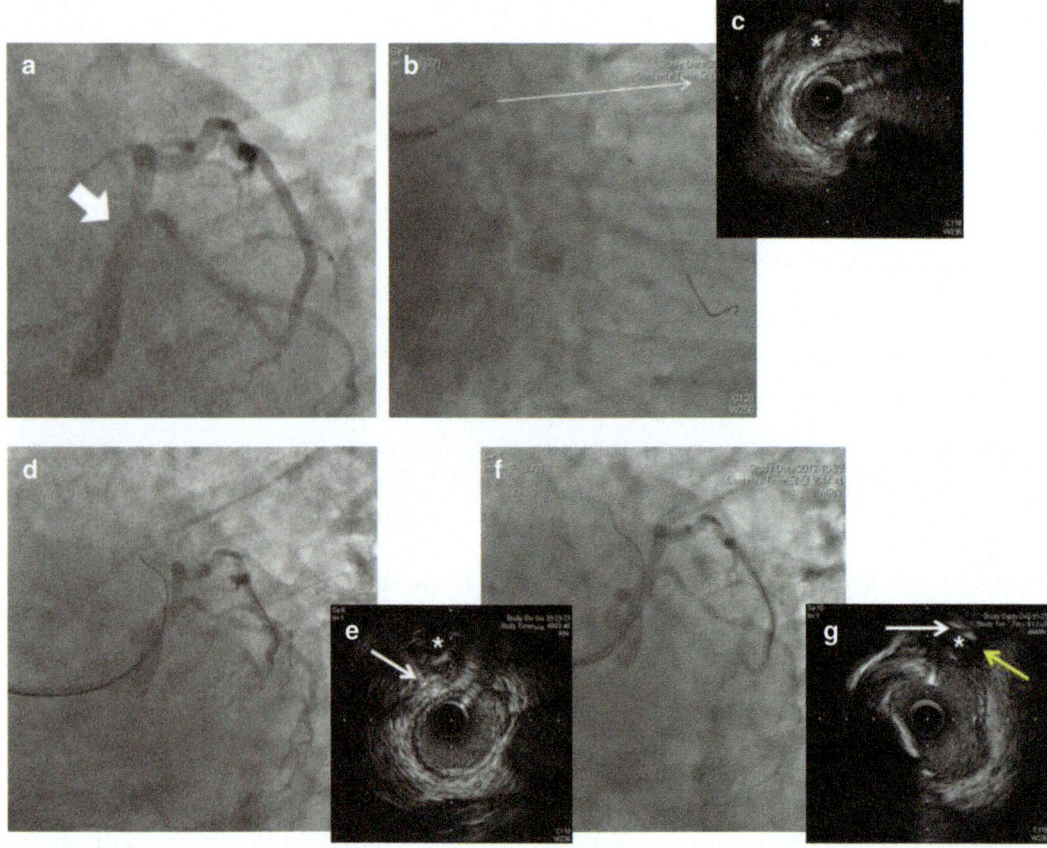

Fig. 10.1 Representative case to find the entrance of the CTO lesion using an IVUS catheter. (**a**) The angiogram shows a stumpless CTO lesion of proximal LAD (white arrow). (**b**) Pullback of an IVUS catheter from the side branch to just at the occlusion of main vessel was performed to identify the entrance of CTO lesion. (**c**) The IVUS imaging provides suspected entry point of CTO lesion of LAD (white asterix). (**d**) Guidewire crossed the suspected entry point of CTO lesion of LAD. (**e**) IVUS image confirmed that guidewire (white arrow) is not in the true lumen (white asterix) but in the subintimal space. (**f**) Second guidewire tried to enter the true lumen of CTO lesion of LAD. (**g**) The IVUS catheter confirmed that 1st guidewire (white arrow) is in the subintimal space, and 2nd guidewire (yellow arrow) is in the true lumen (white asterix)

if the wire is in the subintimal space, IVUS examination should be performed repeatedly to correct wire position.

2. Guidewire Penetration from the Subintimal Space to the True Lumen

    If the guidewire is in the subintimal space, parallel wiring technique should be considered to get into the true lumen. However, angiographic findings may provide limited information about the guidewire position. Therefore, it is difficult to continue subsequent procedure under fluoroscopic guidance. In this case, an IVUS examination can provide useful information to continue next steps. An

IVUS catheter is helpful to discriminate true lumen and false lumen. Moreover, an IVUS catheter can identify whether guidewire is in the true lumen or not and has a benefit to correct guidewire position if the guidewire is in the false lumen. In addition, IVUS can confirm when the guidewire has reentered the true lumen from the false lumen [3, 4].

IVUS-guided wire penetration from the subintimal space to the true lumen is as follows (Fig. 10.2). First, the IVUS catheter is advanced to the subintimal space through the first wire. Enlargement of subintimal space by wiring often collapses the distal true lumen;

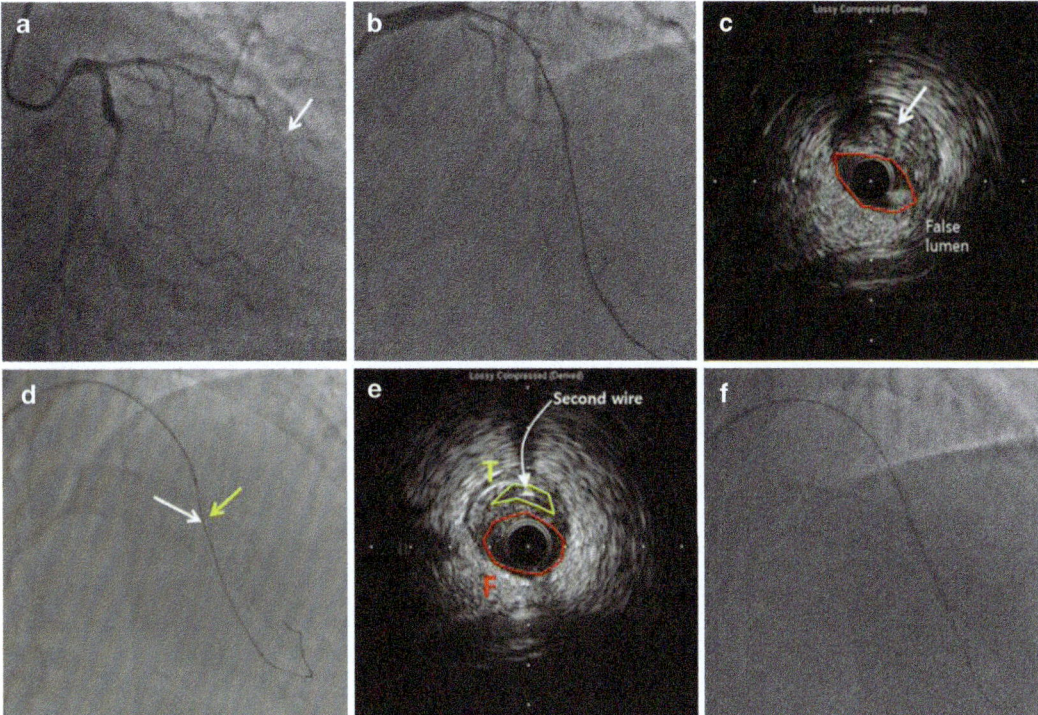

Fig. 10.2 Representative case for guidewire reposition from the subintimal space to the true lumen using an IVUS catheter. (**a**) The angiogram shows a CTO lesion in the mid-LAD (white arrow). (**b**) After guidewires crossed the CTO lesion, angiogram cannot provide exact information about the position of two wires. (**c**) The IVUS catheter clearly demonstrated that the guidewire is not in the true lumen (white arrow) but in the subintimal space (red circle). (**d**) A stiff guidewire was delivered to penetrate the true channel from subintimal space under the IVUS guidance. (**e**) The IVUS image clearly shows that the IVUS catheter is in the subintimal space (red circle; **f**) and 2nd guidewire is in the true lumen (yellow circle; T). (**f**) The wire was carefully advanced to the distal true lumen. And then, long stent implantation was successfully done in the true lumen

therefore, angiography-guided parallel wiring technique would fail to enter true lumen. However, IVUS clearly shows the cross-sectional information which is useful to guide the second wire into the true lumen because negotiation of wire penetration should be performed in true lumen. In this situation, stiff wire should be used as the second wire to penetrate the true channel. Sometimes, balloon dilatation is required to deliver the IVUS catheter into the subintimal space. However, this method should never be performed when guidewire perforation from the subintimal space is suspected or detected. The 8 Fr guiding catheter is required to conduct real-time wiring under IVUS guidance. After successful wiring, multiple or long stent implantation is inevitable to fully cover the enlarged subintimal space [5, 6].

3. Reverse CART Technique with Retrograde Approach

During reverse controlled antegrade and retrograde subintimal tracking (CART) technique, an IVUS catheter is very useful for guidewire tracking and providing important information [7, 8]. Reverse CART technique starts with a retrograde wire crossing through subintimal space after balloon dilatation with an antegrade balloon (Fig. 10.3). When the retrograde wire cannot pass to the proximal true lumen even after dilatation with antegrade balloon, the IVUS should be used to observe vessel size, wire position, and plaque morphology. The benefits of IVUS examination

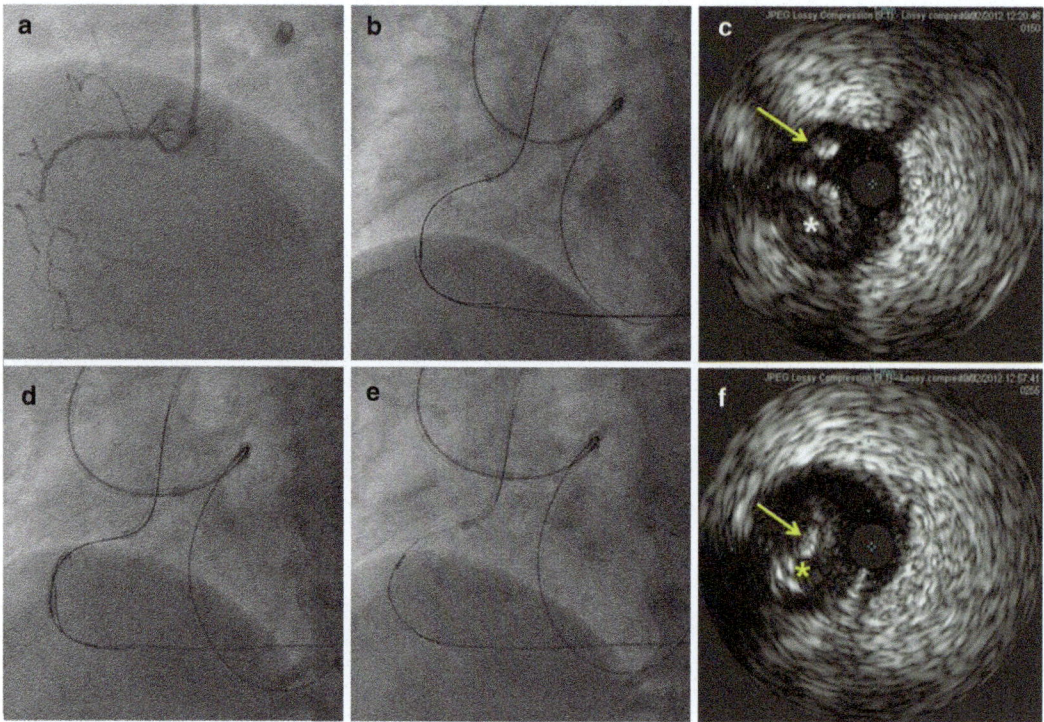

Fig. 10.3 Representative case for reverse CART technique with retrograde approach using an IVUS catheter. (**a**) The angiogram shows a CTO lesion in the mid-RCA. (**b**) Antegrade wire is in the subintimal space, and retrograde wire is in the true lumen. The IVUS catheter is in the subintimal space. (**c**) IVUS imaging clearly shows the position of true lumen (white asterix) and the position of retrograde wire that is in the subintimal space (yellow arrow). (**d**) Balloon dilatation is performed to expand sub- intimal space through antegrade wire to cross the retrograde wire into proximal true lumen. (**e**) Using reverse CART technique, retrograde wire was successfully advanced to RCA guiding catheter. After then IVUS catheter was carefully advanced from proximal to mid-RCA. (**f**) IVUS imaging clearly demonstrated the collapsed subintimal space (yellow asterix) and the position of retrograde wire (yellow arrow) that is in the true lumen

during reverse CART technique are as follows: First, IVUS confirmation of vessel size can allow larger-size balloon dilatation. Second, IVUS can confirm the position of antegrade and retrograde wires for wire tracking. The position of each of the antegrade and retrograde wires could affect the success of the reverse CART technique. When the retrograde wire is in the true lumen and the antegrade wire is in the subintimal space, making connection is key to perform successful reverse CART technique. In this situation, IVUS should be used to evaluate vessel size and plaque morphology. Third, IVUS examination can provide useful information about the appropriated portion that making connection between true lumen and subintimal space.

10.3 Conclusion

The IVUS is very useful imaging modality in various stages of modern CTO algorithm to identify entry point of stumpless CTO lesion in initial antegrade approach, to correct guidewire position from subintimal space to true lumen in failed initial antegrade wiring wire, and to perform reverse CART technique in retrograde approach.

References

1. Waksman R, Saito S, et al. Chronic total occlusion: a guide to recanalization. Hoboken, NJ: Wiley-Blackwell; 2009.
2. Park Y, Park HS, Jang GL, Lee DY, Lee H, Lee JH, Kang HJ, Yang DH, Cho Y, Chae SC, Jun JE, Park

WH. Intravascular ultrasound guided recanalization of stumpless chronic total occlusion. Int J Cardiol. 2011;148:174–8.

3. Stone GW, Colombo A, Teirstein PS, Moses JW, Leon MB, Reifart NJ, Mintz GS, Hoye A, Cox DA, Baim DS, Strauss BH, Selmon M, Moussa I, Suzuki T, Tamai H, Katoh O, Mitsudo K, Grube E, Cannon LA, Kandzari DE, Reisman M, Schwartz RS, Bailey S, Dangas G, Mehran R, Abizaid A, Serruys PW. Percutaneous recanalization of chronically occluded coronary arteries: procedural techniques, devices, and results. Catheter Cardiovasc Interv. 2005;66:217–36.

4. Werner GS, Diedrich J, Schlz KH, Knies A, Kreuzer H. Vessel reconstruction in total coronary occlusions with a long subintimal wire pathway: use of multiple stents under guidance of intravascular ultrasound. Catheter Cardiovasc Interv. 1997;40:46–51.

5. Ito S, Suzuki T, Ito T, Katoh O, Ojio S, Sato H, Ehara M, Suzuki T, Kawase Y, Myoishi M, Kurokawa R, Ishihara Y, Suzuki Y, Sato K, Toyama J, Fukutomi T, Itoh M. Novel technique using intravascular

ultrasound-guided guidewire cross in coronary intervention for uncrossable chronic total occlusions. Circ J. 2004;68:1088–92.

6. Matsubara T, Murata A, Kanyama H, Ogino A. IVUS-guided wiring technique: promising approach for the chronic total occlusion. Catheter Cardiovasc Interv. 2004;61:381–6.

7. Surmely JF1, Tsuchikane E, Katoh O, Nishida Y, Nakayama M, Nakamura S, Oida A, Hattori E, Suzuki T. New concept for CTO recanalization using controlled antegrade and retrograde subintimal tracking: the CART technique. J Invasive Cardiol. 2006;18:334–8.

8. Kimura M, Katoh O, Tsuchikane E, Nasu K, Kinoshita Y, Ehara M, Terashima M, Matsuo H, Matsubara T, Asakura K, Asakura Y, Nakamura S, Oida A, Takase S, Reifart N, Di Mario C, Suzuki T. The efficacy of a bilateral approach for treating lesions with chronic total occlusions the CART (controlled antegrade and retrograde subintimal tracking) registry. JACC Cardiovasc Interv. 2009;2:1135–41.

Jon Suh and Nae Hee Lee

The success rate of the percutaneous coronary intervention for coronary chronic total occlusion (CTO-PCI) was 65–70% when using only the antegrade approach, so it was difficult to expect a high success rate. However, the introduction of the retrograde approach using the native collateral channel has significantly increased the success rate of the procedure. In the early days of the retrograde approach, the complexity and variability of the procedure and the possibility of complications caused practitioners to hesitate to use this method, but thanks to the development of techniques and tools, a recent report suggests that the retrograde approach is used for approximately 30% of all CTO-PCIs [1].

11.1 The Rationale of the Retrograde Approach

- Histologically the distal cap is weaker than the proximal cap, which makes it easy to perform the correct penetration of the retrograde wire when using a retrograde approach.
- In general, the distal cap is tapered. With a convex shape if seen from the proximal end, it may be difficult for the antegrade wire to enter the true lumen. On the other hand, the concave shape if seen from the distal end can prevent

the retrograde wire from entering the false lumen of the CTO lesion.
- As there is an antegrade wire and a retrograde wire simultaneously in one blood vessel, various techniques for crossing occlusion (e.g., CART, reverse CART) can be used.

11.2 Indications of the Retrograde Approach

The retrograde approach can be attempted as a primary approach, and it can also be attempted as a secondary approach when the antegrade approach fails. To date, the success rate of the retrograde approach is 69%, and the final success rate (successful with the antegrade approach when the retrograde approach failed) is 86% (Table 11.1). This means that if the retrograde approach fails, about 54% of them can achieve successful reopening even with the existing antegrade approach [2–5]. This implies that to reduce unnecessary efforts, caution should be exercised when choosing a case in the primary retrograde approach. Although there are no systematic indications yet, for the complex CTOs (such as ostial CTO, long (>30 mm) occlusions, occlusions without a stump, occlusions with large side branches at the proximal cap, occlusions with severe tortuosity or calcification, small or poorly visualized distal vessels, anomalous coronary arteries, and ISR-CTO [6]), which have low suc-

J. Suh · N. H. Lee (✉)
Soon Chun Hyang University, Bucheon Hospital, Bucheon, South Korea
e-mail: naeheelee@schmc.ac.kr

© Springer Nature Singapore Pte Ltd. 2019
Y. Jang (ed.), *Percutaneous Coronary Interventions for Chronic Total Occlusion*,
https://doi.org/10.1007/978-981-10-6026-7_11

Table 11.1 The success rate for CTO-PCIs using the retrograde approach

	Retrograde success rate (%)	Final success rate (%)
Lee NH (n = 24)[a]	70	87
Lei GE (n = 42)[b]	71	88
Saito S (n = 157)[c]	69	83
Rathore S (n = 157)[d]	66	85
Overall (n = 268)	69 (success = 185, fail = 83)	86 (success = 230)

Among the 83 failed retrograde cases, antegrade PCI save 45 cases, which means antegrade approach can save 53% of the failed retrograde cases
[a]Int J Cardiol. 2010;144(2):219–29
[b]Chin Med J. 2010;123(7):857–63
[c]Catheter Cardiovasc Interv. 2008;71:8–19
[d]Circ Cardiovasc Interv. 2009(2):124–32

cess rates by the antegrade approach, a retrograde approach should be considered in the presence of proper native collateral channels, especially if there is a history of failures by the antegrade approach. In addition, a retrograde approach can be attempted as a bail-out approach when severe complications such as vascular dissection or perforation occur during a procedure with the antegrade approach (Fig. 11.1). Making the ad hoc retrograde attempt or waiting a little before any attempt when switching from the antegrade approach to the retrograde approach depends on the amount of radiation exposure (fluoroscopy time <30 min), the amount of contrast dye used, and the experience and fatigue of the operator, but in most cases, it will be more successful and safer to perform it as a second-stage surgery [7].

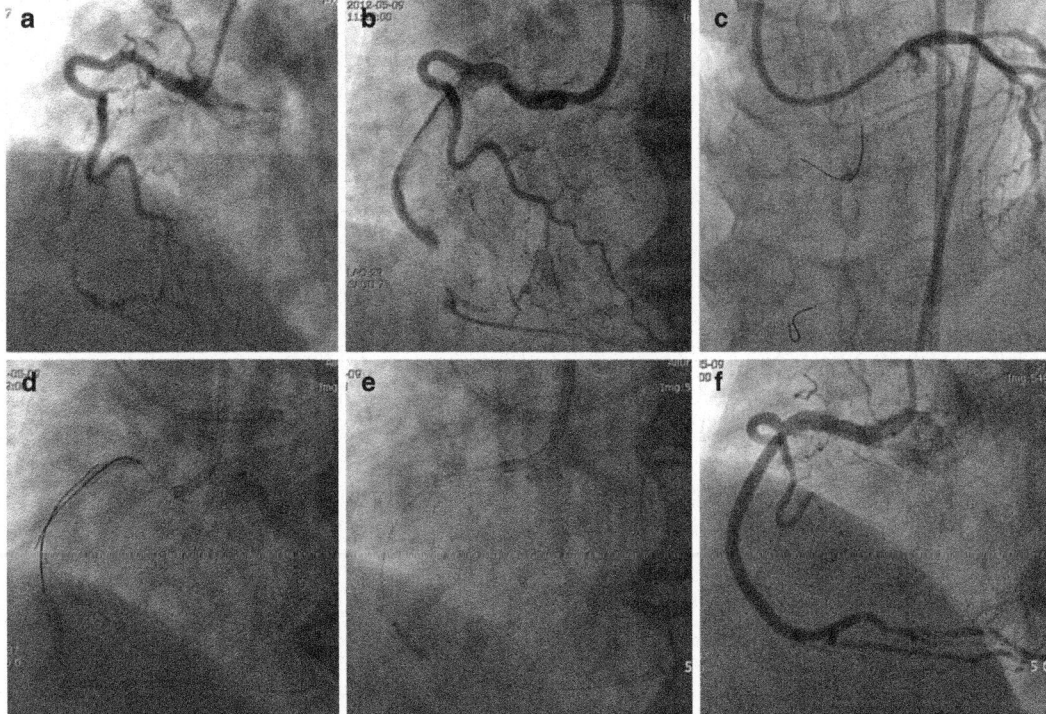

Fig. 11.1 An example of the bail-out ad hoc retrograde approach. (**a**) The baseline angiogram shows a CTO at the proximal RCA. (**b**) Amplatz guiding catheter made severe propagating dissection. (**c**) After failed antegrade wiring, a retrograde approach using septal collateral channel was attempted. (**d**) Reverse CART technique was applied. (**e**) Wire externalization and ballooning. (**f**) Final angiography after multiple stenting

11.3 Vascular Access and Selection of Guiding Catheters

Fundamentally two guiding catheters are needed for the target vessel and the donor vessel. Femoral arteries are preferred because they provide a good support and are less susceptible to patient movements and can use large-sized guiding catheters. If the femoral artery is difficult to use, a radial artery can be used; in this case, a sheathless technique can be used for a large-sized guiding catheter (7 or 8 Fr). As for the collateral donor artery guiding catheter, XB series with 7 to 8 Fr or Amplatz series are used to improve the posterior support, and if the retrograde pathway is considerably long, a guiding catheter is used with its length of 90 cm which is shorter than the conventional guiding catheter of 100 cm in length. If you do not have a short catheter, you can cut the catheter to use it with a smaller sheath. (For a 7 Fr catheter, cut out 10–15 cm from it to connect to a 6 Fr sheath.) In the ipsilateral retrograde approach, only one 8 Fr guiding catheter can be used, and two small diameter catheters can alternatively be used in one vessel at a time (Fig. 11.2)

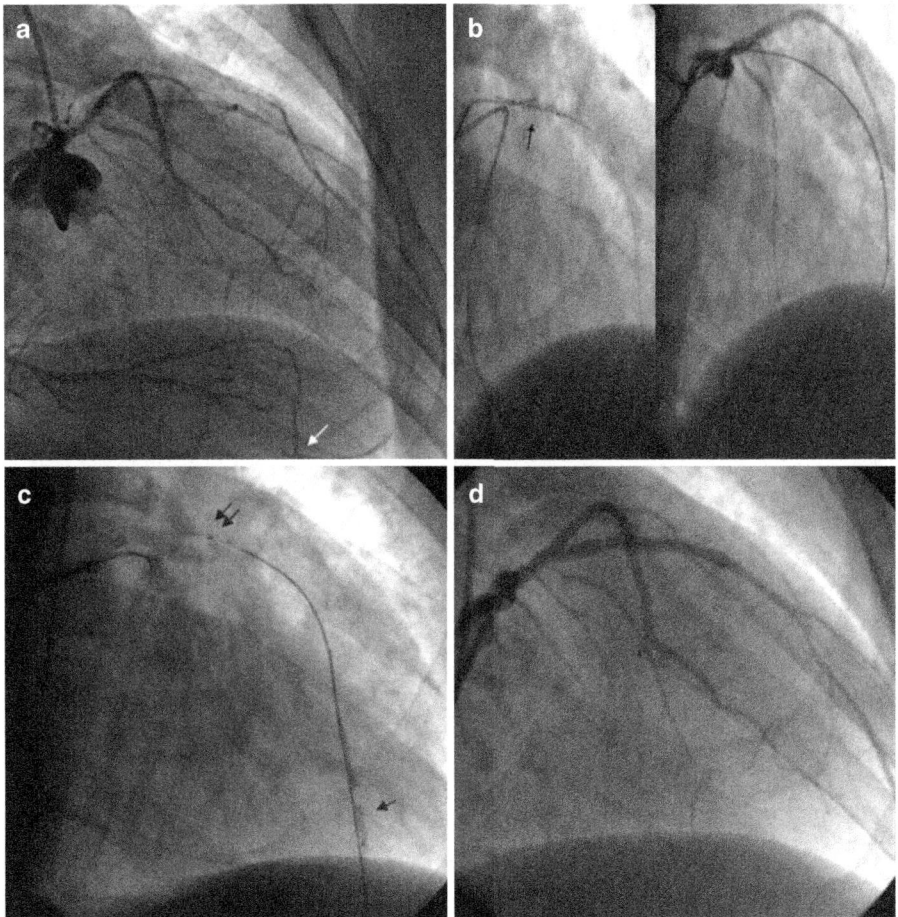

Fig. 11.2 An example of the retrograde approach using two guiding catheters simultaneously in the same coronary artery. (**a**) The baseline angiogram shows a CTO at the trifurcation site of the proximal LAD. An epicardial collateral connection between the distal LCX and distal LAD was observed (arrow). (**b**) Two guiding catheters (a 90 cm 7 Fr AL-1 guiding catheter for retrograde access and another 6 Fr JL-4 guiding catheter for antegrade access) were placed simultaneously in the left main coronary artery. After 2.0 mm retrograde ballooning was performed at the subintimal space of the CTO site, including the site distal to the CTO lesion (arrow), the antegrade wire (Miracle 12g, Asahi Intecc) was passed into the distal true lumen (the CART technique). (**c**) The passed antegrade wire was anchored by retrograde ballooning (arrow) in order to facilitate the antegrade balloon (double arrows) passage (the distal anchoring balloon technique). (**d**) Final angiogram

[8]. In a retrograde approach, large catheters are located in the supply vessels for a long time, which can lead to unexpected thrombotic complications. To prevent this, both vessels should be observed at all times, and ACT should be measured every 30 min and maintained for more than 250–300 s.

11.4 Selection of Native Collateral Channels

This is the most important stage of retrograde interventions, and it is no exaggeration to say that if the wire has passed through the native collateral channels and reached the occlusion of the target vessel, the procedure is successful. The native collateral channels are divided into the epicardial collateral channel and the septal collateral channel, and their size is divided into three categories according to Werner classification (CC0 = no visible connection; CC1 = a continuous, tiny connection; CC2 = a continuous, small vessel-like connection). The epicardial collateral channel may be larger than the septal collateral channel, but in most cases it is difficult to manipulate the wire because of the long tortuous pathways, and even after the wire passes through it, if the diameter is not large enough for the balloon or microcatheter to pass through, trapping may occur. More importantly, perforation, if it ever occurs, can lead to the pericardial tamponade, so a very careful approach is necessary. On the other hand, the septal branch connections are more frequently observed, and the size may be smaller than that of the epicardial collateral connections, but the pathways are short and the degree of bending is not severe, so the wire manipulation is easy. In addition, even if perforation or rupture occurs, the risk of the pericardial tamponade is extremely low, so it can be expanded using small balloons (1.25–1.5 mm), which facilitates the entry and exit of retrograde devices without the risk of trapping [9]. In addition, the advantages of the septal collateral channel are that you can confirm the connection of channels by performing the selective injection of septal perforators to the septal branches using a microcatheter even if it

looks difficult for the wire to pass because of lack of clear channel connection and, without administering contrast dye, you can repeat trial and error to several septal collateral channels with wires to cross them (surfing technique). The recently developed Sion family and Fielder XT-R (Asahi Intecc) have two wire cores called a composite core system unlike the existing wires to prevent wire whipping and maintain wire tip shape very well, so it is used conveniently to pass through severely tortuous or very thin channel. In addition, the Corsair microcatheter [10] has a good supportive capacity and can pass through a thin, highly tortuous channel while providing wider selection of native collateral channels along with the Sion wires (Fig. 11.3). Recently, new developed wire and microcatheter are used at retrograde approach in Japan. The Suoh 03 wire has a very flexible tip, so it may be best suitable for crossing with lower risk of injury in acute bends and continuous tortuosity, such as the epicardial channel. The Caravel microcatheter has a low profile shaft and supreme trackability, so it may be suitable for retrograde approach with tortuous anatomy. However, the desirable native collateral channel for a beginner is a septal collateral channel with a modest degree of tortuousness and a size of CC1 or greater. As for the epicardial native collateral channel, it is safe to access it and has a high success rate, only when the size is CC2. In the case of multiple collateral connections, a channel is selected considering the ease of wire manipulation after passing through the channel (Fig. 11.4).

11.5 CTO Crossing Techniques

The preferred methods to try if the retrograde wire reaches the occlusion site through the native collateral channels are the retrograde wire crossing technique and the kissing wire technique. The retrograde wire crossing technique is a method of directly passing through the occlusion with a retrograde wire; the kissing wire technique uses a retrograde wire as a landmark and passes directly through the occlusion with an antegrade wire (Fig. 11.5). These two methods are relatively

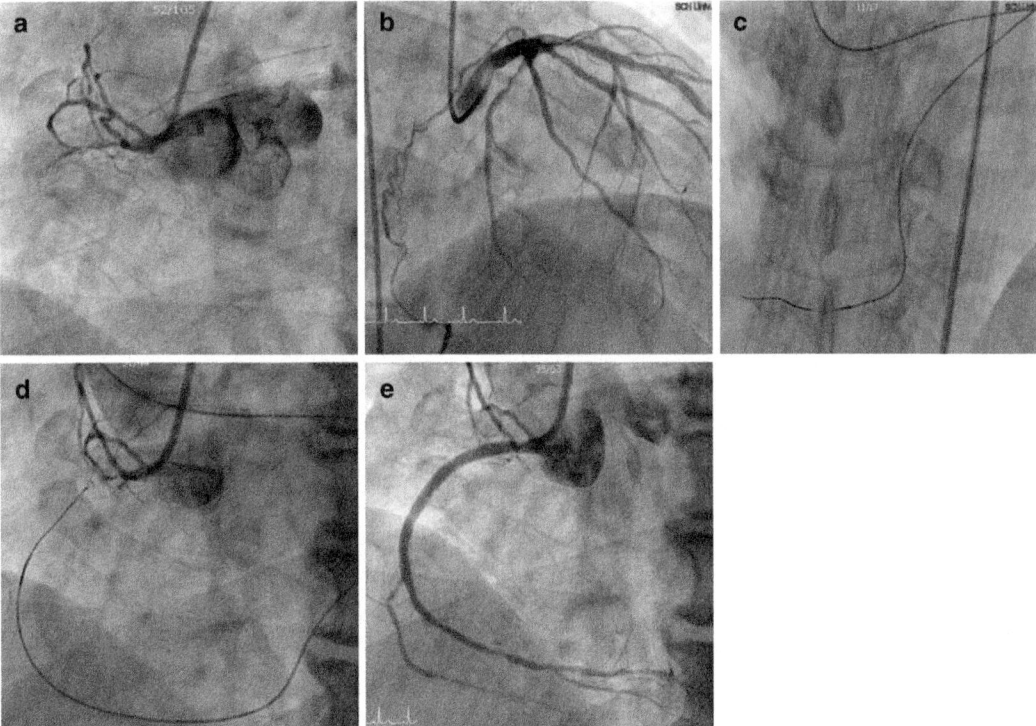

Fig. 11.3 An example of tortuous epicardial channel tracking using Sion wire and Corsair microcatheter. (**a**) The baseline angiogram shows a CTO at the proximal RCA. (**b**) A tortuous epicardial collateral connection between LCX and posterolateral branch was observed. (**c**) A Sion wire with Corsair microcatheter crossed the epicardial channel. (**d**) The retrograde wire crossing technique was successful. (**e**) A final result

simple, but due to the characteristics of retrograde pathways such as the long course and angulations and the complexity of the lesions such as the long occlusion length, calcification, and tortuousness, it is difficult to pass through the lesions with just retrograde wires or antegrade wires. Therefore, a more technically complicated subintimal tracking technique is needed. The CART technique [11] connects the subintimal space of the occlusion site with the distal true lumen by retrograde ballooning and manipulates the antegrade wire located in the subintimal space through the distal true lumen (Fig. 11.6). On the other hand, the reserve CART technique uses antegrade ballooning to connect the subintimal space with the proximal true lumen and manipulates the retrograde wire located in the subintimal space through the proximal true lumen (Fig. 11.7). Attention should be paid to keep the antegrade wire and retrograde wire in

line; expandable balloons of 2–2.5 mm are suitable, and in some cases larger diameter balloons may be used. In the CART technique, the retrograde balloon must enter the lesion through the collateral channel; however, in the reserve CART technique, the retrograde wire only needs to pass through the channel to reach the lesion, and the antegrade balloon enters the lesion instead of the retrograde balloon, so the procedure is easier than in the CART technique and the procedure time can be shortened. In addition, as described earlier, the introduction of the Corsair microcatheter allows the passage through difficult collateral channels (e.g., a thin tortuous epicardial channel) without balloon dilation, which was previously considered impossible, so recently the reserve CART technique is used more frequently. In the reserve CART technique, attention should be paid to the fact that the intentional subintimal dissection of arteries after an antegrade subintimal

J. Suh and N. H. Lee

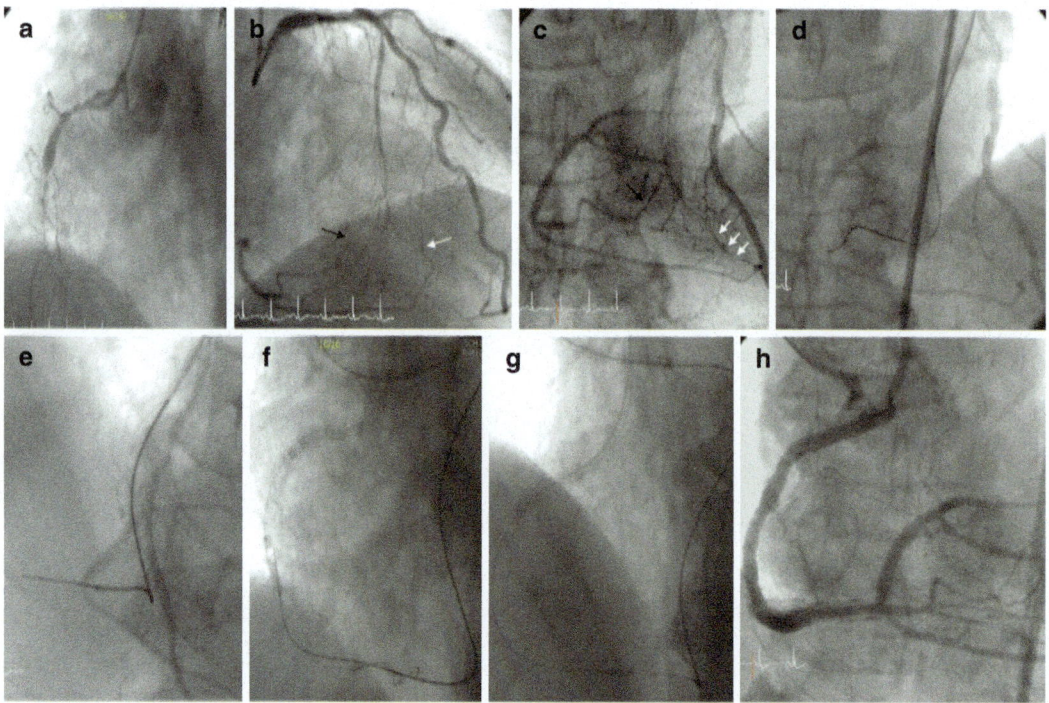

Fig. 11.4 An example of selection of ideal collateral channel among the multiple collateral connections. (**a**) The baseline angiogram shows a CTO at the mid-RCA. (**b**, **c**) There are multiple collateral connections between the LAD and the RCA. The mid-septal collateral connection (white arrow) looks easy for crossing. However, because PDA ostial occlusion site has an acute angle, we selected more tortuous proximally located collateral channel (black arrow) which has a coaxial alignment for the occlusion. (**d**, **e**) The Sion wire with Corsair catheter crossed the channel. (**f**, **g**) Reverse CART technique and wire externalization. (**h**) A final result

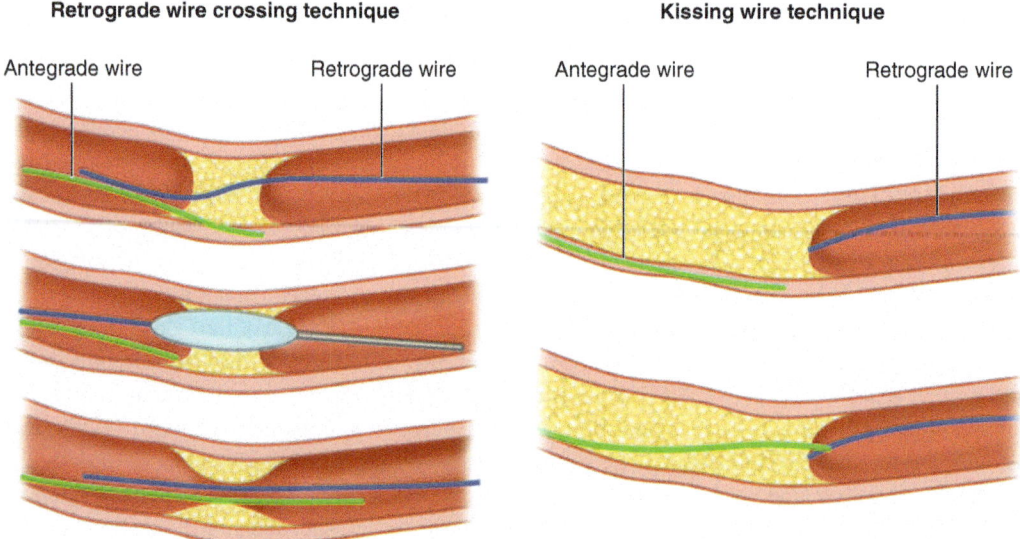

Fig. 11.5 Illustration of the retrograde wire crossing technique and kissing wire technique

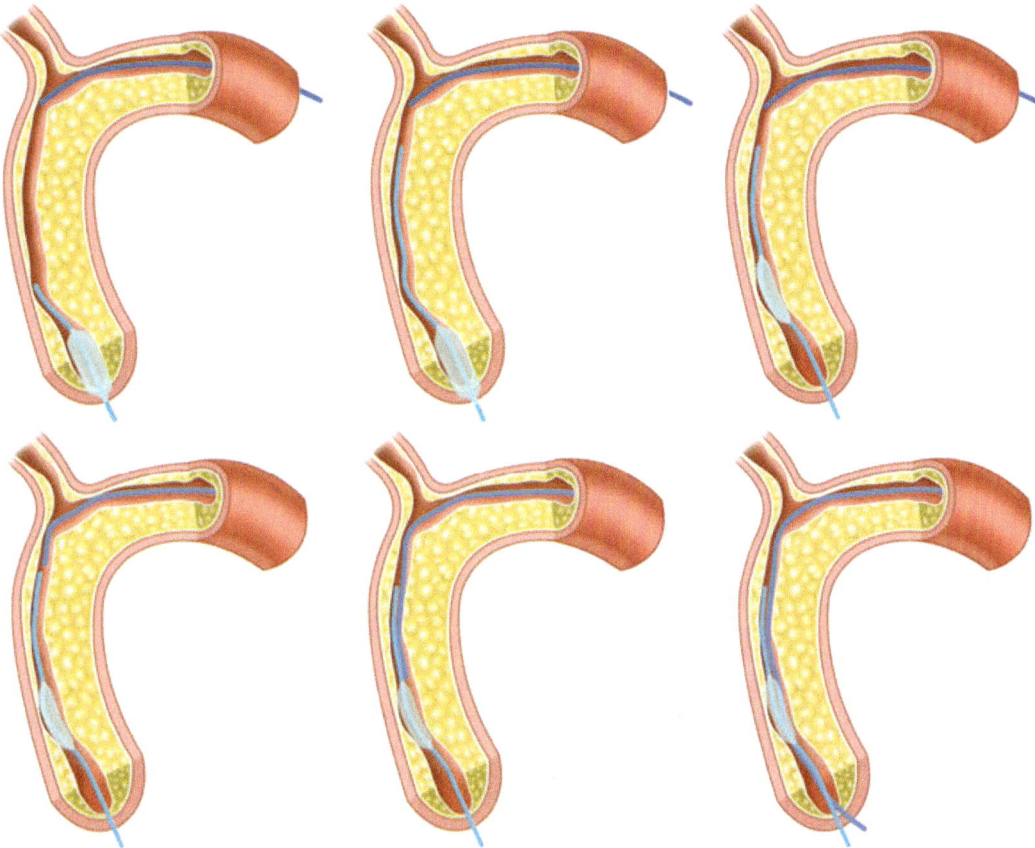

Fig. 11.6 Basic concept of the CART technique

balloon dilation can be worsened by antegrade injection of the contrast dye. Therefore, in the reserve CART technique, IVUS is recommended instead of the contrast dye test to determine the position of the wire, the size of the vessel, and the position of the stent [12].

11.6 Techniques for Facilitating the Passage of Predilatation Balloons

The retrograde approach to the balloon passage after the wire passes through the occlusion has many advantages. This is because various anchoring balloon techniques such as distal anchoring balloon techniques and double anchoring balloon techniques [13] can be used in addition to the proximal anchoring balloon techniques com-

monly used in the conventional antegrade approach, which improves the guiding catheter support by balloon dilation in the branch vessel of the occlusion proximal because an antegrade wire and a retrograde wire are simultaneously present in one vessel (Fig. 11.8). The distal anchoring balloon technique fixes the retrograde wire or antegrade wire which passed through the occlusion to the opposite balloon, facilitating the passage of the balloon (Fig. 11.2). Recently, the wire externalization technique (where after the wire enters the target vessel guiding catheter, it is fixed with a balloon, the microcatheter is introduced into the guiding catheter, and it is replaced with a 300 cm wire, it is taken out of the guiding catheter through which the balloon is dilated, and the stent is inserted) is used when the retrograde wire passes through the occlusion, as in the retrograde wire crossing technique or the reserve

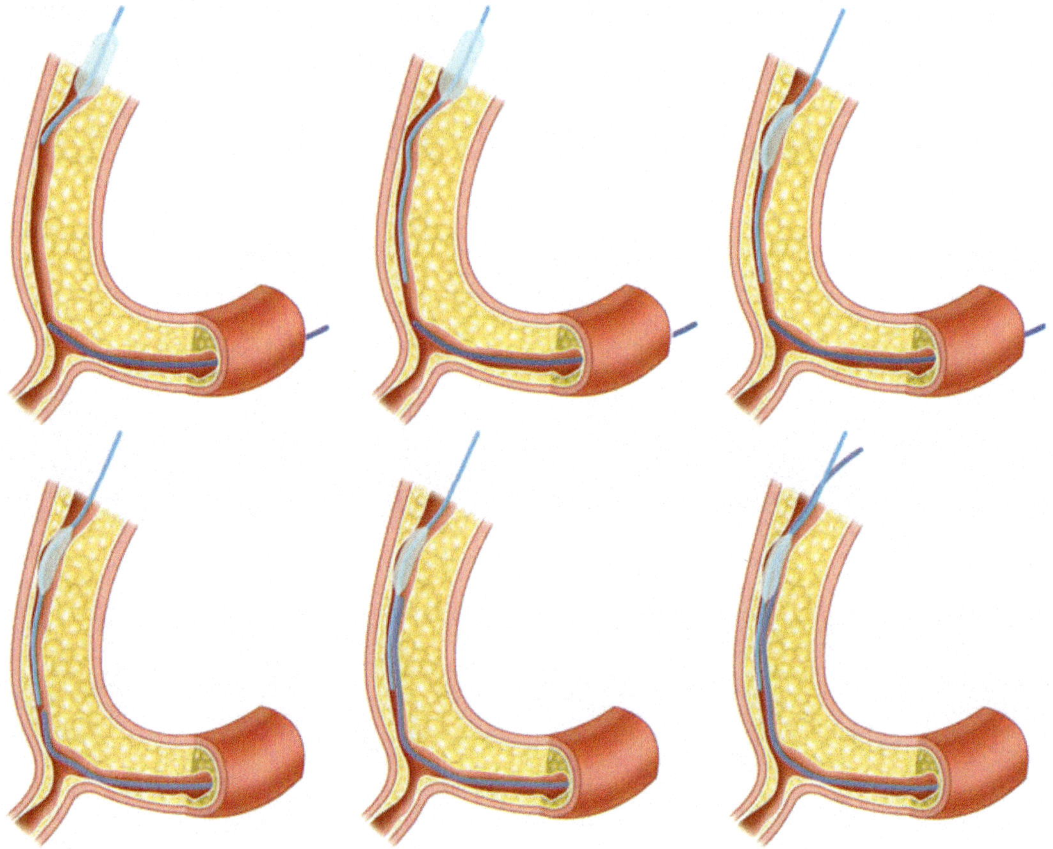

Fig. 11.7 Basic concept of the reverse CART technique

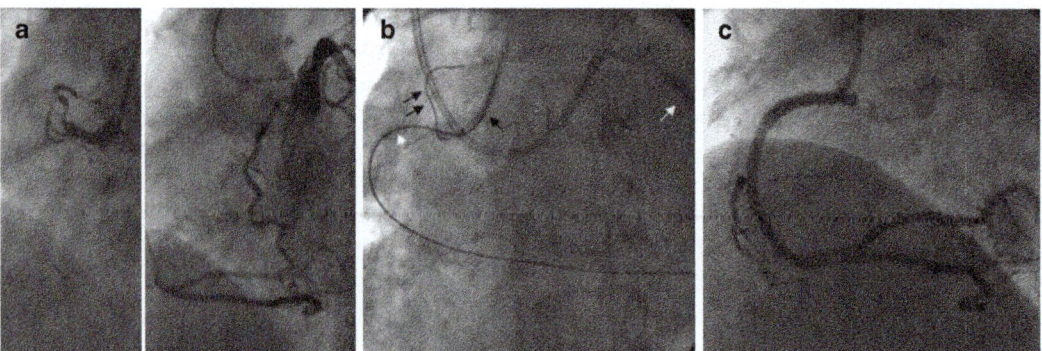

Fig. 11.8 Double anchoring balloon technique to facilitate the passage of the retrograde balloon through the CTO lesion. (**a**) The baseline angiograms show a CTO at the proximal RCA and a well-developed epicardial collateral. (**b**) A Conquest Pro 9g wire crossed the occlusion and entered the donor-guiding catheter. After the distal anchoring balloon technique failed, the addition of the proximal anchoring balloon technique (another balloon inflation at the LCX, white arrow) to the distal anchoring balloon technique (black arrow) provided maximal support for retrograde balloon (white arrow head) passage (the double anchoring balloon technique). Double arrows indicate another wire in the conus branch for IVUS examination to identify whether the cross retrograde wire was placed in the proximal true lumen. (**c**) Final angiogram

CART technique (Fig. 11.9). It should be noted that the microcatheter must continue to be located distal to the target vessel after passing through the native collateral channel, and after the target vessel has been reopened, the retrograde wire must be removed first before you remove the microcatheter. This is because wire entrapment may occur if the retrograde wire is placed in the collateral channel for a long time without the

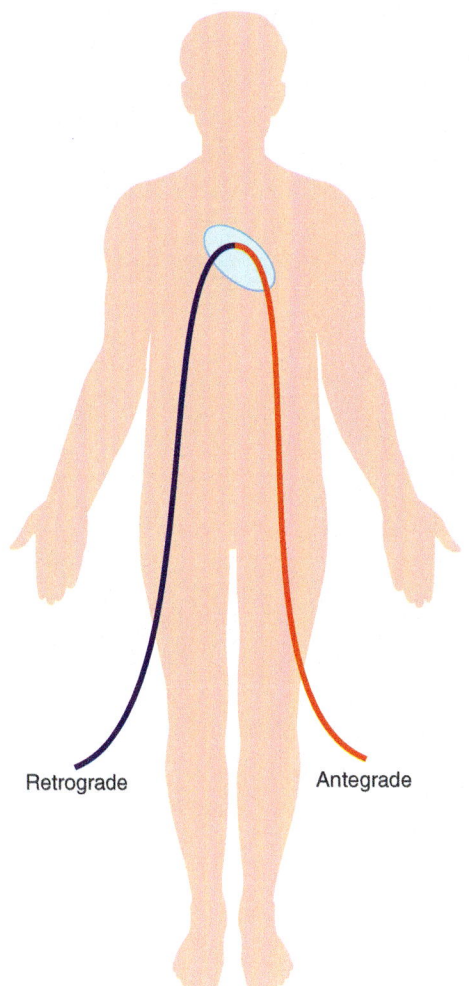

Fig. 11.9 Illustration of the wire externalization. (1) CTO penetration by guidewire through retrograded guiding catheter. (2) Insertion of retrograded guidewire inside antegraded guiding catheter. (3) Insertion of microcatheter over retrograded guidewire into antegraded guiding catheter. (4) Exchange of retrograded guidewire for 300 cm guidewire. (5) Removal of 300cm guidewire from patient's body through antegraded guiding catheter. (6) Proceed on to antegrade angioplasty

microcatheter. The RG3 wire (Asahi Intecc) is a newly developed dedicated externalization wire that greatly facilitates the externalization process.

11.7 Complications of the Retrograde Approach

In addition to the side effects that can occur with the existing antegrade approach, the retrograde approach always has the potential for side effects associated with the collateral donor artery [2, 14]. Dissection of supplying vessels and thrombus formation (Fig. 11.10) can cause ischemic side effects that threaten the patient's life. As previously mentioned, you should try to maintain the ACT for more than 250–300 s and be careful of the entrapment of the retrograde device and the subsequent deep migration of the guiding catheter of the supplying vessel when using the thin, tortuous collateral channels. If the epicardial native collateral channels are used, the native collateral channel impairment along with the pericardial tamponade can lead to severe ischemic side effects if the epicardial native collateral channels are the main source of the target vessels (often observed in the case of the highly developed endocardial native collateral channels), so careful attention should be paid. Because CART or reverse CART techniques are fundamentally subintimal dilatation in or near the lesion, excessive balloon or stent dilation may cause vascular perforation, so if these techniques are used, pay attention to the cardiac tamponade, and it is desirable to observe the situation for several hours in the intensive care unit.

11.8 Predictors of Successful Retrograde Approach

According to a study, successful retrograde approach is predicted if the size of the native collateral channels is greater than CC1, the collateral tortuosity of the native collateral channels is less than 90 degrees, and the angle of the connection between the distal part of the native collateral

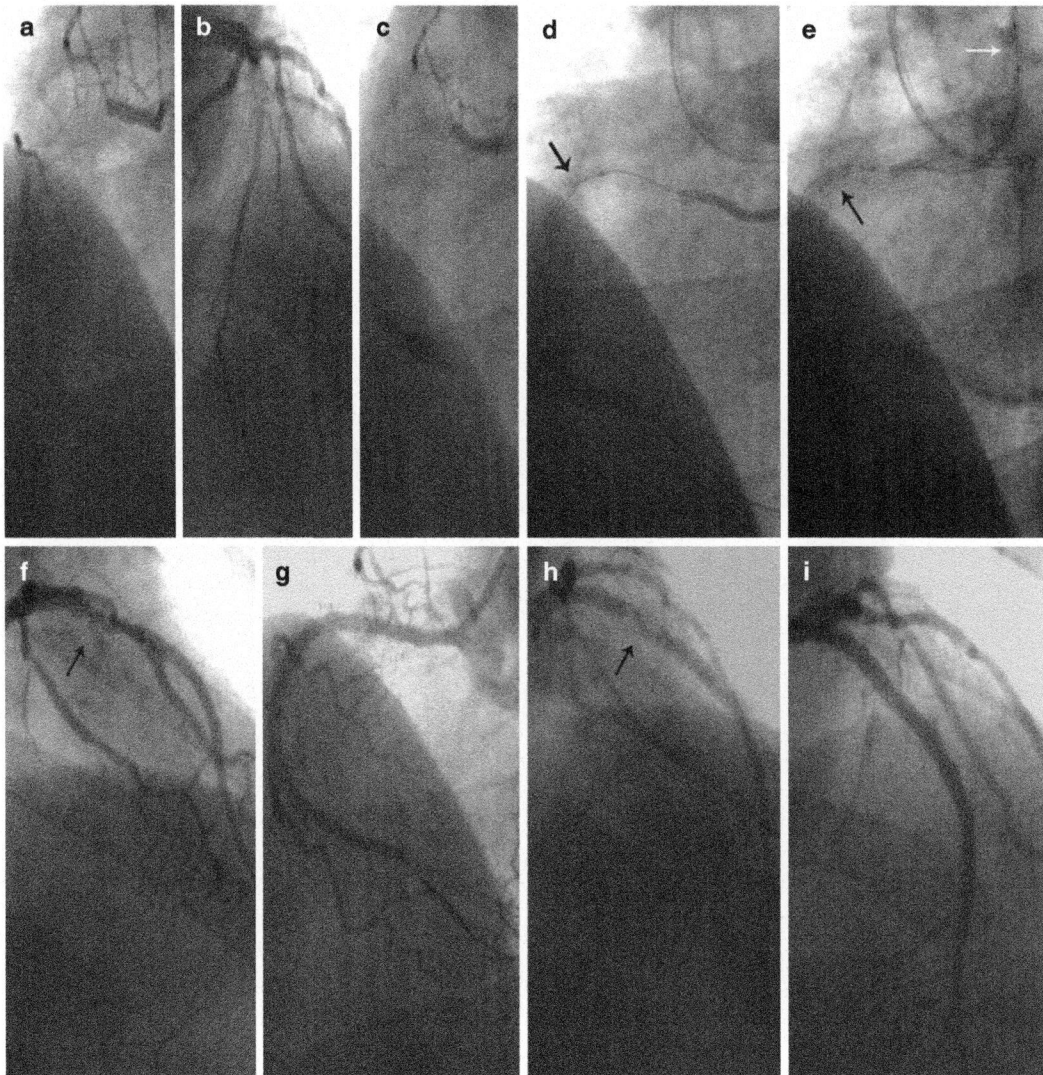

Fig. 11.10 An example of the bail-out reverse CART technique accompanied by multiple donor vessel complications. (**a, b**) Baseline angiograms show multiple CTOs at the proximal RCA and mid-LAD. (**c**) After antegrade recanalization of LAD-CTO, RCA-CTO was attempted with the antegrade approach. However, wire manipulation provoked severe dissection that propagated to the distal RCA. (**d**) The bail-out retrograde approach was tried. After the retrograde wire crossing technique failed, the reverse CART technique with 2.5 mm balloon (arrow) enabled the retrograde wire (choice-PT) passage into the proximal true lumen. (**e**) After the retrograde wire entered the right guiding catheter, it was anchored by antegrade

ballooning in the guiding catheter (white arrow) to facilitate the retrograde balloon passage (black arrow). (**f**) During the removal of the retrograde wire, severe resistance occurred, which made the left guiding catheter move to the mid-LAD segment, resulting in the first complication (distortion of the prior stenting site at the proximal LAD, arrow), which was treated by bail-out stenting. (**g**) Final RCA image after implantation of multiple stents from the distal to the proximal RCA. (**h**) The second complication (acute stent thrombosis, arrow) occurred after RCA stenting which was urgently managed by thrombus suction, abciximab, and high-pressure ballooning. (**i**) Final left coronary angiogram

channel and the recipient vessels is less than 90 degrees, whereas the rate of failure is high when the size of epicardial channel and the native collateral channel is CC0; the angle of the connection between corkscrew channel, the distal part of the native collateral channel, and the target vessel is greater than 90 degrees; and the connection between the distal part of the native collateral channel and the target vessel is not clear. Particularly, factors that were important in the existing antegrade approach such as the degree of bending, length, and calcification of the occlusion didn't have much influence in the retrograde approach [4]. Recently published article showed successful retrograde procedure in CTO was related with Werner's score, diameter of distal CTO segment, and tortuous collateral [15].

11.9 Choosing Between the Antegrade Approach and the Retrograde Approach

After the introduction of the retrograde approach along with the development of technology and instrumentation, the success rate of a skilled physician's CTO-PCI is over 90%. When choosing between the antegrade approach and the retrograde approach, you should consider both safety and ease of the procedure. For example, attempting a retrograde approach from the beginning, thinking that the native collateral channel is fairly good when the difficulty level is not very high is not desirable especially when using the epicardial channels, considering the disadvantages of the retrograde approach (complexity of procedures and unexpected complications). Also, when the antegrade approach fails without the parallel wire technique, you might switch to a retrograde approach; this should be avoided. This is because the parallel wire technique is the key to increasing the success rate of the antegrade approach. On the other hand, if the difficulty level is very high and there is a proper native collateral channel, especially if there is a history of previous failures, it is advisable to attempt the retrograde approach from the beginning. In conclusion, the safety and high success rate of the CTO-PCI can be expected with the proper and complementary use of the antegrade approach based on lesion shapes and the retrograde approach based on native collateral channels (Fig. 11.11).

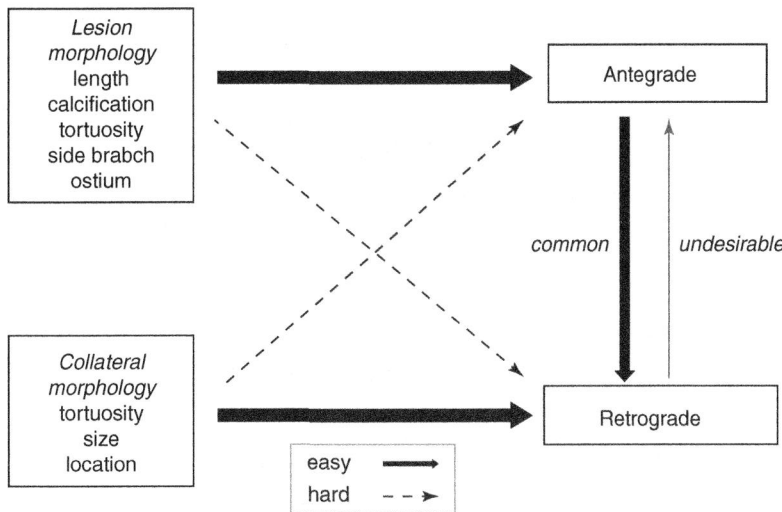

Fig. 11.11 Schema of CTO-PCI

References

1. Muramatsu T, Tsukahara R, Ito Y, Ishimori H, Park SJ, de Winter R. Changing strategies of the retrograde approach for chronic total occlusion during past the 7 years. Catheter Cardiovasc Interv. 2013;81(4):E178–85.
2. Lee NH, Seo HS, Choi JH, Suh J, Cho YH. Recanalization strategy of retrograde angioplasty in patients with coronary chronic total occlusion -analysis of 24 cases, focusing on technical aspects and complications. Int J Cardiol. 2010;144(2):219–29.
3. Saito S. Different strategies of retrograde approach in coronary angioplasty for chronic total occlusion. Catheter Cardiovasc Interv. 2008;71:8–19.
4. Rathore S, Katoh O, Matsuo H, Terashima M, Tanaka N, Kinoshita Y, Kimura M, Tsuchikane E, Nasu K, Ehara M, Asakura K, Asakura Y, Suzuki T. Retrograde percutaneous recanalization of chronic total occlusion of the coronary arteries: procedural outcomes and predictors of success in contemporary practice. Circ Cardiovasc Interv. 2009;2(2):124–32.
5. Ge L, Qian JY, Liu XB, Qin Q, Cui SJ, Yao K, et al. Retrograde approach for the recanalization of coronary chronic total occlusion: preliminary experience of a single center. Chin Med J (Engl). 2010;123(7):857–63.
6. Suh J, Cho YH, Lee NH. Antegrade ballooning with retrograde approach for the treatment of long restenotic total occlusion. J Invasive Cardiol. 2011;23(7):E164–7.
7. Brilakis ES, Grantham JA, Thompson CA, DeMartini TJ, Prasad A, Sandhu GS, Banerjee S, Lombardi WL. The retrograde approach to coronary artery chronic total occlusions: a practical approach. Catheter Cardiovasc Interv. 2012;79(1):3–19.
8. Lee NH, Suh J, Cho YH, et al. Recanalization of a coronary chronic total occlusion by a retrograde approach using ipsilateral double guiding-catheters. Korean Circ J. 2009;39:42–5.
9. Surmely JF, Katoh O, Tsuchikane E, Nasu K, Suzuki T. Coronary septal collaterals as an access for the retrograde approach in the percutaneous treatment of coronary chronic total occlusions. Catheter Cardiovasc Interv. 2007;69:826–32.
10. Tsuchikane E, Katoh O, Kimura M, Nasu K, Kinoshita Y, Suzuki T. The first clinical experience with a novel catheter for collateral channel tracking in retrograde approach for chronic coronary total occlusions. JACC Cardiovasc Interv. 2010;3(2):165–71.
11. Surmely JF, Tsuchikane E, Katoh O, et al. New concept for CTO recanalization using controlled antegrade and retrograde subintimal tracking: the CART technique. J Invasive Cardiol. 2006;18:334–8.
12. Rathore S, Katoh O, Tuschikane E, Oida A, Suzuki T, Takase S. A novel modification of the retrograde approach for the recanalization of chronic total occlusion of the coronary arteries intravascular ultrasound-guided reverse controlled antegrade and retrograde tracking. JACC Cardiovasc Interv. 2010;3(2):155–64.
13. Lee NH, Suh J, Seo HS. Double anchoring balloon technique for recanalization of coronary chronic total occlusion by retrograde approach. Catheter Cardiovasc Interv. 2009;73:791–4.
14. Suh J, Cho YH, Lee NH. Bail-out reverse controlled antegrade and retrograde subintimal tracking accompanied by multiple complications in coronary chronic total occlusion. J Invasive Cardiol. 2008;20:E334–7.
15. Chai W-l, Agyekum F, Zhang B, Liao H-T, Ma D-L, Zhong Z-A, Wang P-N, Jin L-J. Clinical prediction score for successful retrograde procedure in chronic total occlusion percutaneous coronary intervention. Cardiology. 2016;134:331–9.

CART/Reverse CART/ Contemporary Reverse CART for Successful Retrograde PCI

12

Dong-Bin Kim and Hee-Yeol Kim

In a retrograde approach, retrograde wire-crossing or kissing wire technique is firstly preferred. A retrograde wire-crossing technique is a method of direct passage with retrograde wire through CTO, and the kissing wire technique is a method of advancing the antegrade wire, using retrograde wire as a landmark. The two methods are a relatively simple method.

However, it is difficult to pass CTO by simple antegrade and retrograde wire maneuver, because there are long occlusion length, calcification, and tortuousness of CTO lesion. Therefore, a more complex technique of subintimal tracking is required.

In this chapter, we overview the different technique of subintimal angioplasty, especially CART, reverse CART, and contemporary CART, which aim is to create a channel between the intima and the subintimal space using an intentional dissection.

12.1 Controlled Antegrade and Retrograde Subintimal Tracking (CART) Technique

CART technique connected an anterograde wire in proximal occlusion lesion into the distal true lumen by retrograde ballooning.

Both antegrade and retrograde wire is located in subintimal space (Fig. 12.1a). A balloon (1.25–2.5 mm) is positioned in distal portion of the CTO and inflated over the retrograde wire into the retrograde subintimal space (Fig. 12.1b, c). The antegrade wire is manipulated to advanced through the enlarged retrograde subintimal space into distal true lumen (Fig. 12.1d).

However, the use of the CART procedure is sometimes difficult and risky, as there is inherent risk in delivering bulky balloon along fragile collateral channel. Nowadays the classic CART is rarely performed. A reverse CART is a more efficient and safe method.

12.2 Reverse Controlled Antegrade and Retrograde Subintimal Tracking (CART) Technique

The reverse CART has the same basic concept as CART. Reverse CART technique connects a retrograde wire in distal subintimal space into proximal true lumen by anterograde ballooning.

D.-B. Kim
Department of Cardiology, St. Paul's Hospital, The Catholic University of Korea, Seoul, South Korea

H.-Y. Kim (✉)
Department of Cardiology, Bucheon St. Mary's Hospital, The Catholic University of Korea, Bucheon-si, Gyeonggi-do, South Korea
e-mail: cumckhy@catholic.ac.kr

© Springer Nature Singapore Pte Ltd. 2019
Y. Jang (ed.), *Percutaneous Coronary Interventions for Chronic Total Occlusion*,
https://doi.org/10.1007/978-981-10-6026-7_12

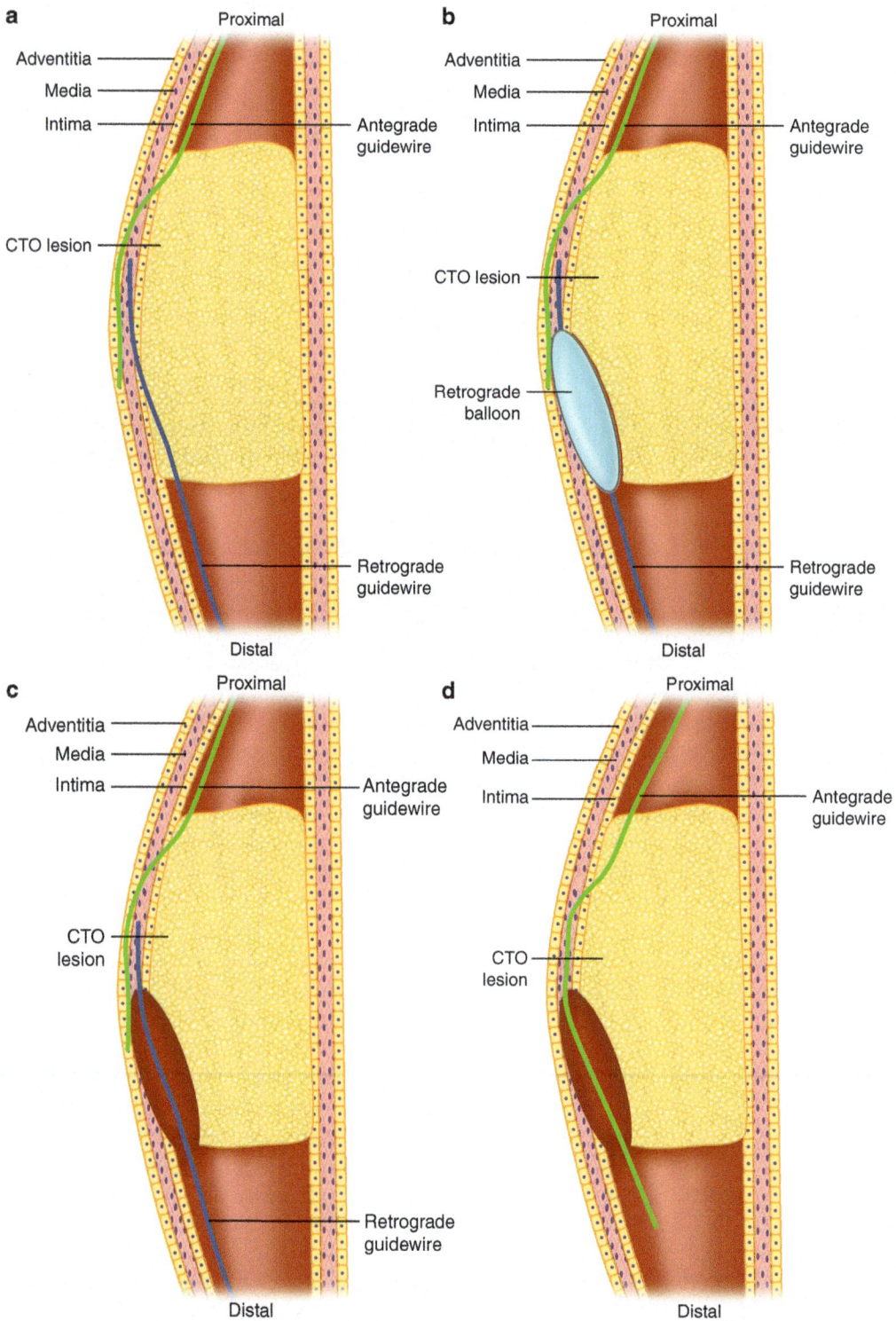

Fig. 12.1 Illustrations of CART. (**a**) An antegrade wire is advanced from the proximal true lumen into the subintimal space and the retrograde wire is delivered into distal true lumen and then into the CTO subintimal space. (**b**) The balloon is advanced through the retrograde wire and

dilated. (**c**) Balloon makes a large dissection in subintimal space of distal lumen. (**d**) An antegrade wire in proximal lumens is advanced into distal dissection space and connects proximal and distal true lumen

In some cases, both wires seem to meet in one view, but, the wires are seen as "parallel" in different views. The wires are in different layers, so it is difficult to meet in the same plane (Fig. 12.2). In this case, the reverse CART is needed.

The CART technique requires a retrograde balloon to pass through a collateral channel, but in a reverse CART technique, only retrograde wire needs to be passed through collateral channels to reach CTO lesion. Therefore, reverse CART technique is easy and short-time procedure compared to CART techniques. Also, the introduction of the Corsair microcatheter makes difficult channel passage possible without balloon dilatation of the collateral channel. The frequency of the reverse CART technique is increasing recently.

The ideal situation for reverse CART is both anterograde and retrograde guidewire in subintimal. After retrograde wire crossing or kissing wire technique fails, intentional penetration of the subintimal space with the antegrade wire followed by balloon inflation may increase success in recanalization of CTO. First, the operator advances antegrade guidewire into subintimal space. Antegrade and retrograde guidewire should be on the same line (Fig. 12.3a). The antegrade balloon is delivery through anterograde guidewire and is ballooned in subintimal space, the expansion balloon is 2–2.5 mm in size, and in some cases, a larger diameter bal-

loon may be used (Fig. 12.3b). The antegrade balloon makes a large dissection space (Fig. 12.3c). The retrograde guidewire is advanced into proximal true lumen through large dissection space (Fig. 12.3d).

In case the retrograde wire is in the subintimal space and the antegrade wire is in the true lumen, the connection between antegrade and retrograde wire is more difficult, because of a large layer of tissue between the two wires. Aggressive anterograde dilatation will be required to create enough dissection space to connect the subintima. The most common reason for reverse CART failure is the use of an undersized antegrade balloon. Inflation with an adequately sized balloon in the antegrade space is important to disturb the body of the CTO and to advancement of retrograde guidewire into antegrade true lumen.

In reverse CART, the operator should be aware of dye injection. A subintimal dissection of an intentionally created vessel after an antegrade subintimal ballooning can be exacerbated if the antegrade injection of contrast dye is performed. Therefore, in the reverse CART technique, IVUS is recommended instead of the contrast agent test to determine wire position, vessel size, and stent position [1]. IVUS usage ensures the proper expansion of the subintimal space and minimizes the risk of perforations.

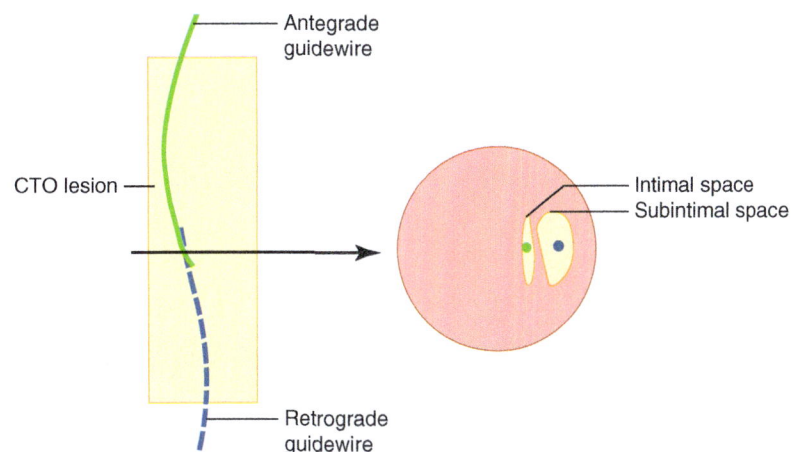

Fig. 12.2 Illustration of guidewires in intima and subintimal space. Antegrade and retrograde guides seem to be near in one projection, but two guidewires are in different layers. In this case, it is difficult to meet two guidewire due to layer resistance

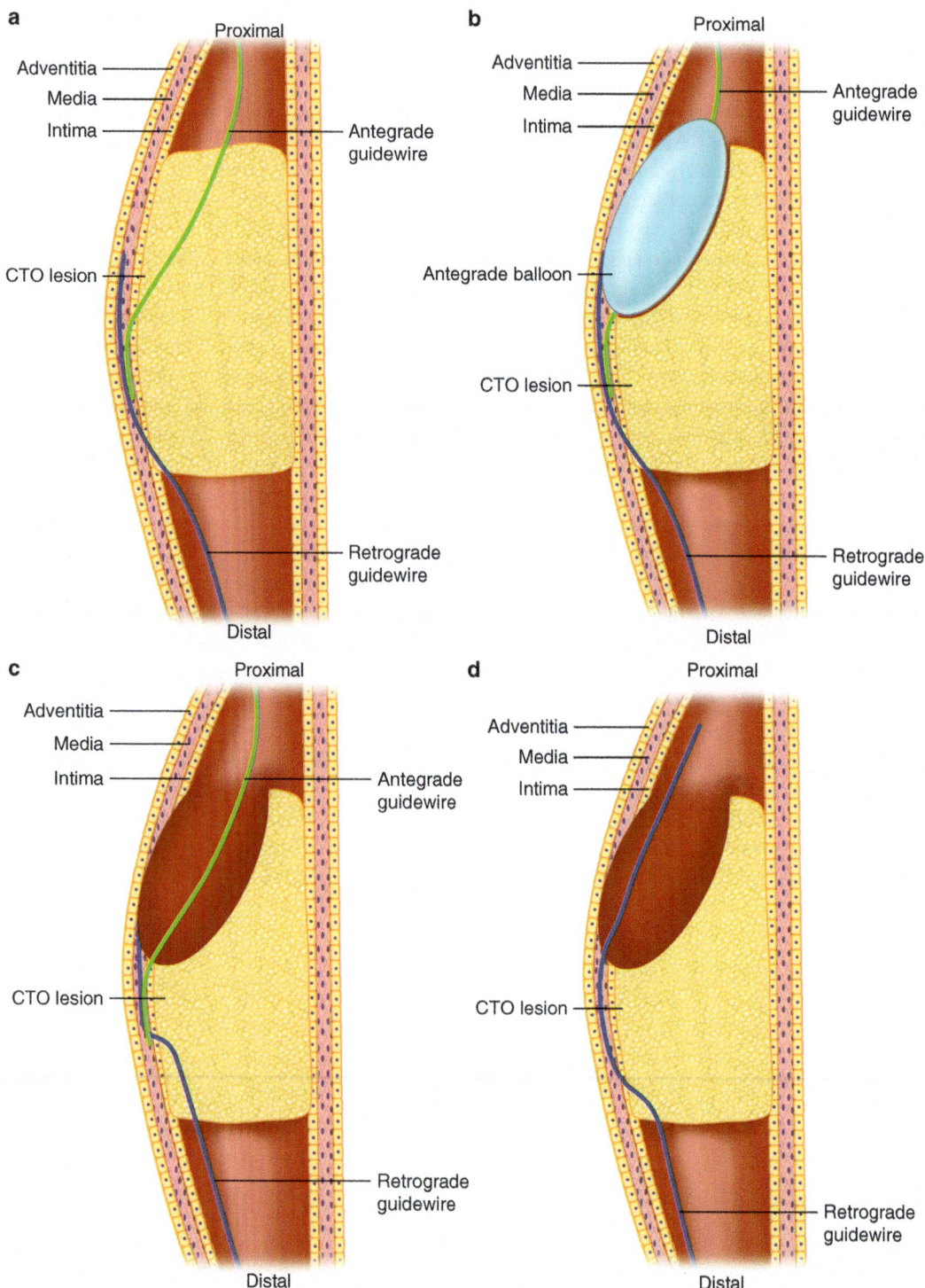

Fig. 12.3 Illustrations of reverse CART. It is similar to the CART technique except that a balloon is advanced over the antegrade guidewire to the proximal part of the occlusion and the retrograde wire crosses into the proximal true lumen. (**a**) the anterograde guidewire is advanced into subintimal space; (**b**) antegrade balloon is delivery through anterograde guidewire and is ballooned in subintimal space; (**c**) balloon makes a large dissection space. (**d**) The retrograde guidewire is advanced into proximal true lumen through large dissection space

12.3   Contemporary Reverse CART Technique

There are essential problems of the conventional reverse CART. In most of the retrograde approaches, the advancement of retrograde wire was the first step for the reverse CART. Recent new guidewire enables the intentional retrograde wire direction control. However, once the retrograde dissection is created, the precise control becomes difficult. Expansion of space around guidewire reduces force component for penetration. As a response to the rotation of CTO wires, semilunar space is created easily due to the layered structure of the fibrous tissue.

In conventional reverse CART, the connection is made at the position of overlapped antegrade and retrograde wires. In contemporary reverse

CART technique, antegrade smaller ballooning is done before retrograde wiring. The purpose of balloon dilatation is not to make a connection in both approaches. The purposes of balloon dilatation in the contemporary reverse CART are to compress the space around the retrograde guidewire and target for a retrograde guidewire. Therefore, it does not need a big balloon to complete contemporary reverse CART. Antegrade preparation for CTO site and IVUS examination should be recommended for the contemporary reverse CART to find a suitable point for penetration of the retrograde wire and to decide antegrade balloon size.

The anterograde guidewire is advanced into subintimal space (Fig. 12.4a). Antegrade balloon is delivery through anterograde guidewire and is ballooned before advancement of retrograde

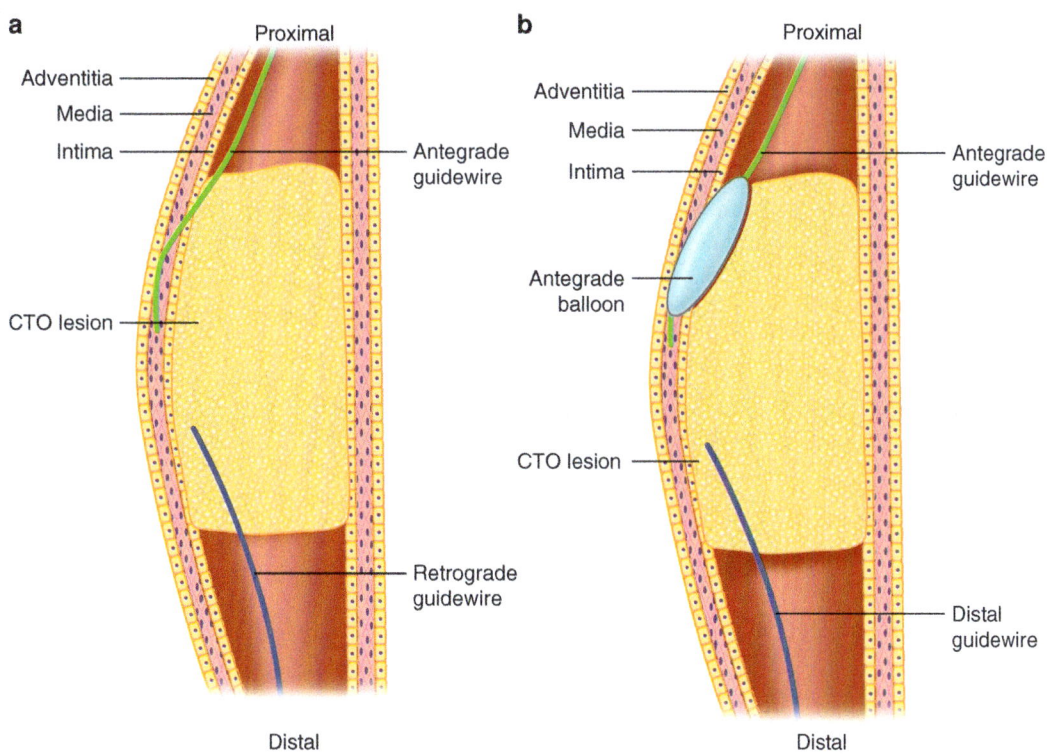

Fig. 12.4 Illustrations of the contemporary reverse CART. Balloon compresses the space around the retrograde guidewire and is a target for a retrograde guidewire. (**a**) the anterograde guidewire is advanced into subintimal space; (**b**) antegrade balloon is delivery through anterograde guidewire and is ballooned in subintimal space

before advancement of retrograde guidewire; (**c**) inflated balloon keeps in dissection space and the retrograde guidewire is advanced to the inflated balloon. (**d**) After deflation of balloon, the retrograde guidewire is advanced into proximal true lumen

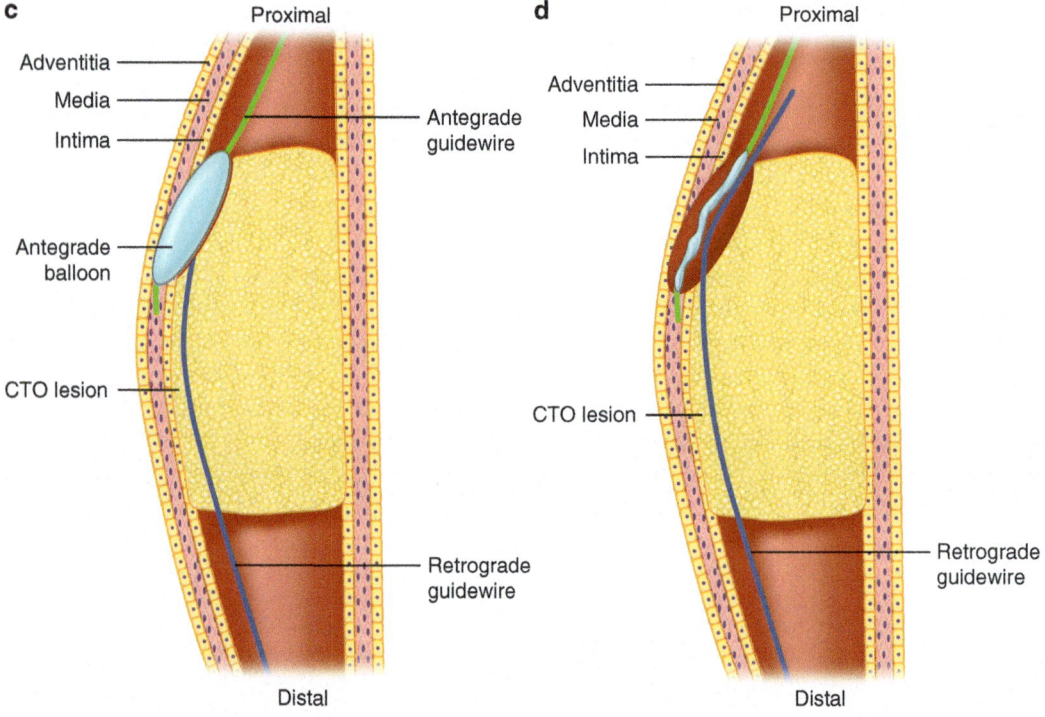

Fig. 12.4 (continued)

wire (Fig. 12.4b). Inflated balloon keeps in subintimal space, and the retrograde guidewire is advanced to the inflated balloon. The inflated balloon should be target of the retrograde wire (Fig. 12.4c). After deflation of balloon, the retrograde guidewire can enter into proximal true lumen (Fig. 12.4d); contemporary reverse CART minimizes the length of subintimal stenting.

12.4 Current Retrograde CTO Crossing Strategy

Advancement of devices and techniques has changed the retrograde CTO crossing strategy., The reverse CART is most frequent method followed by retrograde wire cross [2]. Original CART is rarely used (Fig. 12.5).

Fig. 12.5 Current CTO
crossing strategy in
Japan retrograde summit
registry. *CART*
controlled antegrade and
retrograde subintimal
tracking

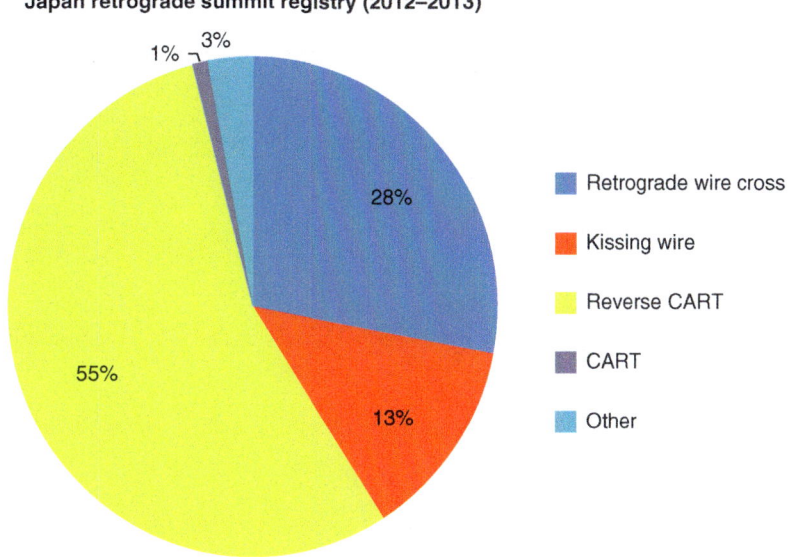

References

1. Rathore S, Katoh O, Tuschikane E, Oida A, Suzuki T, Takase S. A novel modification of the retrograde approach for the recanalization of chronic total occlusion of the coronary arteries intravascular ultrasound guided reverse controlled antegrade and retrograde tracking. J Am Coll Cardiol Cardiovasc Interv. 2010;3:155–64.

2. Habara M, Tsuchikane E, Muramatsu T, Kashima Y, Okamura A, Mutoh M, Yamane M, Oida A, Oikawa Y, Hasegawa K, for the Retrograde Summit Investigators. Comparison of percutaneous coronary intervention for chronic total occlusion outcome according to operator experience from the Japanese Retrograde Summit Registry. Catheter Cardiovasc Interv. (2016);87:1027–35.

Use of Intravascular Ultrasound for Wire-Crossing in Retrograde CTO PCI

Jae-Hwan Lee

Intravascular ultrasound (IVUS) is a very important tool for retrograde CTO intervention. Currently, the reverse CART technique rather than the classic CART technique is used as the main guidewire passage technique for retrograde CTO recanalization (Fig. 13.1) [1, 2]. The IVUS is almost indispensable for its safe and successful performance [3, 4]. When the microcatheter arrives at the distal landing zone of the CTO using a retrograde approach, antegrade and retrograde guidewire should be manipulated to reach as close as possible within the CTO segment [5]. At this time, if the IVUS is inserted into the CTO segment through an antegrade guidewire, the position of antegrade and retrograde guidewires in the CTO segment can be confirmed [3]. If the IVUS catheter is difficult to enter into the CTO segment, it may be possible to enter by expanding the space within the CTO segment using a small balloon of about 1.0–1.5 mm. IVUS provides various information on guidewire location, CTO lesion size, plaque components, and calcium distribution. Such information may minimize complications such as vascular injury, rupture, or subintimal dissection in retrograde CTO interventions [6].

Reverse CART technique is a method for retrograde passage of guidewire through the CTO segment space that underwent antegrade balloon dilatation. IVUS can be used to evaluate the current position of the retrograde guidewire. The location of the guidewire within the CTO segment can be roughly classified into four categories (Figs. 13.1, 13.2, 13.3, and 13.4). First, both guidewires are present in an intraluminal space. Second, antegrade guidewire is positioned in an intraluminal space, and retrograde guidewire is positioned in a subintimal space. Third, antegrade guidewire is positioned in a subintimal space, and retrograde guidewire is positioned in an intraluminal space. Fourth, both exist in a subintimal space.

The operator should choose the appropriate strategy for each situation. If both guidewires are present in the intraluminal space (Fig. 13.1), the reverse CART may be performed immediately. In the second situation, the antegrade guidewire is positioned in the intraluminal space, and the retrograde guidewire is positioned in the subintimal space (Fig. 13.2); the antegrade guidewire can be carefully moved downward to further increase the guidewire entry length to the true lumen and redirect the retrograde guidewire toward the antegrade guidewire, or reverse CART can be performed immediately. In the third situation, antegrade guidewire is positioned in the subintimal space, and retrograde guidewire is positioned in the intraluminal space (Fig. 13.3); IVUS guidance allows the retrograde guidewire to enter a more proximal CTO segment. At this time, the

J.-H. Lee (✉)
Chungnam National University Hospital,
Daejeon, South Korea
e-mail: myheart@cnu.ac.kr

© Springer Nature Singapore Pte Ltd. 2019
Y. Jang (ed.), *Percutaneous Coronary Interventions for Chronic Total Occlusion*,
https://doi.org/10.1007/978-981-10-6026-7_13

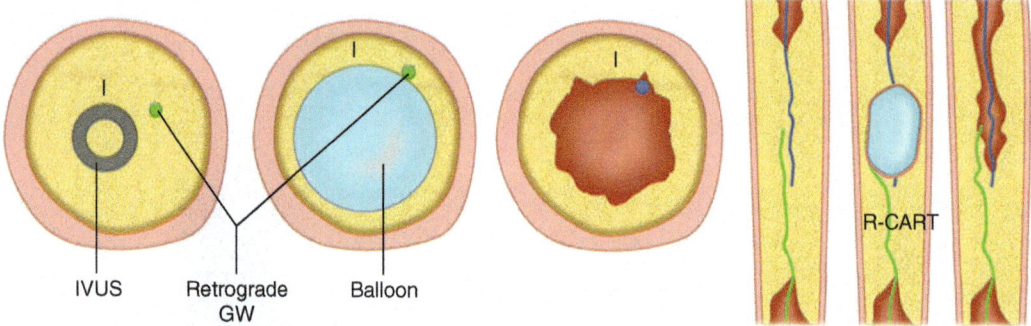

Fig. 13.1 If both guidewires are present in the intraluminal space, the reverse CART may be performed immediately. *IVUS* intravascular ultrasound, *GW* guidewire, *R-CART* reverse controlled antegrade and retrograde subintimal tracking, *I* intima

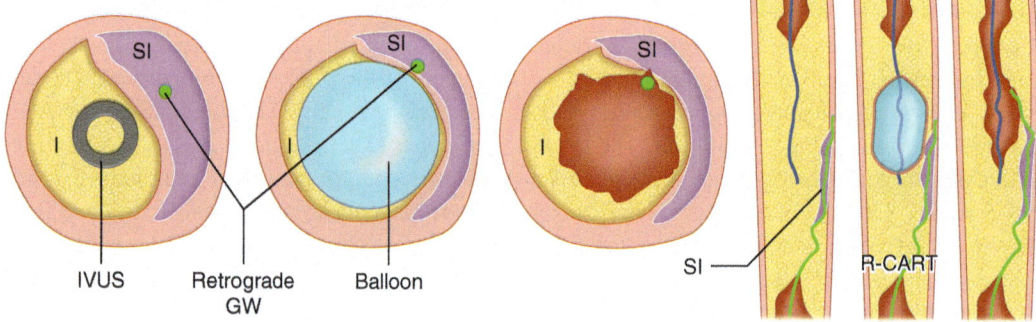

Fig. 13.2 The antegrade guidewire is in the intraluminal space, and the retrograde guidewire is in the subintimal space. In this situation, the antegrade guidewire can be carefully moved downward to further increase the guidewire entry length to the true lumen and redirect the retrograde guidewire toward the antegrade guidewire, or reverse CART can be performed immediately. *IVUS* intravascular ultrasound, *GW* guidewire, *R-CART* reverse controlled antegrade and retrograde subintimal tracking, *I* intima, *SI* subintima

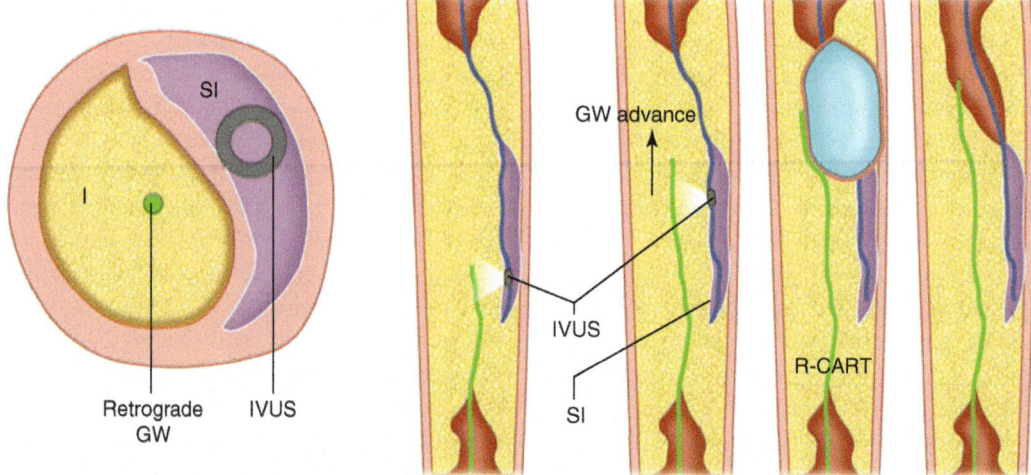

Fig. 13.3 Antegrade guidewire is in a subintimal space, and retrograde guidewire is in an intraluminal space. IVUS guidance allows the retrograde guidewire to enter a more proximal CTO segment. At this time, the retrograde guidewire should be sufficiently rigid and controllable to allow free torque control. *IVUS* intravascular ultrasound, *GW* guidewire, *R-CART* reverse controlled antegrade and retrograde subintimal tracking, *I* intima, *SI* subintima

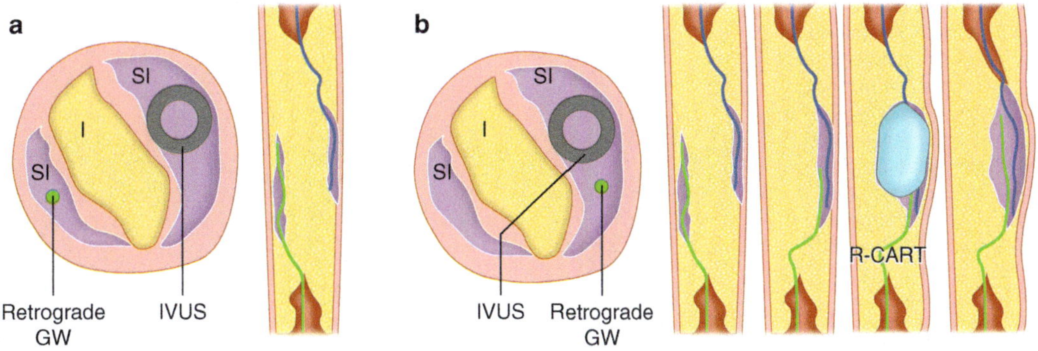

Fig. 13.4 Both guidewires are present in the subintimal space. In this situation, the treatment strategy should be different depending on whether the two guidewires are in the same subintimal space or in completely different subintimal spaces. If two guidewires are in close proximity to the same subintimal space, you can try reverse CART using a balloon of sufficient size (**a**). However, if two guidewires are located far away from each other in a completely different space, it is more likely that the retrograde guidewire will reach the nearest possible space under the supervision of the IVUS and finally complete the reverse CART (**b**). *IVUS* intravascular ultrasound, *GW* guidewire, *R-CART* reverse controlled antegrade and retrograde subintimal tracking, *I* intima, *SI* subintima

retrograde guidewire should be sufficiently rigid and controllable to allow torque control. In the last situation where both guidewires are present in the subintimal space (Fig. 13.4), the treatment strategy should be different depending on whether the two guidewires are in the same subintimal space or in different subintimal spaces. If two guidewires are in close proximity to the same subintimal space, the operator can try reverse CART using a balloon of sufficient size (Fig. 13.4a). However, if two guidewires are located far away from each other in a completely different space, it is more likely that the retrograde guidewire must reach the closest possible space under IVUS supervision and complete the reverse CART (Fig. 13.4b).

If it is confirmed that the two guidewires are located in the same intimal or subintimal space by IVUS or in the close space through a rotational angiogram, the reverse CART technique can be completed by selecting an appropriate size balloon. If the size of the antegrade balloon is small or recoil of the subintimal space occurs after balloon dilation, passage of the retrograde guidewire becomes difficult. Interpretation of IVUS inserted through the antegrade guidewire is helpful in choosing the appropriate balloon size for the size of the vessel and is helpful in determining repeat balloon dilatation or balloon size escalation when recoil occurs.

Despite the reverse CART technique, the retrograde guidewire passage may not be achievable due to the lack of backup support, poor guidewire manipulation, and excessive calcification or bending of CTO segment. In this situation, stent-assisted reverse CART can be performed (Fig. 13.5) [7]. It involves deployment of a stent within the antegradely dissected plane to create open target for retrograde guidewire crossing. At this time, the distal end of the stent should be placed in the same space of the two guidewires, and IVUS helps to determine the proper size, length, and position of the stent.

Currently, contemporary reverse CART technique is one of the preferred technologies (Fig. 13.6). This technique is based on the minimal expansion of the CTO segment using a small antegrade balloon and manipulation of the retrograde guidewire to target it. For the successful result, the retrograde guidewire must have the ability to work as the operator's intention. The Gaia series is preferred guidewire for contemporary reverse CART technique [8]. This technique can reduce unnecessary subintimal space expansion, arterial injury, and the length of subintimal stenting in the CTO segment. This technique can be applied easily if the antegrade balloon is located at the center of the CTO segment (Fig. 13.6a), but it can be applied even if the antegrade balloon is located at the edge of the CTO vessel (Fig. 13.6b).

Fig. 13.5 Stent-assisted reverse CART. Despite the reverse CART technique, the retrograde guidewire passage may not be able because of the lack of backup support, poor guidewire manipulation, or excessive calcification or bending of CTO segment. In this situation, stent-assisted reverse CART can be performed. It involves deployment of a stent within the antegradely dissected plane to create open target for retrograde guidewire crossing. At this time, the distal end of the stent should be placed in the same space of the two guidewires, and IVUS helps to determine the proper size, length, and position of the stent

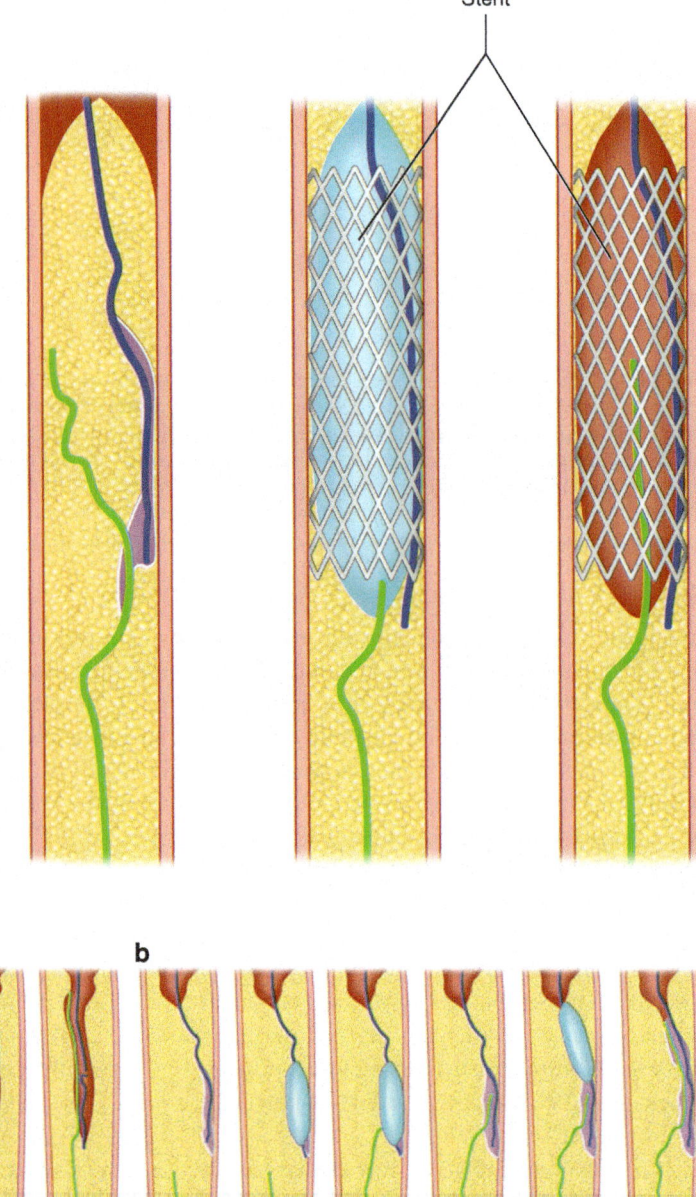

Stent

Fig. 13.6 Contemporary reverse CART technique. This technique minimally expands the CTO segment using a small antegrade balloon and manipulates the retrograde guidewire to target it. For the successful application of this method, the retrograde guidewire must have the ability to operate precisely and intentionally, and the Gaia series is the most appropriate. This can reduce unneces-sary subintimal space expansion, arterial injury, and the length of subintimal stenting in the CTO segment. This method can be applied more easily if the antegrade balloon is located at the center of the CTO segment (**a**), but it can be applied even if the antegrade balloon is located at the edge of the CTO vessel (**b**)

Injecting contrast media through the antegrade guiding catheter should be avoided as far as possible, to avoid flow-induced subintimal dissection. IVUS provides very important clues in the selection of appropriate balloon and stent size. The distal location of the stent can be identified by the distal landing zone observed through contralateral injection, but often it is not possible to obtain sufficient information due to the poor visualization of distal landing zone or other reasons. In this situation, IVUS can be used to accurately identify the size and position of the distal landing zone for stent location [6, 9]. Confirmation of the position of the IVUS catheter in the cine angiogram can be used for determination of stenting location without injecting the contrast agent.

References

1. Surmely JF, Tsuchikane E, Katoh O, Nishida Y, Nakayama M, Nakamura S, Oida A, Hattori E, Suzuki T. New concept for CTO recanalization using controlled antegrade and retrograde subintimal tracking: the CART technique. J Invasive Cardiol. 2006;18:334–8.
2. Hobbs AN, Young RJ. Practical purification of hydrophilic fragments and lead/drug-like molecules by reverse phase flash chromatography: tips, tricks and contemporary developments. Drug Discov Today. 2013;18:148–54.
3. Furuichi S, Satoh T. Intravascular ultrasound-guided retrograde wiring for chronic total occlusion. Catheter Cardiovasc Interv. 2010;75:214–21.
4. Rathore S, Katoh O, Tuschikane E, Oida A, Suzuki T, Takase S. A novel modification of the retrograde approach for the recanalization of chronic total occlusion of the coronary arteriesintravascular ultrasound-guided reverse controlled antegrade and retrograde tracking. JACC Cardiovasc Interv. 2010;3:155–64.
5. Dash D. Retrograde coronary chronic total occlusion intervention. Curr Cardiol Rev. 2015;11(4):291–8.
6. Tsujita K, Maehara A, Mintz GS, Kubo T, Doi H, Lansky AJ, Stone GW, Moses JW, MB L, Ochiai M. Intravascular ultrasound comparison of the retrograde versus antegrade approach to percutaneous intervention for chronic total coronary occlusions. JACC Cardiovasc Interv. 2009;2:846–54.
7. Joyal D, Thompson CA, Grantham JA, Buller CE, Rinfret S. The retrograde technique for recanalization of chronic total occlusions: a step-by-step approach. JACC Cardiovasc Interv. 2012;5:1–11.
8. Khalili H, Vo MN, Brilakis ES. Initial experience with the Gaia composite core guidewires in coronary chronic total occlusion crossing. J Invasive Cardiol. 2016;28:E22–5.
9. Sianos G, Werner GS, Galassi AR, Papafaklis MI, Escaned J, Hildick-Smith D, Christiansen EH, Gershlick A, Carlino M, Karlas A, Konstantinidis NV, Tomasello SD, Di Mario C, Reifart N, Euro CTOC. Recanalisation of chronic total coronary occlusions: 2012 consensus document from the EuroCTO club. EuroIntervention. 2012;8:139–45.

CrossBoss and Stingray System

14

Maoto Habara, Seung-Whan Lee,
and Etsuo Tsuchikane

Over the last decade, interventional cardiologists have globally made tremendous progress in understanding and overcoming conditions associated with chronically occluded coronary arteries. Percutaneous coronary intervention (PCI) of chronic total occlusions (CTO) is a rapidly evolving field. The initial success rate is increasing with the improvements in technology and technique such as the retrograde approach [1]. Recently, antegrade dissection and reentry (ADR) for CTO PCI has also evolved to one of the techniques, especially in USA and Europe [2]. Although there are several ADR techniques including subintimal tracking and reentry (STAR) or the limited antegrade subintimal tracking (LAST) technique, recent ADR can be achieved with the CrossBoss catheter (Boston Scientific, Nattick, Massachusetts) and the Stingray system (Boston Scientific) [3]. In this section, we describe about the CrossBoss and Stingray system designed for CTO crossing and reentry.

The CrossBoss catheter is a stiff, metallic, over-the-wire catheter with a 1 mm blunt, hydrophilic-coated distal tip that can advance

when the catheter is rotated rapidly using a proximal torque device (Fig. 14.1). Figure 14.2 shows the illustration of the Stingray CTO reentry system, with its two components; the Stingray CTO orienting balloon catheter and the Stingray CTO reentry guidewire. At first, the CrossBoss catheter enters the subintimal space and advance through the occlusion length (Fig. 14.3a). It creates a limited dissection plane making reentry into the distal true lumen easier. Then the CrossBoss catheter is retracted leaving the guidewire past the occlusion. The Stingray balloon catheter is advanced and inflated up to 3–4 atm within the subintimal space (Fig. 14.3b). A contralateral angiography is performed to pinpoint balloon-vessel relationship and Stingray guidewire is directed and exited through the luminal port, with a direct puncture technique (stick and drive technique) (Fig. 14.3c). On the other hand, *Stick and Swap technique* is also frequently used. Access the distal vessel with the Stingray wire (Strike across) withdraw and remove (Fig. 14.4a). The Stingray balloon remains aligned with the created channel from false to true lumen. Shape a polymer jacketed wire with a 45°angle mm from the tip. Advance the wire and replicate the reentry steps. If connection was made during the "stick," the polymer wire will follow the channel and be able to navigate the distal vessel (Fig. 14.4b). Stick and Swap technique is usually performed in the presence of tortuosity or atheroma in the

M. Habara · E. Tsuchikane
Department of Cardiology, Toyohashi Heart Center, Toyohashi, Aichi, Japan

S.-W. Lee (✉)
Department of Cardiology, Asan Medical Center, University of Ulsan College of Medicine, Seoul, South Korea
e-mail: seungwlee@amc.seoul.kr

© Springer Nature Singapore Pte Ltd. 2019
Y. Jang (ed.), *Percutaneous Coronary Interventions for Chronic Total Occlusion*,
https://doi.org/10.1007/978-981-10-6026-7_14

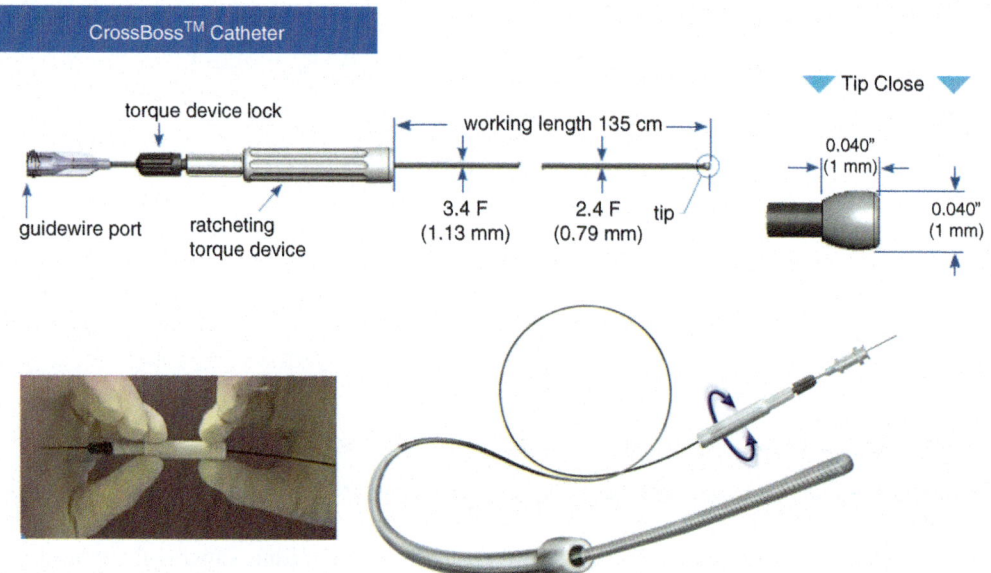

Fig. 14.1 Illustration of the CrossBoss catheter, which is an over-the-wire device with a 1 mm rounded tip, a coiled shaft, and a moveable proximal torque device that releases under high torque to prevent product damage. Fast-spin device allows rapid rotation of the catheter to facilitate crossing. Multi-wire coiled shaft provides precise turn-for-turn torque response. Atraumatic, rounded tip reduces risk of perforation. 0.014 in. (0.36 mm) guidewire compatible. 6Fr (2.0 mm) guide catheter compatible

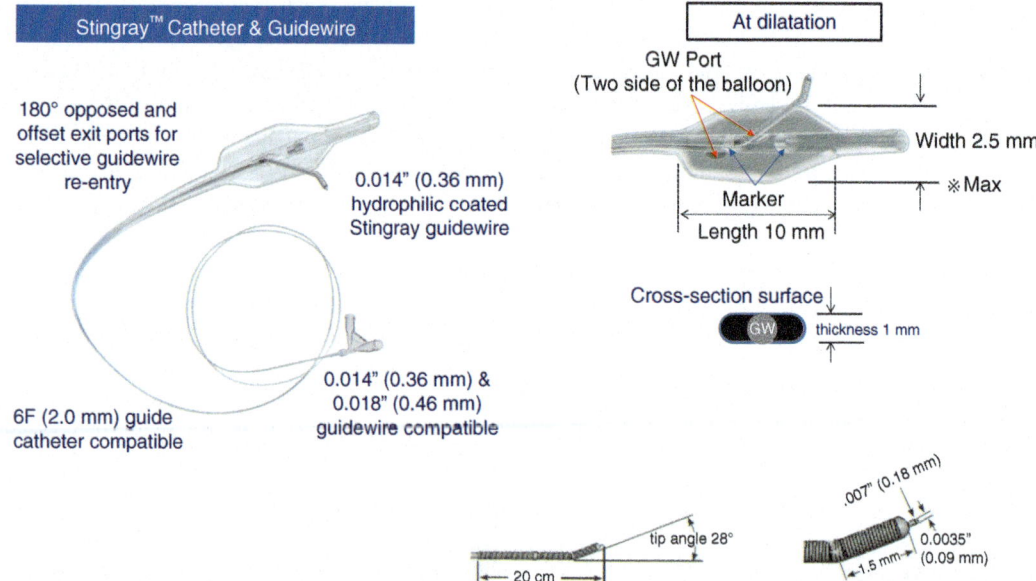

Fig. 14.2 Illustration of the Stingray chronic total occlusion (CTO) reentry system. The system is composed of the Stingray CTO balloon catheter and the Stingray CTO reentry guide wire. The Stingray balloon has two side exit ports located on diametrically opposite balloon surfaces (red allows) immediately proximal to two radiopaque markers (blue allows). The flat shape of the balloon orients one exit port automatically toward the vessel true lumen upon low-pressure inflation (2–4 atm). The Stingray guide wire has a 0.0035 in. distal taper allowing it to reenter the true vessel lumen through the exit port of the Stingray balloon after subintimal passage of the guide wire. Self-orienting, flat balloon hugs the vessel, automatically positioning one exit port toward the true lumen. 180°opposed and offsetting exit ports enable selective guidewire reentry. Stingray guidewire's angled tip and distal probe are designed for facilitated reentry into the true lumen. Two radiopaque marker bands for exact placement

a Advance CrossBoss catheter through occlusion site

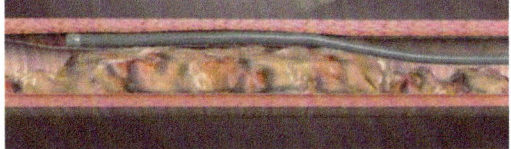

b Advance Stingray balloon and inflated

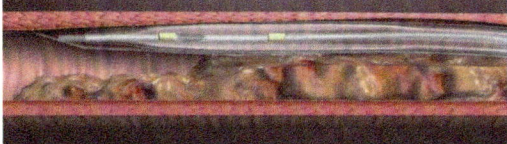

c Access the distal vessel with the Stingray wire

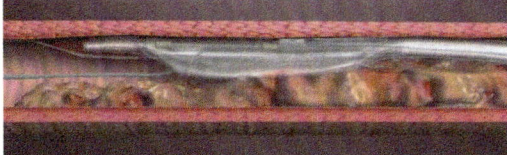

Fig. 14.3 Illustration of The CrossBoss catheter and the Stingray system procedure; stick and drive technique (direct puncture)

reentry zone. We show the typical CTO case succeeded with these devices in Fig. 14.5.

Brilakis et al. described a PCI algorithm for CTO, referred to as the hybrid algorithm [4]. In the hybrid approach to CTO PCI, ADR is recommended as the initial crossing strategy in CTOs with unambiguous proximal cap and good quality distal vessel, when the occlusion length is estimated to be ≥20 mm [5, 6]. Recently RECHARGE registry (n = 1253 CTO PCI) in Europe demonstrated that the adoption of hybrid algorithm improved overall success rate up to 86%, in which ADR (wire-based or device based) was used in 7% (88 cases) as primary strategy and 23% (292 cases) as further strategy including primary (88 cases) and bailout strategy (210 cases). Overall use of controlled ADR using combined CrossBoss-Stingray system was only 7.4% (93/1253), of which 81% were successful [7, 8]. In the meanwhile, although there are many excellent recommendations within the hybrid algorithm, there has

Fig. 14.4 Illustration of stick and swap technique

a Stick   **b** Swap

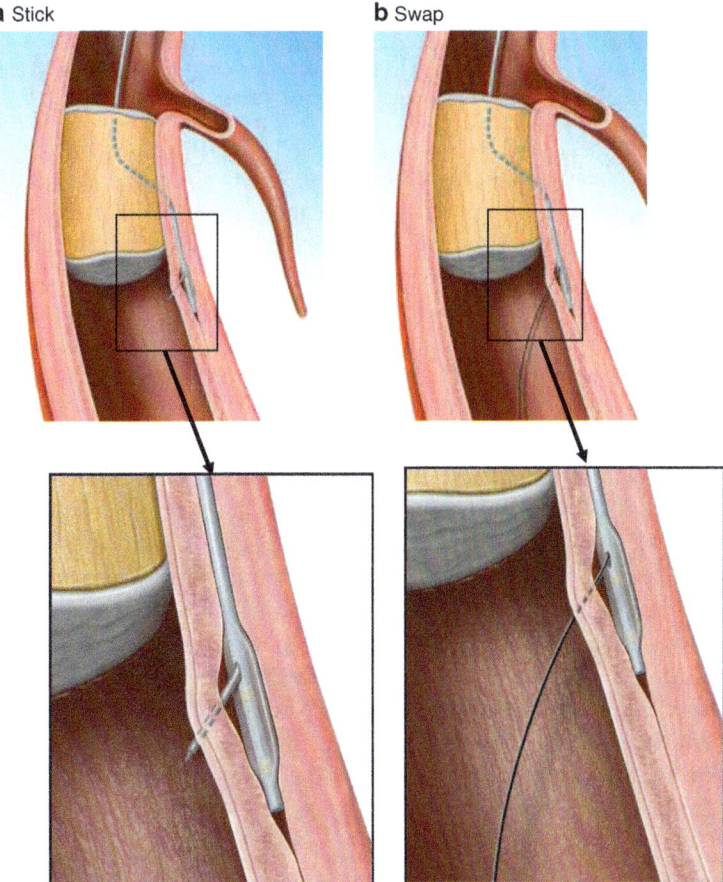

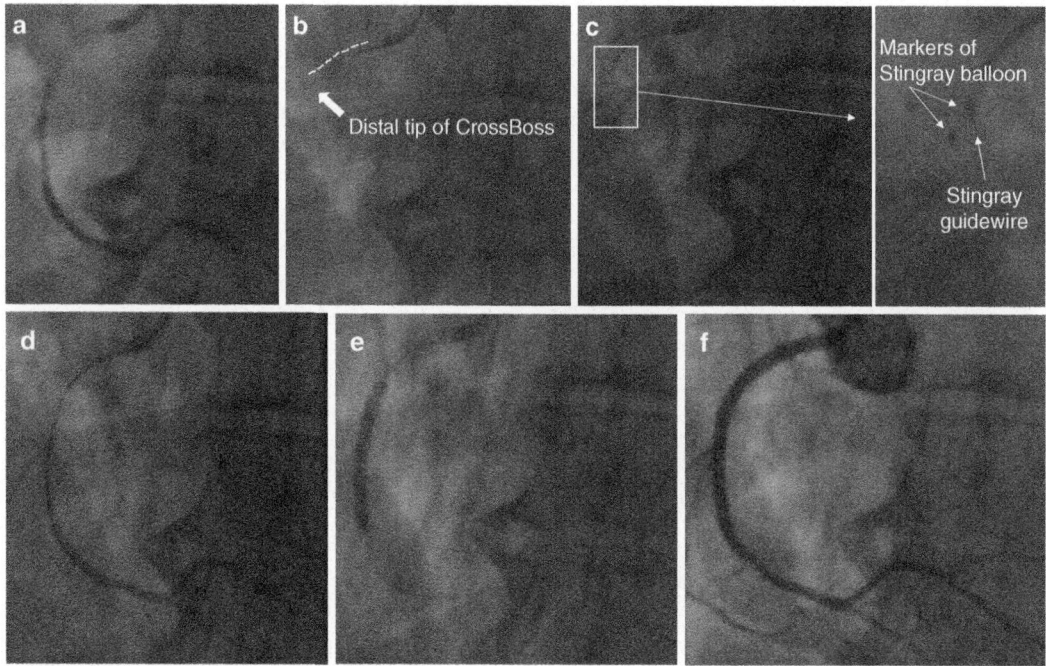

Fig. 14.5 (a) Chronic total occlusion of right coronary artery proximal. (b) CrossBoss catheter was entered into the CTO subintimal space and advanced beyond the CTO site. (c) CrossBoss was removed and changed to the Stingray balloon. The Stingray balloon catheter is advanced and inflated within the subintimal space. (d) A contralateral angiography is performed to pinpoint balloon-vessel relationship, and Stingray guidewire is directed and exited through the luminal port, with a direct puncture technique (stick and drive technique). (e) Implanted stent. (f) Final angiography

been infrequent adoption of that in the Asia Pacific region, because in our region, the traditional wire-based CTO procedure including retrograde approach is dominant and limited access to the CrossBoss and Stingray system which eliminates the ADR arm of the hybrid algorithm. Actually, the success rate of CTO PCI was already about 86–90% without those devices in our region [9, 10, 11]. In addition, although ADR techniques appears safe, they still carry risk for coronary perforation (0.4–14.3%) and periprocedural myocardial infarction because of side branch occlusion (2.4–16.0%) [2]. A certain degree of branch occlusion is another inevitable technique consequence, and branch occlusion-induced myonecrosis can be a source of future adverse events [12]. Especially, CrossBoss sometimes make coronary perforation because the device is usually advanced blindly and go into small side branch (Fig. 14.6). Moreover, there are currently no long-term fol-

low-up data with these devices. Therefore, the use of ADR with the Stingray system may be limited in a new algorithm from the Asia Pacific CTO (AP-CTO) club [13]. In the AP-CTO algorithm, ADR is only recommended when antegrade wire escalation failed and there is no interventional collateral for retrograde approach. Moreover, a relatively disease-free reentry zone, close proximity of the antegrade wire to the distal true lumen, and the absence of severe calcification in the reentry zone might be necessary for success. Hence, CrossBoss catheter may be needed for ADR as the second- or third-line techniques in AP-CTO algorithm. A case with LAD-CTO treated by ADR was shown in Fig. 14.7.

Although CrossBoss might be needed for ADR, the device should be considered as the first-line device for recanalization of occlusive in-stent restenosis in AP-CTO algorithm [13, 14]. The advantage of the CrossBoss is that its blunt

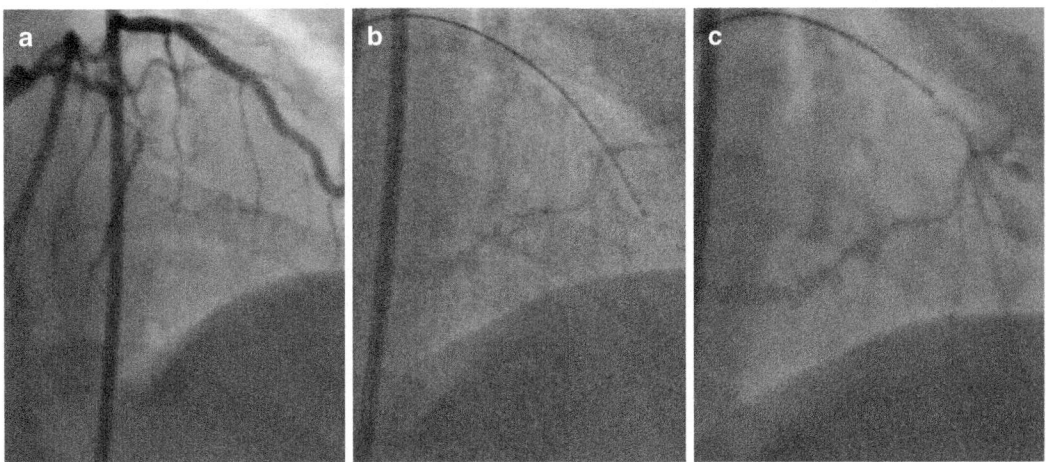

Fig. 14.6 Coronary perforation due to CrossBoss. (**a**) Chronic total occlusion of left anterior descending artery. (**b**) CrossBoss was advanced through CTO site. (**c**) Contralateral angiography revealed coronary perforation

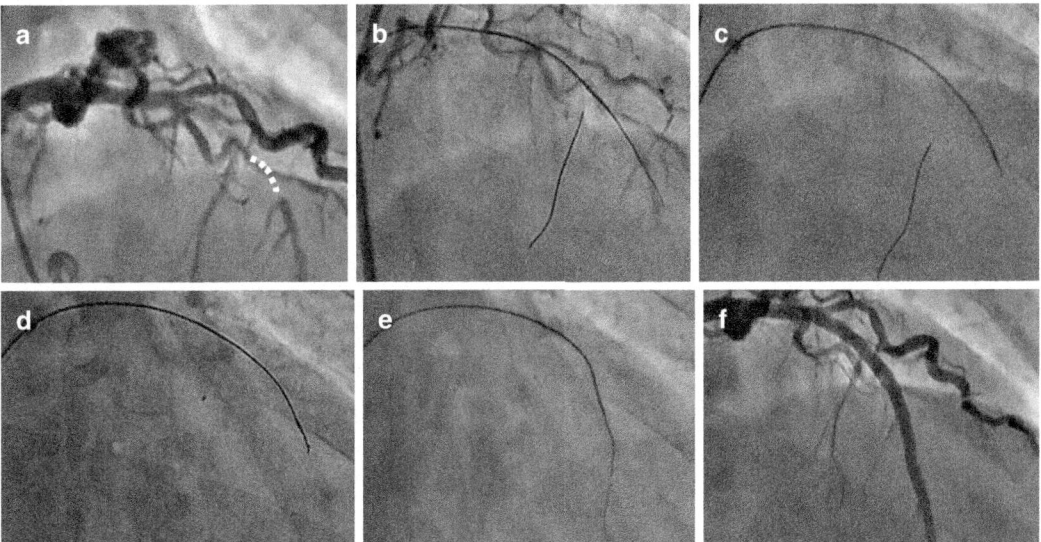

Fig. 14.7 (**a**) Chronic total occlusion of LAD (white line). (**b**) Failure of antegrade wire escalation (Gaia second and third). (**c**) Failure of retrograde approach and advance Corsair micro-catheter instead of CrossBoss. (**d**) Access the distal vessel with the Stingray wire and removed. (**e**) Advance the Fielder XTR wire to navigate the distal vessel through the channel which was made by Stingray guidewire (Stick & Swap). (**f**) Final angiography

rounded tip generally prevents the device from going outside of stent struts, which results in either inability to cross with a devices or deformation of the previously placed stent.

Improving dissection and reentry techniques and successfully adopting them to coronary arteries have undeniably resulted in dealing with more complex CTOs, particularly benefiting some postcoronary artery bypass grafting patients. Thus, this technique should not be abandoned because it is an important addition to the CTO toolbox. However, we need more evidence, particularly long-term evidence, to support its use as a primary strategy.

References

1. Rathore S, Matsuo H, Terashima M, Kinoshita Y, Kimura M, Tsuchikane E, Nasu K, Ehara M, Asakura Y, Katoh O, Suzuki T. Procedural and in-hospital outcomes after percutaneous coronary intervention for chronic total occlusions of coronary arteries 2002 to 2008: impact of novel guidewire techniques. JACC Cardiovasc Interv. 2009;2:489–97.

2. Michael TT, Papayannis AC, Banerjee S, Brilakis ES. Subintimal dissection/reentry strategies in coronary chronic total occlusion interventions. Circ Cardiovasc Interv. 2012;5:729–38.

3. Whitlow PL, Burke MN, Lombardi WL, Wyman RM, Moses JW, Brilakis ES, Heuser RR, Rihal CS, Lansky AJ, Thompson CA, FAST-CTOs Trial Investigators. Use of a novel crossing and re-entry system in coronary chronic total occlusions that have failed standard crossing techniques: results of the FAST-CTOs (Facilitated Antegrade Steering Technique in Chronic Total Occlusions) trial. JACC Cardiovasc Interv. 2012;5:393–401.

4. Brilakis ES, Banerjee S, Karmpaliotis D, Lombardi WL, Tsai TT, Shunk KA, Kennedy KF, Spertus JA, Holmes DR Jr, Grantham JA. Procedural outcomes of chronic total occlusion percutaneous coronary intervention: a report from the NCDR (National Cardiovascular Data Registry). JACC Cardiovasc Interv. 2015;8:245–53.

5. Brilakis ES, Grantham JA, Rinfret S, Wyman RM, Burke MN, Karmpaliotis D, Lembo N, Pershad A, Kandzari DE, Buller CE, DeMartini T, Lombardi WL, Thompson CA. A percutaneous treatment algorithm for crossing coronary chronic total occlusions. JACC Cardiovasc Interv. 2012;5:367–79.

6. Rangan BV, Kotsia A, Christopoulos G, Spratt J, Rinfret S, Banerjee S, Brilakis ES. The hybrid approach for intervention of chronic total occlusions. Curr Cardiol Rev. 2015;11(4):299–304.

7. Maeremans J, Walsh S, Knaapen P, Spratt JC, Avran A, Hanratty CG, Faurie B, Agostoni P, Bressollette E, Kayaert P, Bagnall AJ, Egred M, Smith D, Chase A, McEntegart MB, Smith WH, Harcombe A, Kelly P, Irving J, Smith EJ, Strange JW, Dens J. The hybrid algorithm for treating chronic total occlusions in Europe: The RECHARGE Registry. J Am Coll Cardiol. 2016;68:1958–70.

8. Maeremans J, Dens J, Spratt JC, Bagnall AJ, Stuijfzand W, Nap A, Agostoni P, Wilson W, Hanratty CG, Wilson S, Faurie B, Avran A, Bressollette E, Egred M, Knaapen P, Walsh S, Investigators RECHARGE. Antegrade dissection and reentry as part of the hybrid chronic total occlusion revascularization strategy: a subanalysis of the RECHARGE Registry (Registry of CrossBoss and hybrid procedures in France, the Netherlands, Belgium and United Kingdom). Circ Cardiovasc Interv. 2017;10(6) https://doi.org/10.1161/CIRCINTERVENTIONS.116.004791.

9. Lee PH, Lee SW, Park HS, Kang SH, Bae BJ, Chang M, Roh JH, Yoon SH, Ahn JM, Park DW, Kang SJ, Kim YH, Lee CW, Park SW, Park SJ. Successful recanalization of native coronary chronic total occlusion is not associated with improved long-term survival. JACC Cardiovasc Interv. 2016;9:530–8.

10. Habara M, Tsuchikane E, Muramatsu T, Kashima Y, Okamura A, Mutoh M, Yamane M, Oida A, Oikawa Y, Hasegawa K, Retrograde Summit Investigators. Comparison of percutaneous coronary intervention for chronic total occlusion outcome according to operator experience from the Japanese retrograde summit registry. Catheter Cardiovasc Interv. 2016;87:1027–35.

11. Suzuki Y, Tsuchikane E, Katoh O, et al. Outcomes of percutaneous coronary interventions for chronic total occlusion performed by highly experienced Japanese specialists: the first report from the Japanese CTO-PCI Expert Registry. JACC Cardiovasc Interv. 2017;10(21):2144–54.

12. Lee SW, Lee PH, Kang SH, Choi H, Chang M, Roh JH, Yoon SH, Ahn JM, Park DW, Kang SJ, Kim YH, Lee CW, Park SW, Park SJ. Determinants and prognostic significance of periprocedural myocardial injury in patients with successful percutaneous chronic total occlusion interventions. JACC Cardiovasc Interv. 2016;9:2220–8.

13. Harding SA, Wu EB, Lo S, et al. A new algorithm for crossing chronic total occlusions from the Asia Pacific Chronic Total Occlusion Club. JACC Cardiovasc Interv. 2017;10(21):2135–43.

14. Wilson WM, Walsh S, Hanratty C, et al. A novel approach to the management of occlusive in-stent restenosis (ISR). EuroIntervention. 2014;9:1285–93.

Tips and Tricks of Successful Stent Delivery and Implantation

15

Chang-Hwan Yoon

Chronic total occlusion (CTO) is a challenging lesion to cardiologists with limited success rate. The most difficult procedure is to pass a wire through the occluded lesion [1]. However, it is sometimes difficult to deliver devices along the positioned wire. This chapter overviews tips and tricks of successful stent delivery and implantation for the CTO intervention.

The huddles to interrupt stent delivery and implantation are calcification, tortuosity, poor guiding catheter backup, threaded multiple wires, and presence of previous stent. All of them cause significant resistance and hinder the passage of stent through the lesion.

To overcome the resistance, stronger backup force of guiding catheter is necessary [2]. We can increase the diameter of guiding catheter. For this purpose, femoral approach is better than radial approach because we can use up to 8 Fr. via femoral sheath compared to maximal 6 Fr. via radial sheath or 6.5 Fr. by sheathless radial technique. If JL4 guiding catheter is used, adequate positioning is important to optimize direction to meet coaxial alignment and secondary curve position seated on ascending aortic wall and proper tip engagement into the left main

ostium. Extra-backup (EBU) or Amplatz catheter is a good choice for the strong backup.

Anchor balloon technique is a good option to increase guiding catheter backup force [3]. In RCA intervention, RV branch, sinoatrial node artery, or conus branch can be selected by additional soft tip wire, and 2.0 mm or larger plain balloon is inserted to the distal part of the branch. In left coronary artery intervention, diagonal branch, distal left anterior descending artery, obtuse marginal branch, or distal left circumflex artery can be selected. If there is a previously inserted stent, it is a good anchoring point with the same size balloon catheter. During the balloon inflation, we can check the anchoring force of the balloon by slightly pulling back the balloon catheter. If the anchoring force is sufficient, we can adjust the engagement of a guiding catheter into the ostium and then deliver a stent through the resistant lesion. While delivering the stent, it is important to maintain the anchoring force of the balloon catheter by counterbalancing the pullback force against the pushing force to deliver the stent (Fig. 15.1).

Conventionally mother-and-daughter catheter technique is another way to increase the backup force of the guiding catheter. Especially when the engagement of a guiding catheter is not adjusted and the wire is buckled during pushing the stent hard, deep engagement of a daughter catheter into the target vessel greatly increase backup force and wire support to deliver the stent. Recently, guide extension catheters are available for this purpose. Guidezilla™ from Boston

C.-H. Yoon (✉)
Division of Cardiology, Department of Internal Medicine, Seoul National University Bundang Hospital, Seongnam, South Korea
e-mail: kunson2@snu.ac.kr

© Springer Nature Singapore Pte Ltd. 2019
Y. Jang (ed.), *Percutaneous Coronary Interventions for Chronic Total Occlusion*,
https://doi.org/10.1007/978-981-10-6026-7_15

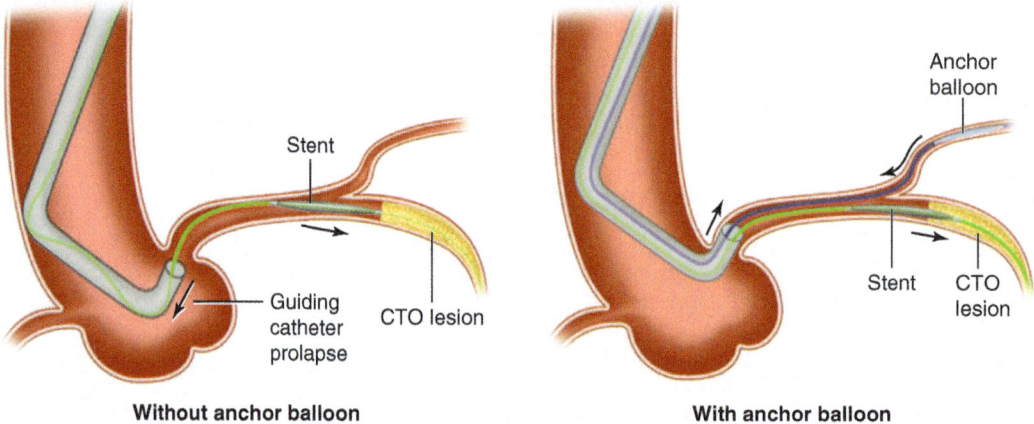

Fig. 15.1 Anchor balloon technique

Scientific and GuideLiner™ from Vascular Solution are designed to access discrete regions of the coronary and/or peripheral vasculature in conjunction with guide catheters and to facilitate placement of interventional devices [4]. We can backload the guide extension catheter onto the guidewire (0.014″) and advance through the hemostasis valve and into the guide catheter. Under fluoroscopy, we advance the guide extension catheter beyond the distal end of the guide catheter and into the desired location within the vessel. And then backload the stent over the in-place guidewire and advance it through guide catheter and the guide extension catheter into the desired lesion [5]. Upon completion of the intervention, we need to remove the guide extension catheter prior to removing the guide catheter from the vessel (Fig. 15.2).

To deliver stent through a heavily calcified lesion, adequate modification of the lesion is essential. Sustained dilation of the stenosis should be gained by predilatation before stent delivery. Repeated and long-term balloon inflation is necessary to modify heavily calcified lesion. Balloon inflation with multiple wires in situ or a cutting balloon help to crack the calcified lesion and obtain an adequate predilatation. Sometimes, lesion dilatation is not possible due to the heavy calcification. In this case, Rotablator is a good option [6]. If small balloon is pas-

saged, then predilatation was done and flow is observed, it is not a hard task to change the passaged wire (0.014″) to Rotablator wire (0.009″). However, if any device was not passed through the lesion except wire, it would be challenging to change the present wire to a Rotablator wire. In addition, rotablation to the occluded lesion is off-label use of Rotablator. But in some case reports, they demonstrated rotablation to the dead-end vessel and then successful stent delivery. Not only undilated lesion but also broken calcification or calcification with abrupt angulation is a difficult lesion through which we had difficulty in delivering stent. In these cases, a Rotablator often successfully modifies the lesions and help to deliver the stent as well as adequately expand the stent within the lesion (Fig. 15.3).

To overcome severe tortuosity, we can use several methods. High backup force using anchor balloon technique or guide extension catheter helps stent delivery. Inserting the second or third wires (buddy wire technique) increase wire support and straighten the tortuous vessel leading to successful stent delivery. We can also change a wire to another wire with higher support power such as Asahi Grand Slam wire and CHOICE Extra Support (ES) wire. A wire with high support power is usually hard to navigate a tortuous vessel. Therefore, it would be better to exchange

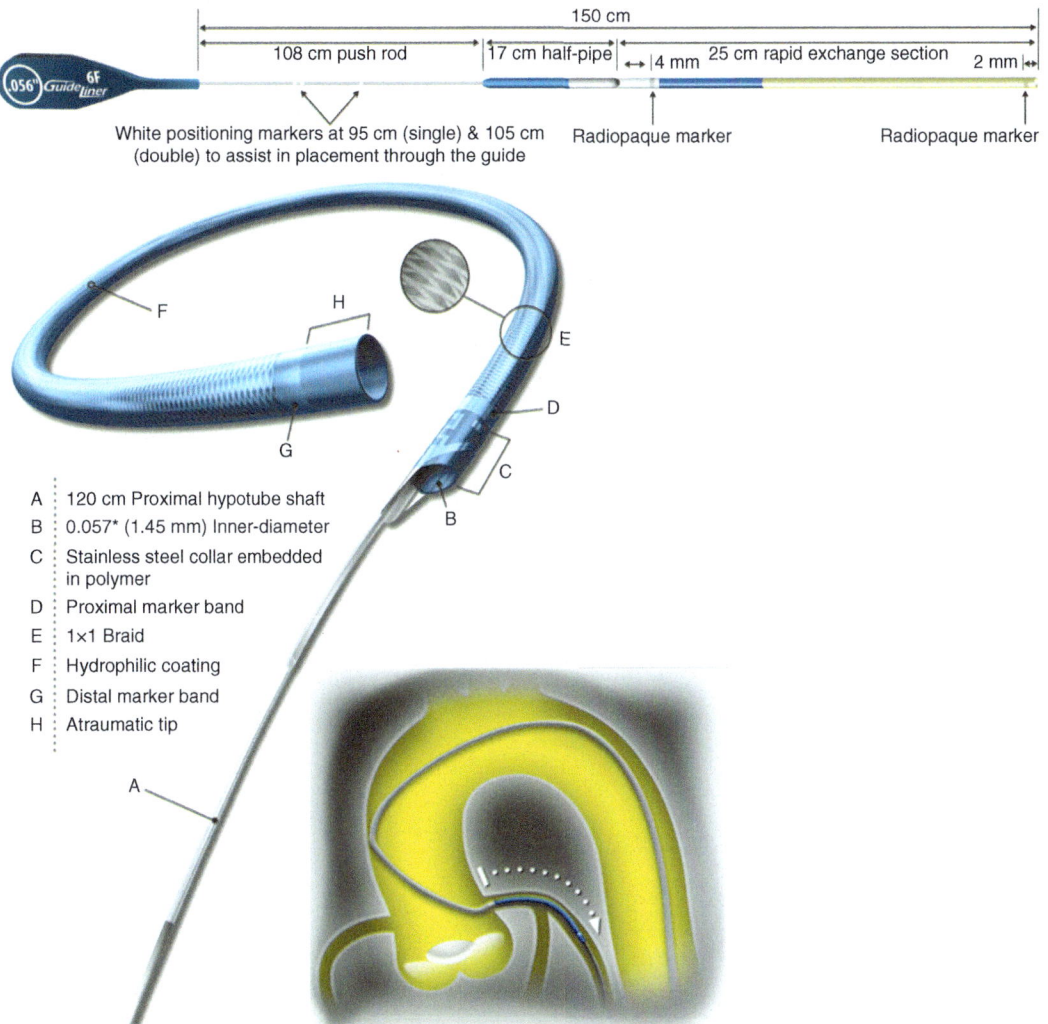

Fig. 15.2 Guide extension catheter

the wire using a microcatheter. If the tortuosity is not severe but hard to deliver a stent because of calcification, it would be better to modify the vessel using Rotablator.

If multivessel procedure is performed with multiple wires, the wires are sometimes threaded tightly and hinder stent delivery through them. In this case, wires should be drawn except the wire in the target lesion. To avoid this situation, one should be careful not to rotate a wire much while inserting a second or a third wire and not to thread the wires during procedure.

If there is a previous stent on the path to the target lesion, a protruded strut into the lumen area is a cause of stent delivery failure. In this case, repeated, high-pressure balloon angioplasty at the highly resistant point in the previous stent is necessary to smoothen the delivery pathway. Too much pushing or retrieving force sometimes peel off the stent from the balloon catheter and lead to a serious complication, stent loss in the coronary artery. Therefore, one should be careful not to exert too much force while passing the previous stent as well as highly calcified lesion.

Fig. 15.3 Rotablator

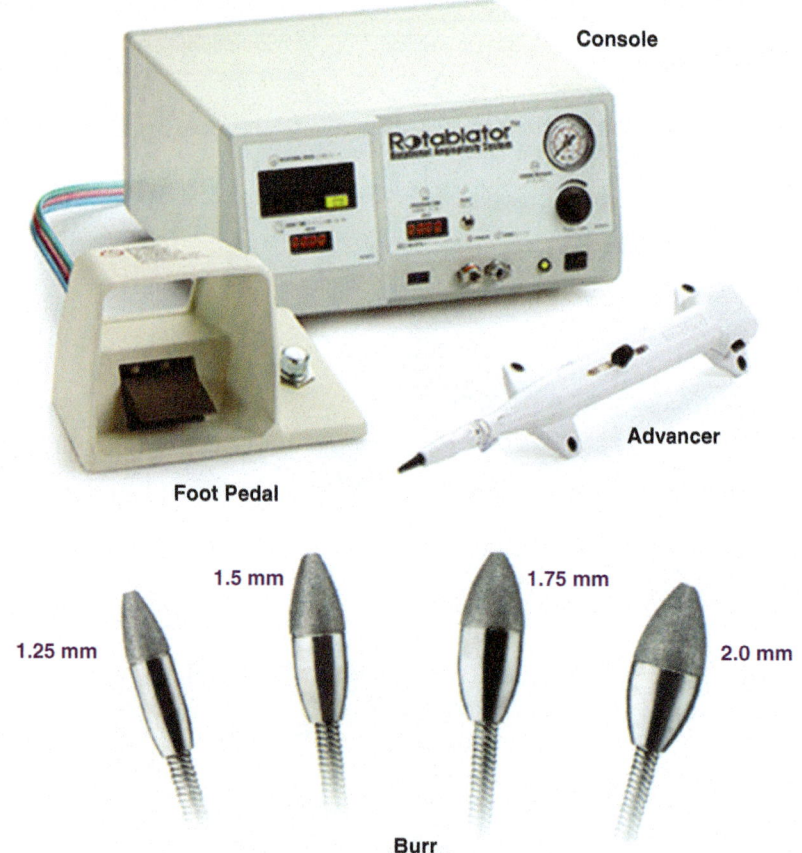

References

1. Harding SA, Wu EB, Lo S, Lim ST, Ge L, Chen JY, Quan J, Lee SW, Kao HL, Tsuchikane E. A new algorithm for crossing chronic total occlusions from the asia pacific chronic total occlusion club. JACC Cardiovasc Interv. 2017;10:2135–43.
2. Yokoi K, Hara M, Ueda Y, Sumitsuji S, Awata M, Salah YK, Kabata D, Shintani A, Sakata Y. Ideal guiding catheter position during bilaterally engaged percutaneous coronary intervention. Am J Cardiol. 2017;119:1518–24.
3. Fujita S, Tamai H, Kyo E, Kosuga K, Hata T, Okada M, Nakamura T, Tsuji T, Takeda S, Bin Hu F, Masunaga N, Motohara S, Uehata H. New technique for superior guiding catheter support during advancement of a balloon in coronary angioplasty: the anchor technique. Catheter Cardiovasc Interv. 2003;59:482–8.
4. Sharma D, Shah A, Osten M, Ing D, Barolet A, Overgaard CB, Dzavik V, Seidelin PH. Efficacy and safety of the guideliner mother-in-child guide catheter extension in percutaneous coronary intervention. J Interv Cardiol. 2017;30:46–55.
5. Yang H, Dai Y, Li C, Lu H, Chang S, Qian J, Ge J. Two cases of successful revascularization of chronic total occlusions by the first use of a new guide extension catheter in unbelievable tortuous right coronary arteries. Int J Cardiol. 2016;223:98–100.
6. Reisman M, Buchbinder M. Rotational ablation. The rotablator catheter. Cardiol Clin. 1994;12:595–610.

Complications of CTO PCI and How to Manage and Prevent

16

Seung-Woon Rha

16.1 Introduction

Many special devices such as dedicated chronic total occlusion (CTO) wires, microcatheters, daughter catheters, tornus, intravascular ultrasound, and rotablators are currently used for the complete recanalization. Further, bigger guiding catheters are frequently used for stronger backup support for the aggressive recanalization. CTO lesion itself is frequently associated with heavily calcified, dense, and hard tissue. All of these components are associated with higher incidence of complications as compared to usual percutaneous coronary intervention (PCI).

In clinical aspects, CTO patients usually have higher incidence of combined coronary risk factors such as diabetes, hypertension, hyperlipidemia, and history of myocardial infarction (MI). CTO patients usually have worse lesion characteristics such as multivessel and multi-lesion disease and reduced ejection fraction (EF). Thus, every operator should understand all the possible complications related to CTO PCI before starting the procedure, should do their best to prevent the complications, and should be ready to safely manage any unexpected complication developed during the CTO PCI.

There are series of complications associated with CTO PCI such as radiation hazard (dermati-

tis and cancer development), contrast nephropathy, and local complications including dissection, perforation, rupture, device entrapment (stent entrapment, migration, and loss), and retrograde CTO PCI-related complications. In this chapter, I would like to focus on the prevention and management of immediate procedure-related complications.

16.2 Dissection

16.2.1 Guiding Catheter-Induced Dissection

Most of the CTO PCI procedures require strong guiding catheter backup support for aggressive CTO wire manipulation and device passage such as balloons and stents. EBU and XB curve for left coronary and AL and RBU curve for right coronary are frequently used. Physicians tend to use bigger diameter guiding catheter such as 7F or 8F for complex CTO PCI, and this larger bore guiding catheter can provide more injury to ostial left main (LM) or ostial right coronary artery (RCA). Because many patients with CTO lesion have multivessel disease including ostial area, forceful guiding manipulation such as "deep intubation" maneuver and subsequent contrast injection can make iatrogenic coronary dissection. Further, side-branch anchoring to enhance guiding catheter support will give more stress to ostial area by

S.-W. Rha (✉)
Korea University Guro Hospital, Seoul, South Korea
e-mail: swrha617@korea.ac.kr

© Springer Nature Singapore Pte Ltd. 2019
Y. Jang (ed.), *Percutaneous Coronary Interventions for Chronic Total Occlusion*,
https://doi.org/10.1007/978-981-10-6026-7_16

guiding catheter. So prevention of guiding catheter or contrast injection induced intimal dissection in risk lesion subset would be particularly important for the safety of CTO PCI.

If unexpected huge dissection developed, how can we manage this complication? All effort to maintain guidewire is important for quick stenting to cover the dissection flap. Full expansion and coverage of dissection entry point is important to prevent further dissection and additional dissection beyond stent struts by contrast injection. If the physician lost the guidewire and the flow limitation developed, this situation would be true emergency. Quick rescue rewiring and subsequent stenting or emergency bypass surgery would be required. Successful rewiring can be done according to my tips based on personal experience (Dr. Rha's tips and tricks).

1. Gentle contrast injection at two different angles from a remote area to see the dissection course.
2. There will be irregular slit-like dense contrast media line, showing intraluminal course.
3. Select hydrophilic well controllable wire such as Sion blue or black to select the true lumen channel.
4. Wiring with two different angle reference views with probing side branch will lead to successful intraluminal wiring. Free distal tip motion without any resistance by dissection flap by tactile sense shows high probability of intraluminal wiring.
5. If antegrade angiography guided rewiring is failed, intravascular ultrasound (IVUS) guided rewiring or reentering to true lumen will be helpful.
6. If antegrade wiring by angiography guided and/or IVUS guided failed, and patient is hemodynamically stable, retrograde intraluminal wiring will ultimately seal all the dissection flap.
7. Once successful wiring is done, IVUS confirmation or small ballooning would be safe to ultimately check the intraluminal wire course before stenting.

Retrograde aortocoronary dissection combined with flow limitation to coronary arteries by dissection flap or acute thrombosis can lead to acute myocardial infarction, cardiogenic shock, and high chance of sudden cardiac death. This situation requires quick LM stenting to secure the distal flow and prevent retrograde aortic dissection progression. However, the following conditions despite of LM stenting would require emergency surgery:

1. Severe aortic regurgitation
2. Involvement of supraaortic vessels
3. Progression of index dissection

16.2.2 Guidewire-Induced Dissection

Dedicated CTO wires have sharp tip with enhanced penetration force which can injure the vessel including intimal dissection and perforation. Recently, the retrograde approach is increasing, and associated collateral channel damage in septal or epicardial channels by guidewires is increasing.

In general, coronary dissection during CTO PCI can be classified as follows (Table 16.1) [1]:

Coronary dissection risk during CTO PCI will be increased if the CTO length is long, tortuous, angulated, and calcified CTO lesion. The stiffer

Table 16.1 National Heart, Lung, and Blood Institute classification system for coronary dissection

Feature	Definition
A	Minor radiolucency within the coronary lumen with minimal or no persistence after dye clearance
B	Parallel track or double lumen separated by a radiolucent area during contrast injection with minimal or no persistence after dye clearance
C	Extraluminal cap with persistence of contrast after dye injection
D	Spiral shape filling defects
E	New persistent intraluminal filling defects
F	Dissection leading to total occlusion without distal antegrade flow

the CTO wire, the dissection extension risk will be increased.

During aggressive antegrade CTO wiring either by single wire or parallel wire technique, antegrade contrast injection should be avoided to prevent further intimal dissection induced by guidewires. Antegrade wiring effectiveness should be guided by contralateral injection. If the guidewire reentry from the dissected false lumen to true lumen is difficult, IVUS-guided reentering might be an excellent strategy.

Regardless of wire-induced dissection extent, prolonged balloon inflation with adequate size will calm down the most of the dissection flap. Sometimes, intimal dissection can cause acute thrombosis or can be associated with acute thrombosis or can be a source of acute thrombosis. So adequate anticoagulation during the procedure is important. Intracoronary thrombolysis can be performed with urokinase if acute thrombosis develop.

If the medical therapy and prolong balloon dilation cannot calm down the wire-induced dissection, subsequent stenting will be necessary. If there is a dissection by balloon dilation or stenting, additional stenting to cover the dissected proximal or distal edge will be recommended when the residual stenosis is more than 50% or the dissection location is in risky area such as LM bifurcation and ostial are.

16.3 Perforation

One of the common complications during CTO PCI is coronary perforation, and the incidence is reported as 2% in CTO PCI [2, 3]. Perforation can be developed during aggressive CTO wiring or by ballooning or stenting.

16.3.1 Guidewire-Induced Perforation

Dedicated CTO wires are frequently used during CTO PCI, and this can be associated with higher incidence of wire-induced perforation during the procedure. Fluoroscopy with better image resolution, coronary MDCT, and IVUS-guided wiring could reduce the wire-induced injury by safe guidance of stiffer CTO wires in contemporary CTO PCI era. However, the longer the target CTO lesion, severely angulated and calcified lesion, still there is an increased risk of wire-induced perforation. Particularly if distal stump is relatively short and narrow, the risk of distal perforation by CTO wire will be increased. If the perforation site is within the main CTO segment or epicardial portion with atherosclerotic plaque burden, prolonged balloon inflation will seal the perforation. However, far distal wire-induced perforation will frequently make pericardial tamponade and need urgent management including emergent pericardiocentesis and hemostasis by coil or gelfoam embolization.

These days, as the number of retrograde CTO PCI is increasing, the wire-induced injury is also increasing. Septal channel injuries by retrograde wires are usually benign and regress spontaneously; however, injury to epicardial channels has higher chance to lead to pericardial tamponade. Too much aggressive wiring through the "corkscrew appearance" epicardial channel tracking would be dangerous.

During and after the wiring, operator should check whether there are wire-induced injuries with adequate amount of contrast injection. If there is suspicious sign of wire-induced extravasation or perforation, careful hemodynamic monitoring and bedside echocardiography examination are essential to confirm.

How can we manage the wire-induced perforation?

First of all, adjustment of medication is important. Antithrombotics should be discontinued, and protamine sulfate, reversal for heparin, should be given. Protamine sulfate 1 mg/25 unit of heparin for the first 4 h and then 25–50 mg/h to achieve the ACT level less than 150 s.

1. Epicardial artery perforation
   Immediate prolonged balloon inflation at perforation site usually can seal the wire-induced perforation. Prolonged inflation at 2–6 atm with

balloon/artery ratio = 0.9–1.0 for at least 10 min is recommended. If the perforation is not completely sealed, more ballooning using "perfusion balloon" for more than 20 min and recheck. Unfortunately, the perfusion balloon is not available in Korea. If the injured epicardial artery reference is bigger than 2.75 mm and balloon tamponade is not successful, immediate graft stenting would be required for ultimate hemostasis.

2. Distal artery, retrograde channel, and side branch injury

   Because ballooning cannot be done in small distal epicardial artery or side branches, immediate embolization using coils, gelfoam, or even autogenous fat tissue harvested at groin puncture area can be effective.

3. Hemodynamic monitoring and periodic bedside echocardiography examination

   During the perforation management, operator should closely monitor the vital signs, and quick bedside echocardiographic examination is essential to confirm the amount of hemopericardium. If the amount is large enough to drain, I strongly recommend the "autotransfusion," immediate infusion of drained blood into femoral vein route (5F short sheath to femoral vein). This will improve hemodynamic instability and will minimize the risk of multiple transfusion.

16.3.2 Balloon- or Stent-Associated Perforation

Despite successful CTO wiring with fluoroscopic guidance, the wire course is not always in intraluminal area. If the wire course is partly in subintimal route and the CTO segment has multiple irregular calcification, the aggressive ballooning and stenting with bigger size can lead to major perforation or rupture.

Other risk factors are elderly patients, female gender, very tortuous and irregular calcified lesion, use of rotational or directional atheroablative device, and IVUS-guided stenting to achieve maximal acute lumen gain.

If the wire course is not absolutely sure, it would be safe to start predilation with small balloon less than 1.5 mm without high pressure. Best confirmation is to examine by IVUS before aggressive ballooning or stenting. Table 16.2 shows the perforation risks during ballooning or stenting.

Once the coronary perforation occurs, the prognosis is related to perforation class, grade of renal insufficiency, and use of GP IIb/IIIa receptor blocker. Javid et al. reported clinical outcomes according to perforation class. Class 1 perforation was not associated with pericardial tamponade or inhospital mortality. In class 2 perforation, the incidence of pericardial tamponade was 12%, inhospital mortality 3%, and emergent coronary artery bypass graft (CABG) was 27%. In class 3

Table 16.2 Risk factors of coronary perforation

1. Oversizing balloon (balloon-artery ratio >1.2)
2. High-pressure balloon inflation outside the stent
3. Stenting of tapering vessel
4. Stenting of contained perforations from other devices
5. Stenting of lesions that are recrossed after severe dissection or abrupt closure
6. Stenting of total occlusion when there has been unrecognized subintimal passage of the wire
7. Stenting of small vessels (<2.5 mm)

Ellise et al. reported three different classes of coronary perforation (Table 16.3) [6]

Table 16.3 Classification according to coronary perforation severity grade

Class	Definition	Risk of tamponade
Class I	Extraluminal crater without extravasation	8%
Class II	Pericardial or myocardial blush without contrast jet extravasation	13%
Class III	Extravasation through a frank (≥1 mm) perforation or cavity spilling into an anatomic cavity chamber	
	A. Directed toward the pericardium	63%
	B. Cavity spilling into coronary sinus, myocardium, etc.	0%

perforation, the incidence of pericardial tamponade was 63%, inhospital mortality 44%, and emergent CABG 60% [3].

Most of class 1 or 2 perforation can be treated with prolonged balloon inflation with heparin reversal. In case of ballooning or stenting associated perforation or rupture (class 3), there will be severe chest pain and dyspnea, abrupt drop of blood pressure, and will lead to very unstable hemodynamic status. Immediate IV fluid loading, inotropic support, and quick balloon tamponade are essential to save the patient. Immediate bedside echocardiographic assessment is essential, and in most of the severe perforation with unstable vital sign state, urgent pericardiocentesis is needed to stabilize the patient. As soon as pericardial blood is drained, quick autotransfusion will help to minimize the chance of additional transfusion. As soon as hemodynamic stability is maintained, ultimate sealing can be achieved by graft stenting [2, 4, 5, 7, 8]. PTFE-covered stent (polytetrafluoroethylene, graft stent) is available from 2.75 mm, larger than 2.75 mm can be treated with graft stent, but smaller than 2.75 mm may need prolonged balloon inflation with heparin reversal. If balloon tamponade is not successful, the operator should consider surgical management or embolization by coil, gelfoam, autogenous fat, platelet infusate, polyvinyl alcohol form (PVA), or local thrombogenic molecules. The following successful graft stenting, adequate dual antiplatelet with high-intensity statin maintenance will be important because of higher incidence of restenosis and thrombosis. Case 1 is a typical class 3 perforation managed by PTFE-covered graft stent (Fig. 16.1).

Case 2 is a typical perforation by ballooning without confirmation of distal CTO wire location in true lumen (Fig. 16.2).

16.4 Device Entrapment, Dislodge (Loss), or Migration

CTO lesion frequently has dense calcium, irregular, diffuse long lesion which is not easy to deliver any device even after the successful CTO wiring. CTO wires, balloons, and stents can be entrapped,

destroyed, migrated, and lost in very tough CTO lesion.

Small wire tip disconnection may not cause immediate hemodynamic instability; however, bigger device such as balloon shaft and unexpanded entrapped stent may cause acute thrombosis, and flow limitation and may cause acute myocardial infarction, lethal ventricular tachyarrhythmia, acute heart failure, and sudden cardiac death. Thus, prevention of device-related complication and immediate management will be essential for safe CTO PCI.

16.4.1 A. Stent Entrapment or Stent Loss (Dislodge)

Stent loss (SL) is defined as the undeployed, unexpanded stent remained in unexpected location during stent positioning, and this is the most common complication in device entrapment. Unlike old-generation bare metal stent, current-generation drug-eluting stent (DES) has smaller profile and stronger stent retention force (SRF) to reduce stent entrapment. However, still the incidence of stent loss is reported from 0.32 to 3.4%. Higher risk of SL includes stent delivery without adequate lesion preparation in very dense, hard, calcified, and angulated lesion with forceful push/pull of the undeployed stent. During pullback of the stent, two main mechanisms of SL are (1) entrapped in tight target CTO lesion and (2) stent edge deformity caused by tip of guiding catheter and finally pulled off from the delivery balloon (Fig. 16.3).

How to manage the SL? Immediate and prompt management is important to prevent hemodynamic instability (Fig. 16.4) [9–15].

1. Small balloon technique; deliver the new 1.5 mm small balloon, cross the undeployed stent, inflate, and pull back with the stent.
2. Two wire twisting technique; insert another new wire and twisting 15–20 times and carefully pull back.
3. Lost stent deployed by sequential balloon dilation; if the stent size is too small for larger

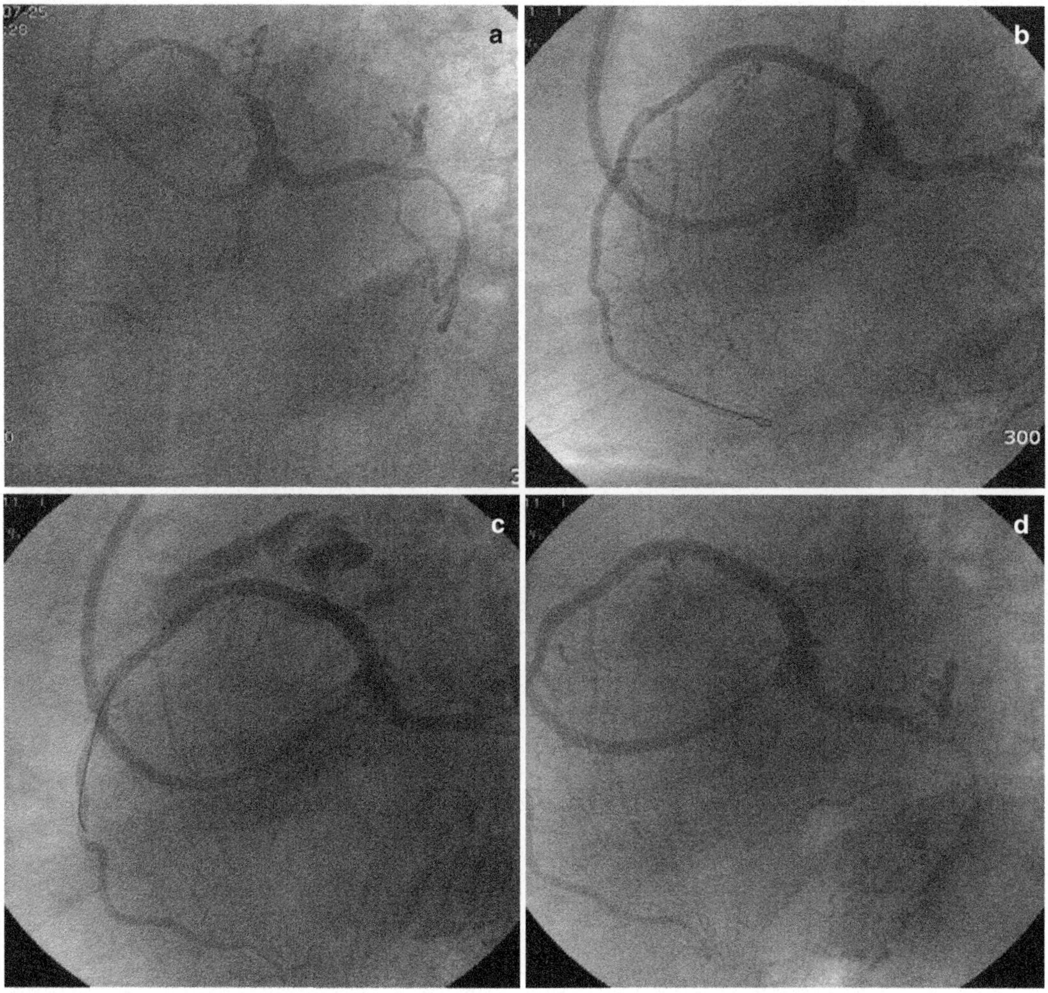

Fig. 16.1 Typical Ellis class 3 epicardial coronary artery perforation managed by graft stenting. Proximal left anterior descending artery (LAD) was successfully predilated with 2.0 mm small balloon following CTO wiring: (**a**) three Taxus stents were deployed by overlapping stenting (**b**), sudden coronary perforation (type 3) developed following aggressive adjuvant post-dilation using bigger non-compliant balloon (**c**), and successfully sealed coronary perforation using PTFE-covered stent graft (JOSTENT 3.5 × 16 mm) (**d**)

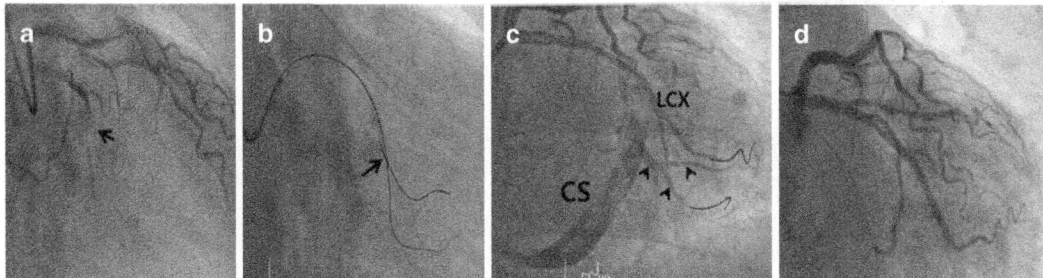

Fig. 16.2 Iatrogenic arteriovenous (AV) fistula during left circumflex artery (LCX) CTO intervention. Baseline angiography showed CTO lesion in mid-LCX artery (**a**). Predilation with small balloon was performed after fielder XT wire crossing the CTO lesion without confirmation of distal wire location by collateral angiography (**b**). Abrupt coronary sinus (CS) was observed through the posterior vein of left ventricle with side branched (arrows, (**c**). Polytetrafluoroethylene-covered stent (3.0 × 19 mm) was implanted to seal off the AV fistula (**d**)

Stent
deformed
Stent stripped
off at guide
Balloon
Stent stuck
on lesion

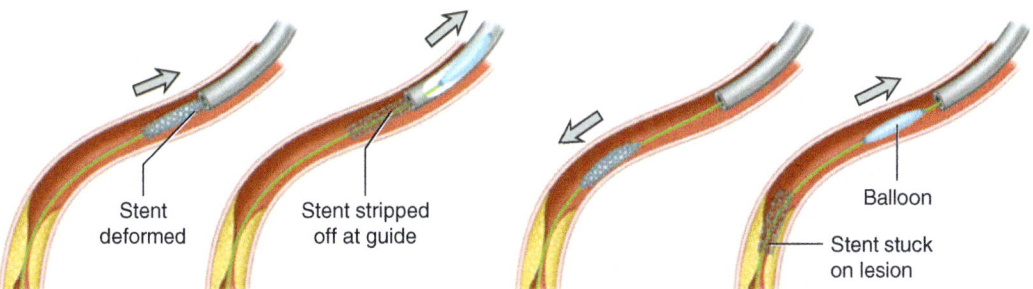

Fig. 16.3 Two main mechanisms of stent loss

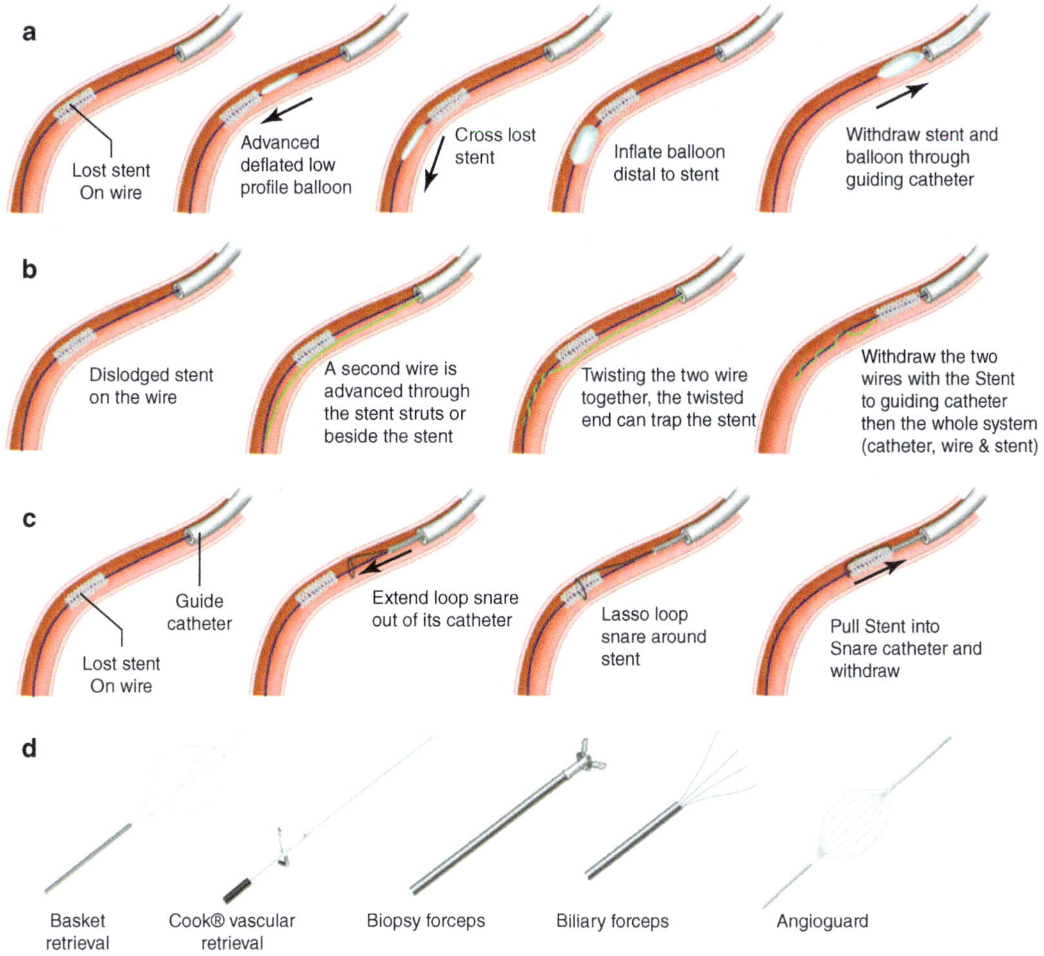

a
Lost stent
On wire
Advanced
deflated low
profile balloon
Cross lost
stent
Inflate balloon
distal to stent
Withdraw stent and
balloon through
guiding catheter
b
Dislodged stent
on the wire
A second wire is
advanced through
the stent struts or
beside the stent
Twisting the two wire
together, the twisted
end can trap the stent
Withdraw the two
wires with the Stent
to guiding catheter
then the whole system
(catheter, wire & stent)
c
Guide
catheter
Lost stent
On wire
Extend loop snare
out of its catheter
Lasso loop
snare around
stent
Pull Stent into
Snare catheter and
withdraw
d
Basket
retrieval
Cook® vascular
retrieval
Biopsy forceps
Biliary forceps
Angioguard

Fig. 16.4 Management of stent loss. Small balloon technique (**a**), two wire twisting technique (**b**), snaring (**c**), other foreign body removal devices (**d**)

reference vessel diameter, another new adequate sized stent deployment should be considered.

4. If wire was lost and could not do rewiring, just new wiring parallel to dislodged stent, sequential balloon crushing and final new stenting should be considered.

   Other foreign body removal devices can be useful in many cases; snare (loop, goose), multipurpose basket, myocardial biopsy forcep, 5F Alligator forcep, 6F bioptome forcep, and angioguard distal protection device [16–19].

5. Finally, if all the percutaneous procedures failed, surgical approach should be considered.

Figure 16.5 showed typical SL case during calcified and angulated CTO PCI. Dislodged stent was retrieved by snare but guiding catheter-induced

left main (LM) dissection was developed which was safely managed by rescue LM stenting.

Figure 16.6 showed failed retrieval by small balloon technique and finally deployed at the entrapped area by sequential balloon dilation.

16.4.2 Balloon Catheter Break and Entrapment

During aggressive manipulation of pre-/post-dilation balloon, and stent delivery balloon, sometimes balloon catheter tip and shaft break and entrapment can be developed. Because the balloon catheter is not easily visible on the fluoroscopy and balloon tip marker can be seen, retrieved catheter length should be checked with

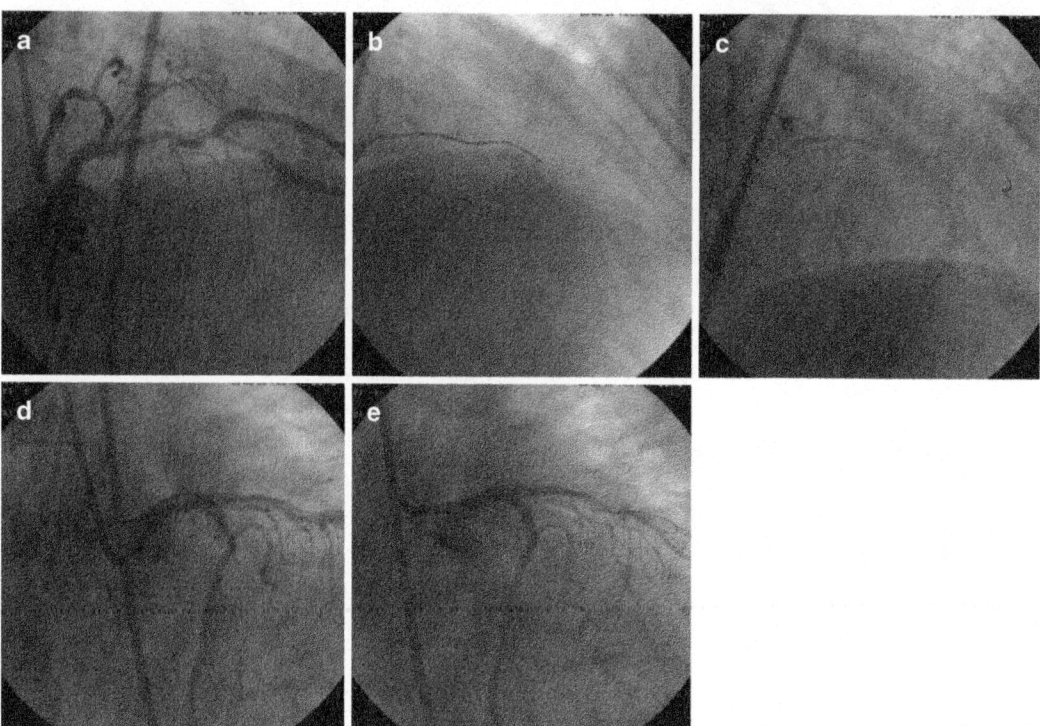

Fig. 16.5 Typical stent loss (SL) retrieved by snare device. Baseline angiography after predilation in mid-LAD CTO which is dense calcified and angulated lesion (**a**). Cypher 2.5 × 33 mm stent could not pass the target lesion and SL developed during pullback for further predilation. Undeployed stent remained from LM to proximal LAD, and immediate rewiring was done (**b**). Dislodged stent was successfully removed by gooseneck loop snare (**c**). However, guiding catheter-induced LM dissection was developed during stent removal (**d**). Immediate recue LM stenting was done (**e**)

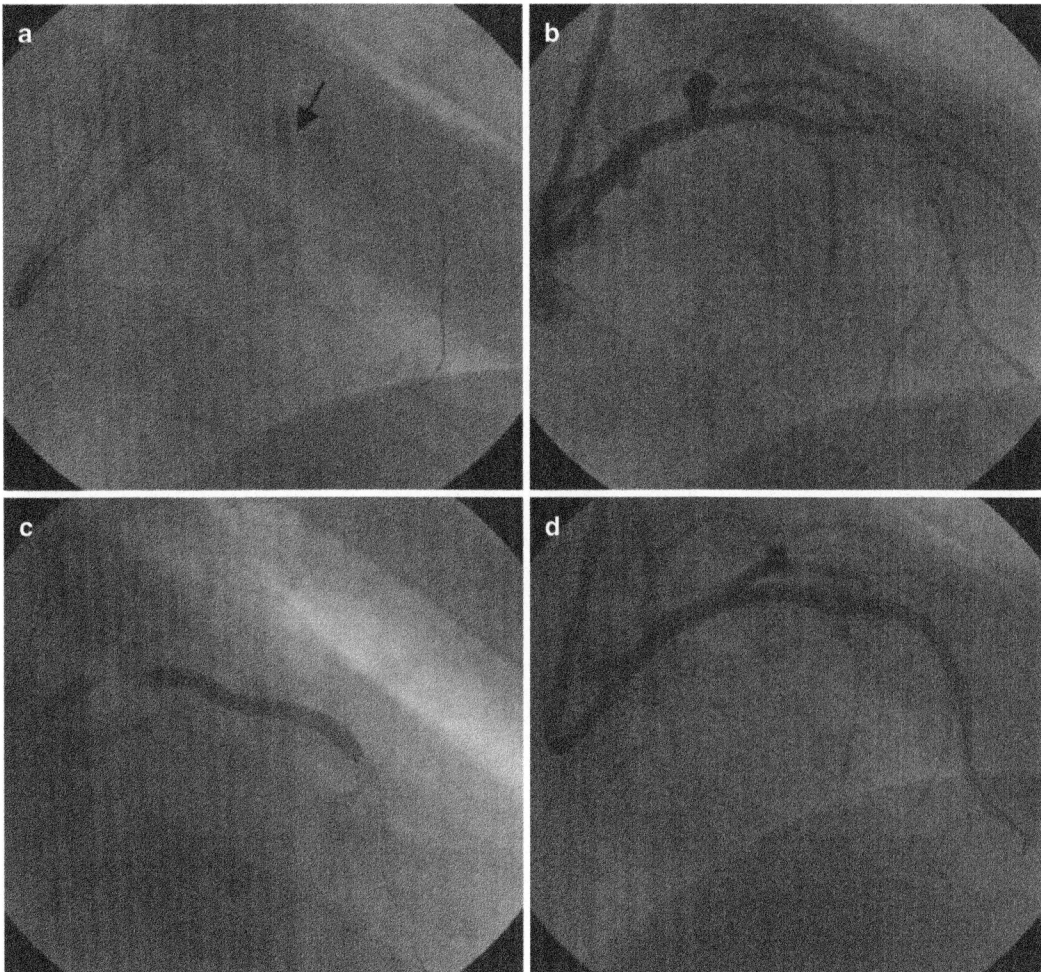

Fig. 16.6 Failed small balloon technique treated by sequential balloon expansion of dislodged stent. Dislodged Taxus 2.5 × 16 mm stent retrieval was failed by small balloon technique (arrow, **a**), and the stent was partially expanded due to inflated 1.5 mm balloon. Further dilation was done using 2.5 × 20 mm plain balloon (**b**). Two overlapping Taxus stents (2.75 mm) were deployed in prox to mid-LAD (**c**). Final angiography showed good distal run-off (**d**)

same balloon catheter so that the operator can assess how much longer catheter remained in the coronary system.

How to manage the entrapped broken balloon catheter? First of all, operator can use any device for foreign body removal such as snares and forceps. If it fails, the most common easy way is to use the "balloon trapping technique." Enough size balloon (2.0–2.5 mm for 6F guiding catheter, 2.5–3.0 for 7F guiding catheter) with longer length will be safe to trap the broken catheter inside of guiding catheter. Whole system can be retrieved with guiding catheter and restart the procedure. The following case is atypical case of broken balloon catheter after adjuvant ballooning. Retrieval was initially failed by snaring, and finally balloon trapping technique was used to remove the broken balloon catheter (Fig. 16.7).

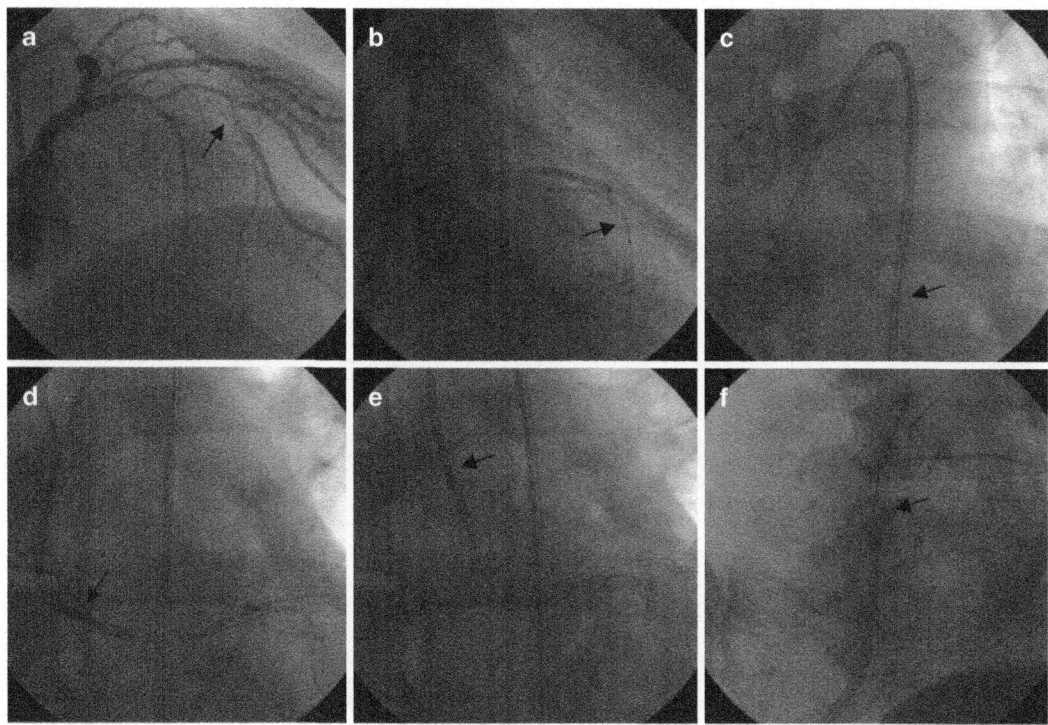

Fig. 16.7 Stent balloon catheter breaks case. Predilation angiography in mid-LAD CTO showed tortuous and angulated mid-LAD lesion (**a**). After balloon anchoring to diagonal branch using "side branch anchor balloon technique," Taxus 2.5 × 33 mm stent could not cross the target lesion (**b**). For further lesion preparation, stent was pulled back but stent delivery catheter was broken, and snaring by 2.8F amplatz gooseneck loop snare (Microsnare) was attempted to remove but failed (**c**). Finally balloon trapping technique using Quantum Maverick balloon 3.0 × 8 mm was successful to retrieve the broken catheter (**d, e, f**)

16.4.3 Guidewire Entrapment or Fracture

Prolonged dynamic CTO wiring can lead to wire fatigue, mechanical stress to wire shaft and ultimately can be broken. Any CTO wire can be broken, but relatively higher incidence of Gaia wire series is being reported. Too much forceful single wire manipulation in dense calcified CTO lesion may cause wire fracture and disconnection. Sometimes, forceful retrograde wiring through corkscrew, tiny collateral channels also can damage the wire. Remained disconnected wire can cause restenosis, late perforation, tachyarrhythmia, and thrombosis. If the small distal tip is broken and remained in side branch or CTO segment, that will not be harmful after successful recanalization. However, longer remained wire segment should be removed at any effort to prevent broken wire-related complications.

The following are the strategies to remove the broken wire fragment (Fig. 16.8):

1. Double or triple wire technique
2. Double wedging of guiding catheter and traction of the system
3. Retrieval by balloon trapping technique (if the wire is remained inside of guiding catheter)
4. Retrieval by snare loop
5. Retrieval using microcatheter
6. Extraction by forcep
7. Stenting against arterial wall
8. Surgical removal

The following case shows retrograde wire fracture and broken wire associated with hemopericardium (Figs. 16.9, 16.10, 16.11, and 16.12).

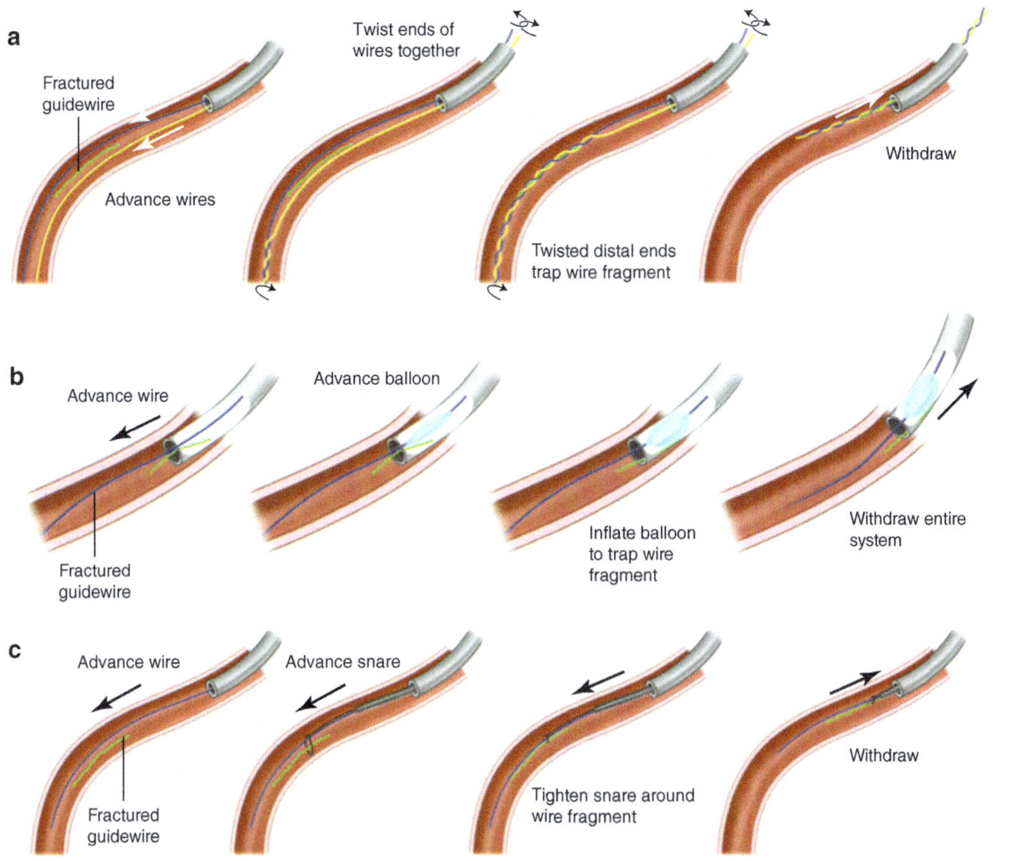

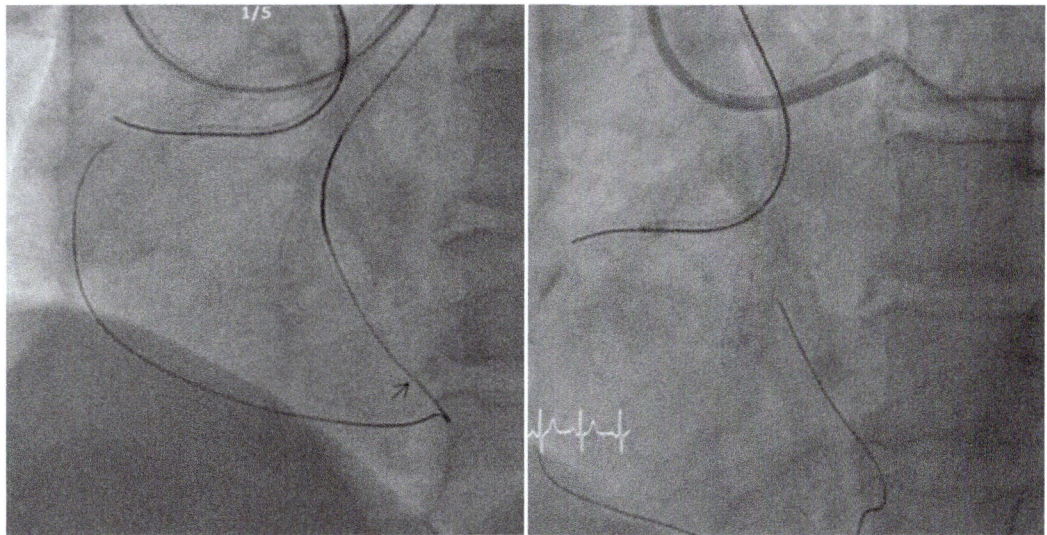

Fig. 16.8 Sample illustration showing wire fragment removal by double or triple wire technique (**a**), balloon trapping technique (**b**) and snaring technique (**c**)

Fig. 16.9 Retrograde Fielder XT-R guidewire got fracture (arrow), broken, and remained in the septal route. Fractured wire remains in the septal route and whole RCA was stented, and remained retrograde septal wire was embedded into arterial wall by long RCA overlapping stenting

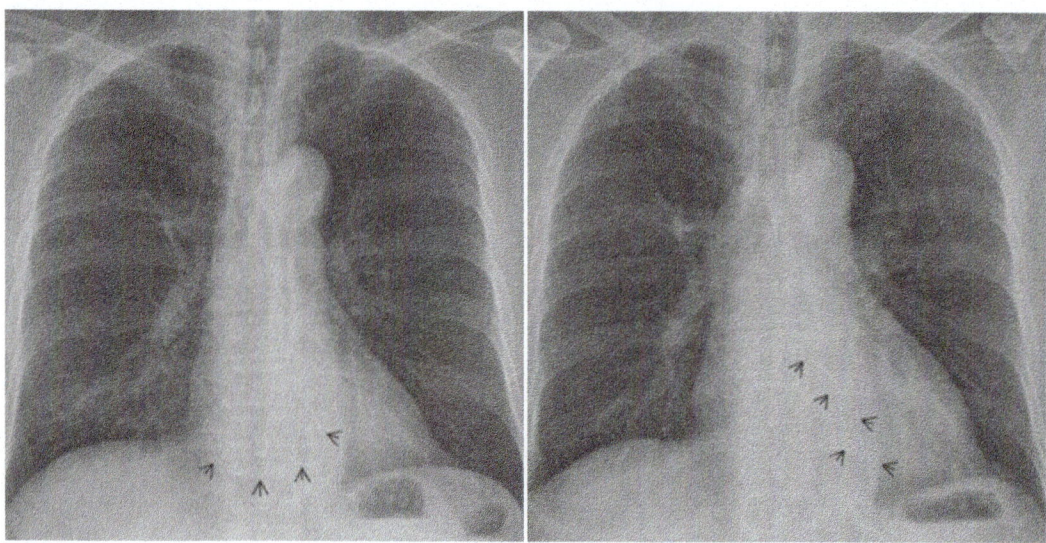

Fig. 16.10 Chest X-ray after 4 days and 11 days from index procedure, guidewire migration, and cardiomegaly was observed

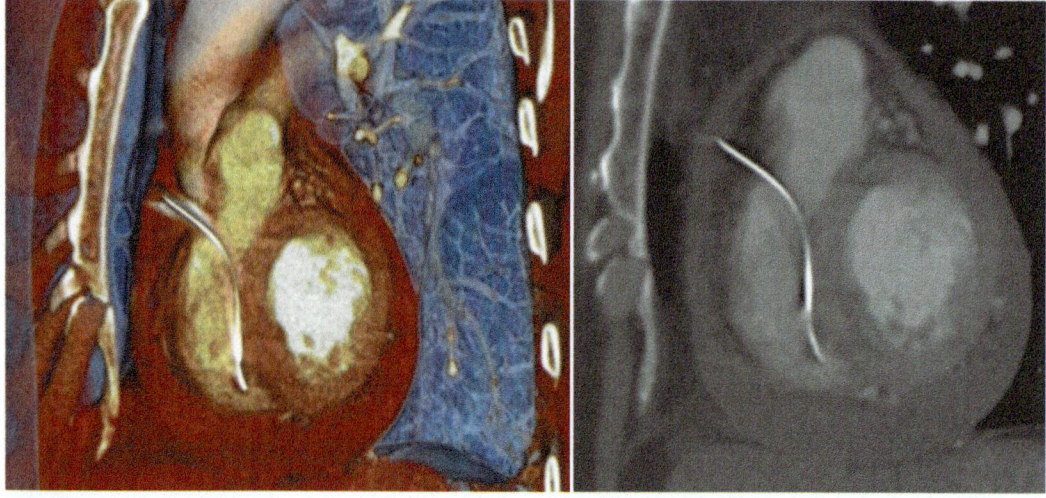

Fig. 16.11 Chest CT showed hemopericardium and the fracture wire penetrated and migrated via septum and right ventricle

16.5 Retrograde CTO PCI-Related Complications

The more aggressive CTO PCI is widely being performed worldwide by retrograde approach to improve the success rate. The more the difficult CTO cases, the prolonged attempt by ipsilateral and retrograde approach will increase the incidence of unexpected complications. The fol-

lowing are the typical retrograde approach-specific complications which should be prevented and managed [20–29]:

1. Donor artery spasm, dissection, and thrombosis
2. Myocardial damage due to prolong ischemia by retrograde microcatheter insertion and manipulation

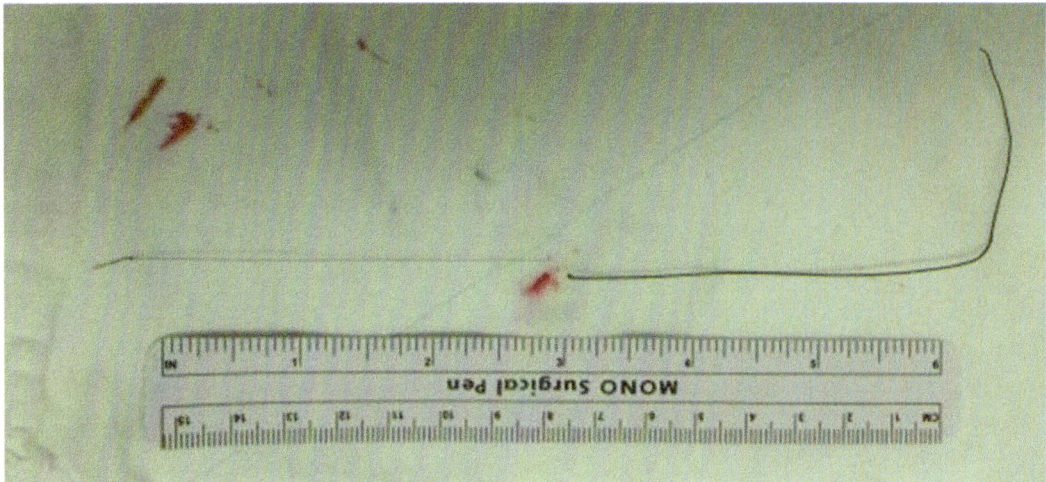

Fig. 16.12 Surgically removed the broken Fielder XT-R wire

3. Collateral channel damages including dissection, extravasation, perforation, septal hematoma, thrombosis, pericardial effusion, and tamponade
4. Retrograde LM dissection and aortic dissection by retrograde wiring and ballooning
5. Chronic aneurysm formation and late stent malapposition

16.5.1 Donor Artery Thrombosis

Among these retrograde approach-specific complications, donor artery thrombosis can be fatal. So prevention is very important for patient's safety during retrograde approach. ACT level should be maintained above the 350 s by every 1 h monitoring to maintain adequate anticoagulation during the retrograde approach. Frequent flushing of retrograde guiding catheter, contrast filling during the retrograde wiring, and disengagement of guiding catheter from coronary ostium for better antegrade flow to minimize thrombosis are my tips and tricks to prevent donor artery thrombosis. If there is previously implanted stents in donor artery, it will be better to avoid to cross the stent strut with retrograde microcatheter. It will be safer to choose other collateral channels than selected stented channels.

If the donor artery thrombosis developed, the following are essential points for prompt management:

1. Removal of retrograde system and quick rewiring for donor artery treatment.
2. Quick thrombus aspiration with aspiration catheter or daughter catheter such as 5F Heartrail catheter in case of huge proximal new thrombi.
3. Active pharmacologic interventions with intracoronary GP IIb/IIIa receptor blocker, thrombolytics, and additional heparinization.
4. If there is an evidence of mechanical injury such as dissection, stenting should be considered.
5. If there is residual slow flow/no reflow, intracoronary nicorandil, nitroglycerin should be given with systemic inotropic support and atropine injection.

Figure 16.13 shows a typical case of donor artery thrombosis which developed during retrograde approach through the previously stented mid-LAD lesion to recanalize RCA CTO.

16.5.2 Transient Myocardial Ischemia

Transient myocardial ischemia and focal myocardial damage (cardiac enzyme elevation) can

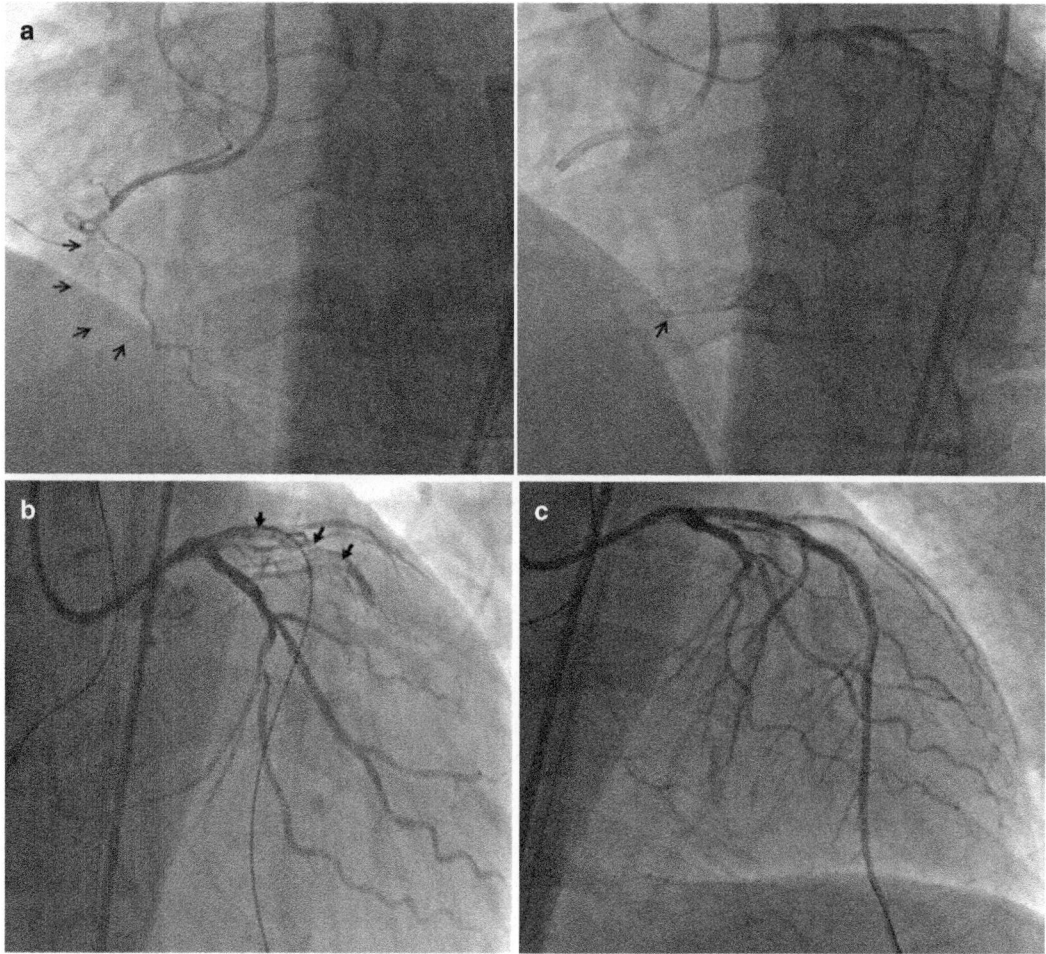

Fig. 16.13 Typical donor artery thrombosis case during retrograde CTO PCI. Proximal RCA CTO lesions without definite distal stump and longer CTO segment at baseline angiography (**a**). Acute donor artery thrombosis (LAD) was developed during retrograde approach through previously stented LAD segment (arrow, **b**), active thrombus aspiration and pharmacologic therapy restored LAD flow without residual thrombosis (**c**)

be occurred during prolonged retrograde approach especially when the retrograde microcatheter is inserted via big collateral channel. Particularly, single big epicardial channel negotiation will have more risk to have ischemic insult. In this aspect, trans-septal approach would be safer than choosing bigger epicardial channel.

16.5.3 Collateral Channel Damages

With the increased retrograde approach, many collateral damage reports are increasing. In general, septal route is safer than epicardial route in terms of minimizing the risk of pericardial tamponade. Retrograde channel track wires such as Sion, Sion blue, Fielder XT-R, and other associated injuries include septal extravasation, perforation, or hematoma. Usually these injuries will be healed spontaneously except huge growing septal hematoma which needs selective embolization by coils or gelfoam. The mocrocatheter should protect entire collateral channel until removal of retrograde wire to protect entire collateral channels. Sometimes, channel dilation with small balloon (1.0–1.2 mm) to deliver microcatheter in very tight collateral channels can lead channel damages. Instead of channel thickness, it's better to select straight channel than tortuous but larger channel. "Surfing" to septal channels can be feasible, but "surfing" to epicardial channels can be dangerous. With the close observation of selective channel injection epicardial channel image, careful selective epicardial channel wiring is important for safe retrograde wiring instead of rough blind retrograde wiring.

If the epicardial channel perforation develops, there will be high chance of pericardial tamponade. Maintaining negative pressure through microcatheter will minimize bleeding into pericardial space. In general, coils or gelfoam cannot be delivered with Corsair microcatheter but can be delivered through Finecross microcatheter. Quick exchange to Finecross and coil embolization will be safe to achieve complete hemostasis. Bedside echocardiographic examination and pericardiocentesis set should be ready in case of unstable hemodynamic status. Sometimes, antegrade flow can contribute bleeding through other ipsilateral collateral channels. Thus, after quick retrograde channel embolization, antegrade channels should be carefully observed to see the presence of residual bleeding focus.

16.5.4 Retrograde LM and Aortic Dissection

If there is an ostial CTO in LAD, LCX, and RCA CTO, single retrograde wire technique to cross the culprit ostial CTO can lead to LM dissection or aortic dissection. If the retrograde wire cannot be reentered into distal LM or ostial RCA, it's better to reverse CART first to confirm the retrograde wire position. IVUS confirmation by antegrade preparation will confirm the retrograde wire position to prevent LM or aortic dissection. Once the LM dissection occurs, it is inevitable to do LM stenting to fully cover the dissected flap to prevent further progression for dissection [21].

16.5.5 Chronic Aneurysm Formation and Late Stent Malapposition

Because of the aggressive procedure by multiple CTO wiring, reverse CART or CART, and use of

drug-eluting stent, there is a report of retrograde approach-related chronic coronary aneurysm development and late stent malapposition. One report with 560 CTO patients reported that chronic artery aneurysm formation was observed in 7.3% of retrograde approach and 2.6% of antegrade approach. Late stent malapposition would contribute this phenomenon. Long-term prognosis of this phenomenon is not known yet.

References

1. Huber M, Mooney J, Madison J, Mooney M. Use of a morphologic classification to predict clinical outcome after dissection from coronary angiography. Am J Cardiol. 1992;19:926–35.
2. Suh SY, Rha SW, Jin Z, Minami Y, Chen K, Na JO, Choi CU, Kim JW, Kim EJ, Park CG, Seo HS, Oh DJ. Unexpected coronary perforation following adjunctive balloon postdilation after overlapping drug-eluting stent implantation rescued by successful stent graft implantation. Int J Cardiol. 2009;132(1):e11–3.
3. Stankovic G, Orlic D, Corvaja N, Airoldi F, Chieffo A, Spanos V, Montorfano M, Carlino M, Finci L, Sangiorgi G, Colombo A. Incidence, predictors, in-hospital, and late outcomes of coronary artery perforations. Am J Cardiol. 2004;93:213–6.
4. Lansky AJ, Yang YM, Khan Y, Costa RA, Pietra C, Tsuchiya Y, Cristea E, Collins M, Mehran R, Dangas GD, Moses JW. Treatment of coronary artery perforation complicating percutaneous coronary intervention with a polytetrafluoroethylene-covered graft. Am J Cardiol. 2006;98:370–4.
5. Briguori C, Nishida T, Anzuini A, Di Mario C, Grube E, Colombo A. Emergency polytetrafluoroethylene-Covered stent implantation to treat coronary ruptures. Circulation. 2000;102:3028–31.
6. Ellis SG, Ajluni S, Arnold AZ, Popma JJ, Bittl JA, Eoger NL, Cowley MJ, Raymond RE, Safian RD, Whitlow PL. Increased coronary perforation in the new device era. Incidence, classification, management and outcome. Circulation. 1994;90:2725–30.
7. Ly H, Awaida JP, Lesperance J, Bilodeau L. Angiographic and clinical outcomes of polytetrafluoroethylene-covered stent use in significant coronary perforations. Am J Cardiol. 2005;95:244–6.
8. Gercken U, Lansky AJ, Buellesfeld L, Desai K, Badereldin M, Mueller R, Selbach G, Leon MB, Grube E. Result of the Jostent coronary stent graft implantation in various clinical settings: procedural and follow-up results. Cathet Cardiovasc Intervent. 2002;56:353–60.
9. Eggebrecht H, Haude M, von Birgelen C, Oldenburg O, Baumgart D, Herrmann J, Welge D, Bartel T, Dagres N, Erbel R. Nonsurgical retrieval of embolized coronary stents. Catheter Cardiovasc Interv. 2000;51:432–40.

10. Brilakis ES, Best PJM, Elesber AA, Barsness GW, Lennon RJ, Holmes DR Jr, Rihal CS, Kirk N. Garratt Incidence, retrieval methods, and outcomes of stent loss during percutaneous coronary intervention: a large single-center experience. Catheter Cardiovasc Interv. 2006;66:333–40.

11. Cantor WJ, Lazzam C, Cohen EA, et al. Failed coronary stent deployment. Am Heart J. 1998;136:1088–95.

12. Alfonso F, Martinez D, Hernandez R, et al. Stent embolization during intracoronary stenting. Am J Cardiol. 1996;78:833–5.

13. Elsner M, Peifer A, Kasper W. Intracoronary loss of balloon-mounted stents: successful retrieval with a 2 mm-Microsnare-device. Cathet Cardiovasc Diagn. 1996;39:271–6.

14. Patterson M, Slagboom T. Intracoronary stent dislodgment: updated strategy enabled by the new generation of materials. Catheter Cardiovasc Interv. 2006;67:386–90.

15. Foster-Smith KW, Garratt KN, Higano ST, Holmes DR Jr. Retrieval techniques for managing flexible intracoronary stent misplacement. Cathet Cardiovasc Diagn. 1993;30:63–8.

16. Kim MH, Cha KS, Kim JS. Retrieval of dislodged and disfigured transradially delivered coronary stent: report on a case using forcep and antegrade brachial sheath insertion. Catheter Cardiovasc Interv. 2001;52:489–91.

17. Eeckhout E, Stauffer JC, Goy JJ. Retrieval of a migrated coronary stent by means of an alligator forceps catheter. Cathet Cardiovasc Diagn. 1993;30:166–8.

18. Berder V, Bedossa M, Gras D, Paillard F, Le Breton H, Pony JC. Retrieval of a lost coronary stent from the descending aorta using a PTCA balloon and biopsy forceps. Cathet Cardiovasc Diagn. 1993;28:351–3.

19. Khattab AA, Geist V, Toelg R, Richardt G. AngioGuard: a simplified snare? Int J Cardiovasc Intervent. 2004;6(3-4):153–5.

20. Herman WR, Foley DP, Rensing BJ, et al. Usefulness of quantitative and qualitative angiographic lesion morphology, and clinical characteristics in predicting major adverse cardiac events during and after native coronary balloon angioplasty. Am J Cardiol. 1993;72:14–20.

21. Dunning DW, Kahn JK, Hawkins ET, O' Neill WW. Iatrogenic coronary artery dissections extending into and involving the aortic root. Cathet Cardiovasc Intervent. 2000;51:387–93.

22. Hiroshi KM. Complications of CTO intervention. Coronary Intervention. 2008;4(4):27–32.

23. Waksman R, Saito R. Chronic total occlusion, a guide to recanalization. 1st ed. Hoboken: Blackwell Publishing Ltd; 2009. p. 167–77.

24. Saito S, Nguyen TN, Colombo A, Dayi H, Grines CL. Practical handbook of advanced interventional cardiology, tips and tricks. 3rd ed. Hoboken: Blackwell Publishing Ltd; 2008.

25. Park SJ, Jang YS, Yoon JH, et al. The manual of interventional cardiology. 1st ed. Seoul: Korean Society of Interventional Cardiology; 2004.

26. Norell MS, Perrins EJ. Essential interventional cardiology. 1st ed. Philadelphia: W.B. Saunders; 2001.

27. Tanaka H, Kadota K, Hosogi S, et al. Mid-term angiographic and clinical outcomes from antegrade versus retrograde recanalization for chronic total occlusions. J Am Coll Cardiol. 2011;57:E1628.

28. Al-Moghairi AM, Al-Amri HS. Management of retained intervention guide-wire: a literature review. Curr Cardiol Rev. 2013;9:260–6.

29. Ellis SG, Holmes DR, et al. Strategic approaches in coronary intervention. 3rd ed. Philadelphia: Lippincott Williams & Wilkins; 2006.

How to Minimize Radiation Hazard and Prevent Contrast-Induced Nephropathy

17

Sang Min Park and Jung Rae Cho

17.1 Radiation Hazard

17.1.1 Introduction

Coronary angiography and intervention with a radiation generation device is the gold standard for diagnosing and treating coronary artery obstructive disease. The acquisition of a qualified image is considered the cornerstone for making an exact diagnosis and successful interventional procedure [1]. From the aspect of image quality, the general rule of X-ray is that the higher the dose, the better the image quality. However, higher radiation is limited by safety concerns [2]. There are numerous kinds of radiation toxicities related to exposure or susceptibility to radiation: skin erythema, cataracts, bone marrow suppression, sterility, and development of cancer or other adverse genetic alterations. For these reasons, radiation hazard has become an emerging health issue in the area of interventional cardiology. Especially during the percutaneous coronary intervention (PCI) of chronic total occlusion (CTO), both the medical staff and patients would inevitably be at risk to higher radiation exposure than simple and less complicated interventional procedures. Multiple factors influence radiation exposure to medical staff: procedure complexity, radiation protection employed, individual patient's anatomy, physician's experience and habits, as well as vascular access site [3–6]. In addition, there might be a considerable difference in emitted radiation dose between the type of angiography equipment including mainly X-ray machines and dose protocol. Therefore, an effort by the operators to reduce excessive radiation dose to a level that gives appropriate diagnostic image quality without excessive exposure is beneficial [7].

17.1.2 Radiation Hazard Type and Characteristics

Previous studies showed that interventional cardiologists have higher levels of somatic DNA damage compared with clinical cardiologists. The amount of this damage is directly correlated to the duration of professional exposure to radiation [3]. The stochastic effect is considered an all-or-none effect that results in DNA injury [8]. The effect is being seen with increasing frequency as the cumulative radiation exposure increases. The representative example of the effect is cancer or other genetic defects. Cancer is the most important somatic risk of low-dose ionizing radiation. The overall cancer risk of

S. M. Park
Division of Cardiology, Chuncheon Sacred Heart Hospital, Hallym University College of Medicine, Chuncheon, South Korea

J. R. Cho (✉)
Division of Cardiology, Kangnam Sacred Heart Hospital, Hallym University College of Medicine, Seoul, South Korea
e-mail: jrjoe@hallym.ac.kr

© Springer Nature Singapore Pte Ltd. 2019
Y. Jang (ed.), *Percutaneous Coronary Interventions for Chronic Total Occlusion*,
https://doi.org/10.1007/978-981-10-6026-7_17

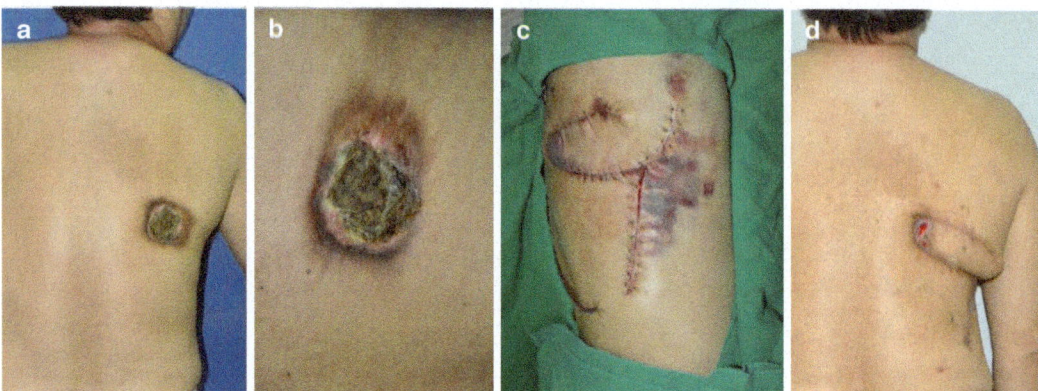

Fig. 17.1 Examples of deterministic skin injuries. (**a**, **b**) radiation-injured skin; (**c**) immediate postoperative status after skin graft surgery; (**d**) 2 months postoperative status (Courtesy of Dr. Jihoon Ahn)

20% for the US population has been well documented. Studies from Hiroshima et al. suggested that the risk of fatal cancer due to whole-body X-ray exposure is approximately 0.004% per 10 mSv. They also proposed that if one cardiologist is exposed to 500 mSv in a lifetime, the estimated risk of cancer is 22% [8, 9]. On the other hand, the deterministic effect is associated with dose-dependent phenomenon and results from cell death. Skin is commonly affected by deterministic type of radiation hazard. Common skin problem includes erythema and desquamation (Fig. 17.1 and Table 17.1). Fair skin may be more susceptible to radiation than darker skin tones. In addition, cataracts, bone marrow suppression, organ atrophy, gonadal injury and/or sterility, and fibrosis are also well known for the deterministic radiation hazards. Elderly patients with collagen vascular disease, diabetes, and hyperthyroidism might be also susceptible to radiation hazards. Some drugs such as actinomycin D, Adriamycin, and methotrexate are known to be associated with radiation susceptibility [10].

17.1.3 Radiation Dose Parameters

It is important to monitor and detect the radiation dose to patients and medical staff. Table 17.2 shows the relevant nomenclature for radiation exposure [11]. Dose-area product (DAP) and air kerma (AK) are commonly used in assessing radiation exposure levels during diagnostic and therapeutic angiographic procedures including

Table 17.1 Threshold of radiation hazard for deterministic and stochastic effect to skin

Effect of single dose	Threshold (Gy)	Onset
Early transient erythema	2	Within hours
Main erythema	6	~10 days
Temporary (permanent) epilation	3 (7)	~3 weeks
Dry (moist) desquamation	14 (18)	~4 weeks
Secondary ulceration	24	>6 weeks
Ischemic dermal necrosis	18	>10 weeks
Dermal atrophy	10	>1 year
Late dermal necrosis	>12	>1 year
Skin cancer	Stochastic	>5 years

CTO intervention. DAP (unit, μGym^2) is a quantity used in assessing the radiation risk from diagnostic X-ray examinations and interventional procedures [12]. This parameter is defined as the absorbed dose multiplied by the area irradiated and correlates well with effective dose. Another important parameter AK is the kinetic energy released per unit mass (unit, mGy), which means kerma in a given mass of air. DAP is calculated by multiplying the KAP and (1-g) where g is the fraction of energy of liberated charged particles that is lost in irradiative processes in the material. Scattered radiation is roughly proportional to the DAP and decreases with distance squared from the location the scatter is generated. That is, twice the distance results in a quarter of the scattered radiation [10, 13, 14]. For the

Table 17.2 Relevant nomenclature for radiation exposure

Terminology	Measuring object	Measure unit	Unit conversion
Exposure	Produced ionization by X-ray	R (Roentgen) or coulomb/kg	$1R = 2.58 \times 10^{-4}$ coulomb/kg
Air K	Kinetic energy released in a given mass of air		
Absorbed dose	Imparted energy by ionizing radiation per unit mass at the point of interest	Rad, or Gy (gray)	100 Rad = 1 Gy
Effective dose	Estimated total body radiation dose	REM or Sv (sievert)	1 Rad = 10 mGy

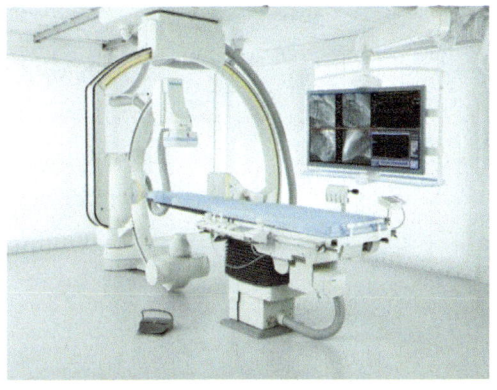 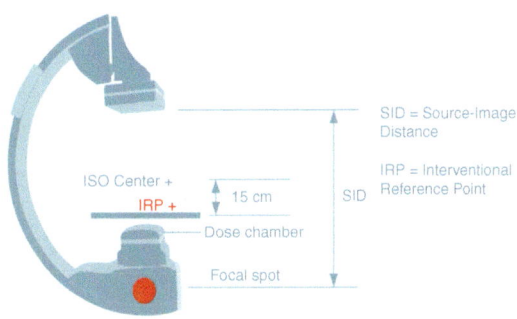

Fig. 17.2 An example of angiography machine and the concepts of isocenter, IRP, and SID

reference point of dose measurement, interventional reference point (IRP) is 15 cm beneath the isocenter. IRP is assumed to be the skin entrance point and does not change with table height. IRP does not change with table height. Source to image distance (SID) is also an important concept to reduce radiation exposure. SID is assumed to be the distance from X-ray generator to image intensifier (Fig. 17.2). Figure 17.3 shows example of real-time radiation dose during procedure and radiation dose report.

17.1.4 General Principles of Reducing Radiation Hazard

The dose delivered to the patient depends on the following three factors: (1) type and setting of the Xray equipment, (2) patient size, and (3) physician conduct [9]. Besides the factors of equipment and patient, physicians have to perform fluoroscopically guided invasive procedures to optimize patient safety and image quality [9, 11, 15]. They also should apply all efforts to reduce their expo-

sure to radiation dose at a level that is "As Low As Reasonably Achievable" (ALARA principle) [16–18]. This principle confers to physicians the responsibility for reducing as much as possible the dose of radiation during cardiovascular procedures to minimize the radiation injury hazard to patients, to professional staff, and to themselves. However, to make an exact diagnosis, additional fluoroscopy and cineangiography were performed by the physician's decision without any limitations [18, 19]. The operators were encouraged to perform the coronary angiography according to the standard technical recommendations for reducing radiation dose as follows [11, 20]:

1. Apply collimation to minimize exposed skin area. In addition, low magnification and low frame rate (e.g., 7.5 frames/s) would be helpful to reduce radiation exposure [2, 21].

2. Avoid steep angle angiography because steeper angle during angiography can cause larger exposed radiation dose. Especially, LAO cranial view with steeper angle delivers the largest radiation dose.

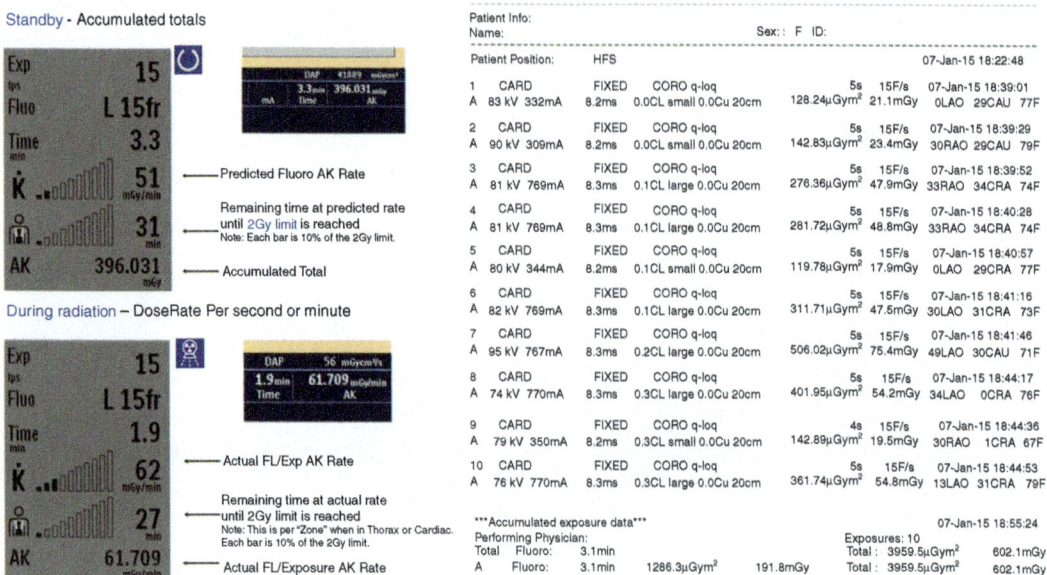

Fig. 17.3 An example of real-time radiation dose during procedure and radiation dose report after procedure

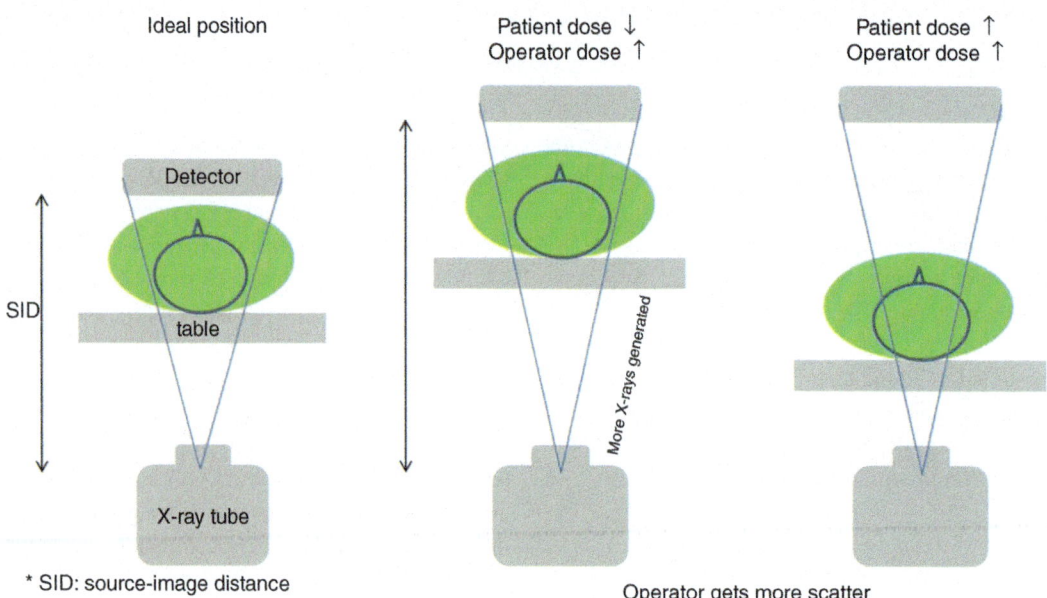

Fig. 17.4 Different radiation dose according to the table height and SID

3. Perform physical examination including skin inspection before and after CTO PCI.
4. Reduce SID and distance between patient's body (table) and image intensifier. Increase the distance between X-ray tube and table as much as possible (Fig. 17.4).
5. Wear protective garment (such as goggle and thyroid protector), and apply the appropriate shield around the table.
6. Monitor your exposed radiation dose such as DAP or AK at the end of the procedure.

In addition, quitting smoking is very important to prevent DNA damage by stochastic effect according to previous research [22].

17.1.5 Example of Specific Preventive Care Plan for Patients and Medical Staff During Angiography

Some investigators proposed that low radiation dose protocol (LDP) would be helpful to protect the patients and operators from unnecessarily excessive radiation hazards in an observational study. In this study, 103 consecutive patients [66.2 ± 12.3 years old, 46 women (44.7%) who undertook diagnostic coronary angiography using Artis Zee™ angiography system (Siemens Health Care, München, Germany)] were divided as conventional radiation dose protocol (CDP) versus LDP group and image interpretability as well as radiation dose-related parameters were compared. The LDP consists of 10-frame rate (FR) per second during fluoroscopy and 40% reduced dose of conventional dose during cineangiography, whereas CDP maintained 15-FR per second during fluroscopy and no reduction of radiation dose during cineangiography. There is no significant interference to evaluate the coronary artery status by visual estimation between both groups. Body weight is well correlated with the level of DAP and AK ($\gamma = 0.27$, $p = 0.006$,

and $\gamma = 0.29$, $p = 0.008$, respectively). There was a markedly reduced effective radiation dose in the LDP group compared to the CDP group (DAP, 1087.8 ± 612.5 vs. 2188.2 ± 949.4 µGym²; AK, 171.5 ± 111.6 vs. 348.1 ± 178.3 mGy, $p < 0.001$), while showed the similar total radiation exposure time (50.7 ± 21.1 vs. 52.0 ± 19.6 s, $p = 0.739$), FR (662.2 ± 197.0 vs. 685.6 ± 211.1, $p = 0.695$), and image counts (10.1 ± 2.0 vs. 10.7 ± 3.5 images). From this study, the use of low-dose radiation protocol was associated with a nearly 50% reduction in exposure to patients undergoing diagnostic angiography without any significant loss of diagnostic information by visual estimation. It might provide another strategy to protect the patients and medical workers from potential radiation hazard in the catheterization room [23] (Fig. 17.5).

17.1.6 Pending Issues for Prevention and Future Direction

Currently, the US Food and Drug Administration (FDA) has set an upper limit to "tabletop" fluoroscopic exposure rate of 10R/min for systems with automatic exposure control; however, there are no regulatory limits on cine exposure rates [24]. In Korea's Ministry of Food and Drug Safety, there is also no specific safety guideline or regulation except for guidance levels about the radiation exposure to adult patients during cardiovascular

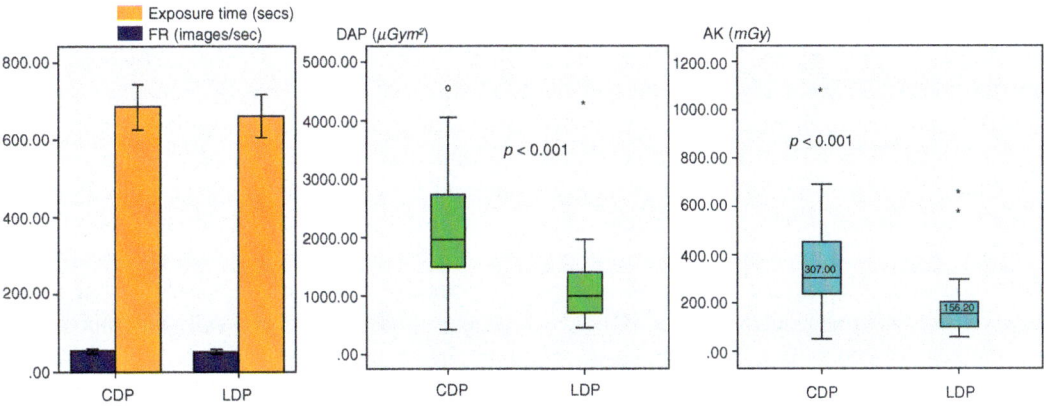

Fig. 17.5 Difference of radiation dose between conventional vs. low-dose protocol

angiography and intervention. Neither safety guidelines nor protective care systems are established for medical staff either, for which lots of efforts should be undertaken [20].

To reduce the radiation hazard to medical staff, some investigators are evaluating the performance of robotics and a suspended lead suit during PCI [25].

17.1.7 Conclusion

Radiation exposure during coronary angiography or PCI is relatively higher compared to other radiologic examinations, and it is considered to be potentially harmful to both the operator and patient. Therefore, operators should take steps to reduce the radiation hazard to prevent the patient and medical staff from future complications. In patients with low body weight, the use of low-dose radiation protocol with a 50% reduction in dose during angiography could be applied to successful CTO intervention without any significant loss of diagnostic information or procedural complication.

17.2 Contrast-Induced Nephropathy

17.2.1 Introduction

Contrast-induced nephropathy (CIN) or contrast-induced acute kidney injury (CI-AKI) is one of the important causes of morbidity and mortality in patients undergoing percutaneous coronary intervention (PCI). According to the most recent guideline (the Kidney Disease: Improving Global Outcomes, KDIGO), CIN is defined as (1) serum creatinine rise by ≥ 0.3 mg/dL within 48 h or (2) serum creatinine rise $\geq 150\%$ from baseline value within 1 week or (3) urine output <0.5 mL/kg/h for >6 consecutive hours [26]. Because of its negative impact on patient outcome after PCI, several scoring systems have been proposed to estimate the risk of CIN post-PCI. Among them, the most commonly used one is Mehran score, which categorized the risk of CIN as low (7.5%),

medium (14.0%), high (26.1%), and very high (57.3%) according to the total score [27] (Fig. 17.6). The predictors of CIN include (1) advanced age, (2) anemia, (3) diabetes, (4) severe heart failure or hypotension, (5) pre-existing chronic kidney disease (CKD), and (6) large volume of contrast agent [27]. Among those, pre-existing CKD is known to be the most critical predictor. In order to prevent CIN, Cigarroa et al. postulated the empirical formula to calculate the maximum allowable contrast dose (MACD) (MACD = 5 mL × weight (kg)/baseline serum creatinine (mg/dL)). By doing this, the operators will be able to limit the amount of contrast agent during coronary angiogram [28]. More recently, a ratio of less than 3.7 for the contrast volume (cc) to creatinine clearance has been proposed as a stricter limit [29].

However, in patients undergoing CTO-PCI, the prevalence of CIN varies from 0.9 to 5.4% in the literature including large-scale registries and meta-analyses which have been published from 2010 to 2014. These reports suggest that in the contemporary patient subsets undergoing CTO-PCI with most advanced PCI techniques, the real-world prevalence of CIN is not very high as it seems to be [30]. Aguiar-Souto et al. retrospectively analyzed the patients who underwent CTO-PCI according to CIN occurrence post-PCI. The half of the patients (55%) was at low-risk group according to Mehran score, and the baseline characteristics were well balanced with overall prevalence of CIN was 6.16% in the study cohort. Interestingly, the patients with CIN used numerically higher amount of contrast agent during PCI than those without (312 mL (210–400) vs. 260 mL (200–345), $p = 0.14$); it could not reach statistical significance [31]. In line with this, the patients who received >400 mL of contrast agents showed twofold higher incidence of CIN compared with those who received <400 mL (10.2% vs. 5.31, $p = 0.27$) without significance. From this study, we can speculate that in low-risk group patients undergoing CTO-PCI, the amount of contrast was not correlated with the incidence of CIN occurrence. On the other hand, the investigators led by Lin et al. categorized 516 patients in CTO-PCI cohort according to Mehran risk score.

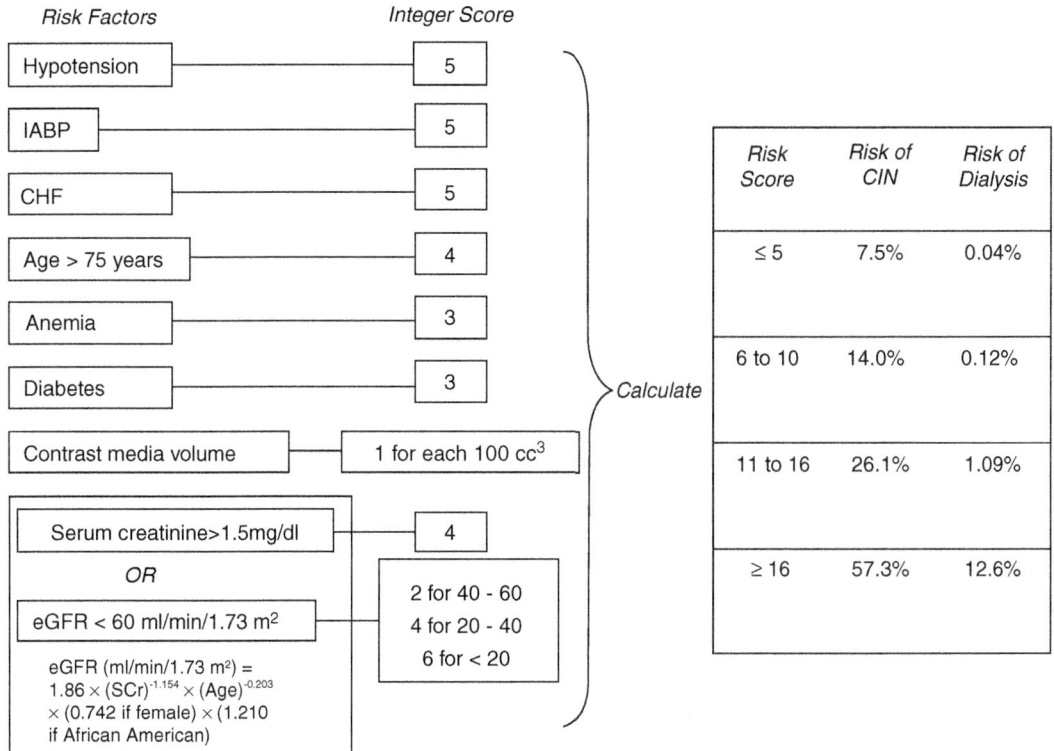

Fig. 17.6 Scheme to define CIN risk score (Mehran risk score)

The incidence of CIN was like this: 0.6% (low-risk group), 3.4% (moderate-risk group), 15.9% (high-risk group), and 37.5% (very high-risk group). In multivariate analysis, the high-risk and the very high-risk groups were predictors of CIN (OR 27.022, 95% CI 2.787–262.028, $p = 0.004$; OR 32.512, 95% CI 2.149–491.978, $p = 0.012$), suggesting that higher Mehran risk score has undeniable impact on the occurrence of CIN in this setting [32]. In case of performing CTO-PCI in patients with higher Mehran score, extra caution should be taken to prevent CIN.

17.2.2 Prevention of CIN in CTO-PCI

1. Hydration

   Hydration with intravenous infusion of 0.9% saline in the periprocedural period may be considered for all risk categories. However, especially for those with estimated glomerular filtration rate (eGFR) less than 60 mL/ min/1.73 m³, saline hydration should strongly be considered before and after CTO-PCI. The infusion rate is usually 1 mL/kg/h for 24 h, beginning 12 h before the use of contrast agent, to maintain urine output >150 mL/h. In patients with lower ejection fraction (EF), 0.45% saline could be used as alternative.

2. N-acetylcysteine (NAC)

   Traditionally, NAC has been believed to act as reno-protective agent against CIN and widely used in the clinical practice. Even though the large-scale randomized clinical trial (ACT trial) failed to demonstrate its efficacy [33], NAC might be still considered when needed.

3. Reduction of contrast volume

   Although there have been conflicting results on the association between the amount of contrast agent and the occurrence of CIN, there is no question for the operators to take every single efforts to reduce the amount of contrast agents during CTO-PCI. To minimize the contrast load, we need to (1) take as less angiogram as possible only in necessary projections, with a good-quality contrast injection (completely fill the coronary tree with the following until micro- or collateral channels are adequately visualized), (2) take super-selective angiogram via micro-catheter when appropriate (e.g., in case of collateral fed from branch vessel), (3) do staged intervention only for CTO in case of PCI for non-CTO lesions, and (4) utilize contemporary guidewire techniques and consider the use of IVUS. In most of the cases, bilateral angiogram is of utmost importance for eventually saving the contrast amount because it could facilitate guidewire passages in the right direction by visualizing the distal true lumen fed by retrograde collaterals, thereby improving the procedural outcome and reducing the whole procedure time and contrast amount. In case of antegrade-only approach, repetitive antegrade injection of contrast with its hydraulic pressure might cause large dissection and intramural hematoma leading to procedural failure. The contemporary guidewire technique includes CART, reverse CART, contemporary reverse CART, and several other techniques which maximize the wire passage in the CTO lesion and has been adopted by many experienced CTO operators to minimize contrast load as well as increase success rate. IVUS-assisted (or guided) approach is also useful to reduce contrast agents due to its visualization of guidewire whether it stays inside true or false lumen without using contrast. In a case report by Uehara et al., CTO-PCI for RCA in patient with chronic kidney disease (serum Cr 3.21 mg/dL) was performed using only 10ml of contrast under IVUS guidance, which highlights the usefulness of IVUS in this situation. In summary, the operator always needs to pay attention to the total amount of contrast used during CTO-PCI whether it becomes too much. However, in case of any instability of patient's symptoms, vital signs, or ECG changes, angiogram should be taken without hesitation to check for any problem happening during the procedure.

17.2.3 Conclusion

Proper assessment of the potential risk and adequate preventive measures could reduce the occurrence of CIN during CTO-PCI.

References

1. Plourde G, Pancholy SB, Nolan J, Jolly S, Rao SV, Amhed I, et al. Radiation exposure in relation to the arterial access site used for diagnostic coronary angiography and percutaneous coronary intervention: a systematic review and meta-analysis. Lancet. 2015;386(10009):2192–203.
2. Hwang J, Lee SY, Chon MK, Lee SH, Hwang KW, Kim JS, et al. Radiation exposure in coronary angiography: a comparison of cineangiography and fluorography. Korean Circ J. 2015;45(6):451–6.
3. Sciahbasi A, Rigattieri S, Sarandrea A, Cera M, Di Russo C, Fedele S, et al. Operator radiation exposure during right or left transradial coronary angiography: a phantom study. Cardiovasc Revasc Med. 2015;16(7):386–90.
4. Liu H, Jin Z, Jing L. Comparison of radiation dose to operator between transradial and transfemoral coronary angiography with optimised radiation protection: a phantom study. Radiat Prot Dosimetry. 2014;158(4):412–20.
5. Georges JL, Livarek B, Gibault-Genty G, Aziza JP, Hautecoeur JL, Soleille H, et al. Reduction of radiation delivered to patients undergoing invasive coronary procedures. Effect of a programme for dose reduction based on radiation-protection training. Arch Cardiovasc Dis. 2009;102(12):821–7.
6. Maccia C, Malchair F, Gobert I, Louvard Y, Lefevre T. Assessment of local dose reference values for recanalization of chronic total occlusions and other occlusions in a high-volume catheterization center. Am J Cardiol. 2015;116(8):1179–84.
7. Deseive S, Chen MY, Korosoglou G, Leipsic J, Martuscelli E, Carrascosa P, et al. Prospective randomized trial on radiation dose estimates of CT angiography applying iterative image reconstruction: The PROTECTION V Study. JACC Cardiovasc Imaging. 2015;8(8):888–96.
8. Roguin A, Goldstein J, Bar O, Goldstein JA. Brain and neck tumors among physicians performing interventional procedures. Am J Cardiol. 2013;111(9):1368–72.
9. De Ponti R. Reduction of radiation exposure in catheter ablation of atrial fibrillation: lesson learned. World J Cardiol. 2015;7(8):442–8.
10. Hildick-Smith DJ, Walsh JT, Lowe MD, Shapiro LM, Petch MC. Transradial coronary angiography in patients with contraindications to the femoral

approach: an analysis of 500 cases. Catheter Cardiovasc Interv. 2004;61(1):60–6.

11. Bashore TM, Balter S, Barac A, Byrne JG, Cavendish JJ, Chambers CE, et al. ACCF Task Force Members. 2012 American College of Cardiology Foundation/ Society for Cardiovascular Angiography and Interventions expert consensus document on cardiac catheterization laboratory standards update: a report of the American College of Cardiology Foundation Task Force on Expert Consensus documents developed in collaboration with the Society of Thoracic Surgeons and Society for Vascular Medicine. J Am Coll Cardiol. 2012;59(24):2221–305.

12. Kallinikou Z, Puricel SG, Ryckx N, Togni M, Baeriswyl G, Stauffer JC, et al. Radiation exposure of the operator during coronary interventions (from the RADIO Study). Am J Cardiol. 2016;118(2):188–94.

13. Brueck M, Bandorski D, Kramer W, Wieczorek M, Höltgen R, Tillmanns H. A randomized comparison of transradial versus transfemoral approach for coronary angiography and angioplasty. JACC Cardiovasc Interv. 2009;2(11):1047–54.

14. Shah B, Burdowski J, Guo Y, Velez de Villa B, Huynh A, Farid M, et al. Effect of left versus right radial artery approach for coronary angiography on radiation parameters in patients with predictors of transradial access failure. Am J Cardiol. 2016;118(4):477–81.

15. Bracken JA, Mauti M, Kim MS, Messenger JC, Carroll JD. A radiation dose reduction technology to improve patient safety during cardiac catheterization interventions. J Interv Cardiol. 2015;28(5):493–7.

16. Geijer H, Beckman KW, Andersson T, Persliden J. Radiation dose optimization in coronary angiography and percutaneous coronary intervention (PCI). I. Experimental studies. Eur Radiol. 2002;12(10):2571–81.

17. Geijer H, Beckman KW, Andersson T, Persliden J. Radiation dose optimization in coronary angiography and percutaneous coronary intervention (PCI). II. Clinical evaluation. Eur Radiol. 2002;12(11):2813–9.

18. National Council on Radiation Protection and Measurements. Implementation of the principle of as low as reasonably achievable (ALARA) for medical and dental personnel. Bethesda (MD): NRCP report no. 107. http://www.ncrponline.org/Publications/ Press_Releases/107press.html

19. Kastrati M, Langenbrink L, Piatkowski M, Michaelsen J, Reimann D, Hoffmann R. Reducing radiation dose in coronary angiography and angioplasty using image noise reduction technology. Am J Cardiol. 2016;118(3):353–6.

20. Korean Society of Interventional Radiology. Guideline for reducing radiation exposure during interventional procedure. Korean Food and Drug Administration. 2014.

21. Ebrahimi R, Uberoi A, Treadwell M, Sadrzadeh Rafie AH. Effect of low-frame invasive coronary angiography on radiation and image quality. Am J Cardiol. 2016;118(2):195–7.

22. Boyaci B, Yalçin R, Cengel A, Erdem O, Dörtlemez O, Dörtlemez H, et al. Evaluation of DNA damage in lymphocytes of cardiologists exposed to radiation during cardiac catheterization by the COMET ASSAY. Jpn Heart J. 2004;45(5):845–53.

23. Park SM, Cho JR, Choi JH, Son JW, Hong KS. Comparison of effective radiation dose between low- and conventional-dose protocols in patients undergoing diagnostic coronary angiography (Poster Presentation in ESC 2016). Eur Heart J. 2016;37:191–598.

24. Kato M, Chida K, Sato T, Oosaka H, Tosa T, Munehisa M, et al. The necessity of follow-up for radiation skin injuries in patients after percutaneous coronary interventions: radiation skin injuries will often be overlooked clinically. Acta Radiol. 2012;53(9):1040–4.

25. Madder RD, VanOosterhout S, Mulder A, Elmore M, Campbell J, Borgman A, et al. Impact of robotics and a suspended lead suit on physician radiation exposure during percutaneous coronary intervention. Cardiovasc Revasc Med. 2017;18(3):190–6.

26. KDIGO clinical practice guideline for acute kidney injury. Kidney Int Suppl. 2012;2:8–12.

27. Mehran R, Aymong ED, Nikolsky E, Lasic Z, Iakovou I, Fahy M, et al. A simple risk score for prediction of contrast-induced nephropathy after percutaneous coronary intervention: development and initial validation. J Am Coll Cardiol. 2004;44(7):1393–9.

28. Cigarroa RG, Lange RA, Williams RH, Hillis LD. Dosing of contrast material to prevent contrast nephropathy in patients with renal disease. Am J Med. 1989;86(6 Pt 1):649–52.

29. Laskey WK, Jenkins C, Selzer F, Marroquin OC, Wilensky RL, Glaser R, et al. Volume-to-creatinine clearance ratio: a pharmacokinetically based risk factor for prediction of early creatinine increase after percutaneous coronary intervention. J Am Coll Cardiol. 2007;50(7):584–90.

30. Pavlidis AN, Jones DA, Sirker A, Mathur A, Smith EJ. Prevention of contrast-induced acute kidney injury after percutaneous coronary intervention for chronic total coronary occlusions. Am J Cardiol. 2015;115(6):844–51.

31. Aguiar-Souto P, Ferrante G, Del Furia F, Barlis P, Khurana R, Di Mario C. Frequency and predictors of contrast-induced nephropathy after angioplasty for chronic total occlusions. Int J Cardiol. 2010;139(1):68–74.

32. Lin YS, Fang HY, Hussein H, Fang CY, Chen YL, Hsueh SK. Predictors of contrast-induced nephropathy in chronic total occlusion percutaneous coronary intervention. EuroIntervention. 2014;9(10):1173–80.

33. ACT Investigators. Acetylcysteine for prevention of renal outcomes in patients undergoing coronary and peripheral vascular angiography: main results from the randomized Acetylcysteine for Contrast-induced nephropathy Trial (ACT). Circulation. 2011;124(11):1250–9.

The manufacturer's authorised representative in the EU is Springer
Nature Customer Service Centre GmbH, Europaplatz 3, 69115 Heidelberg,
Germany. If you have any concerns regarding our products, please
contact ProductSafety@springernature.com

Printed and bound by CPI Group (UK) Ltd, Croydon, CR0 4YY
29/04/2026
02099466-0012